American Association of Critical-Care Nurses

Core Review for Critical Care Nursing

5th Edition

Edited by

JoAnn Grif Alspach, RN, MSN, EdD, FAAN

Consultant, Staff Development and Competency-Based
Performance Appraisal Systems

Editor, *Critical Care Nurse*
Annapolis, Maryland

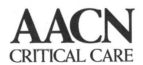

W.B. SAUNDERS COMPANY
A Division of Harcourt Brace & Company
Philadelphia London Toronto Montreal Sydney Tokyo

W.B. SAUNDERS COMPANY
A Division of Harcourt Brace & Company

The Curtis Center
Independence Square West
Philadelphia, Pennsylvania 19106

Library of Congress Cataloging-in-Publication Data

Core review for critical care nursing / [edited by] JoAnn Grif Alspach —5th ed.

p.   cm.

"American Association of Critical-Care Nurses."

Includes bibliographical references and index.

ISBN 0–7216–5232–8

1. Intensive care nursing—Examinations, questions, etc.   I. Alspach, JoAnn.
   II. American Association of Critical Care Nurses.

[DNLM: 1. Critical Care examination questions.   2. Critical Care nurses'
instruction.   WY 18.2 C7975 1998]

RT120.I5C67 1998   610.73′61—dc21

DNLM/DLC   98-9756

CORE REVIEW FOR CRITICAL CARE NURSING, Fifth Edition   ISBN 0–7216–5232–8

Copyright © 1998, 1991, 1985 by W.B. Saunders Company.

Printed in the United States of America.

Last digit is the print number: 9   8   7   6   5   4   3   2   1

This edition of the
Core Review for Critical Care Nursing
is dedicated to the memory of our AACN colleague and friend,
Sharon Connor.

Contributors

NEUROLOGIC
Randy M. Caine, EdD, RN, CS, CCRN, ANP-C
Professor of Nursing
California State University, Long Beach
Long Beach, California

CARDIOVASCULAR
Karen L. Cooper, MSN, RN, CCRN, CNA
Administrative Supervisor
Kaiser Permanente Medical Center
Managed Care Specialist
Zurich Insurance
Director of Education
Stat Nursing Services
San Francisco, California

PULMONARY
Kathleen Ellstrom, RN, CS
Pulmonary Clinical Nurse Specialist
Pulmonary and Critical Care Division
UCLA Medical Center
Los Angeles, California

HEMATOLOGY/IMMUNOLOGY
Elisabeth L. George, MSN, RN, CCRN
Clinical Coordinator, Thoracic Surgery
University of Pittsburgh Medical Center
Pittsburgh, Pennsylvania

RENAL
Ann E. Keane, MSN, RN, MA, CCRN
Director of Nursing, Acute Care Services
Sound Shore Medical Center of
Westchester
New Rochelle, New York

MULTISYSTEM
Melva Kravitz, PhD, RN
Director, Research and Education
Yale–New Haven Hospital
Associate Professor
Yale School of Nursing
New Haven, Connecticut

ENDOCRINE
Margaret M. McNeill, BSN, RN, MS, CCRN
Major, Nurse Corps
United States Air Force
Langley Air Force Base, Virginia

GASTROINTESTINAL
Barbara C. Opperwall, MSN, RN, CS
Nurse Practitioner
Allergy Care for Children and Young
Adults
Grand Rapids, Michigan

Reviewers

CARDIOVASCULAR
Anita M. Bush, RN, PhD, CCRN, CNRN
Affiliate Assistant Professor, University of
Alaska School of Nursing, Fairbanks, Alaska

ENDOCRINE
Caleb A. Rogovin, CRNA, MS, CCRN, CEN
Staff Nurse Anesthetist, Department of
Anesthesiology and Pain Management,
Cook County Hospital, Chicago, Illinois

GASTROINTESTINAL
Jeanne M. Maiden, RN, MS, CCRN
Professional Development Specialist, Tri-City
Medical Center, Oceanside, California

HEMATOLOGY/IMMUNOLOGY
Margo A. Halm, RN, MA, CCRN
Cardiac Advanced Practice Nurse, United
Hospital, St. Paul, Minnesota

MULTISYSTEM
Katherine E. Slaughter, MSN, RN, CCRN
Assistant Nurse Manager, Surgical Intensive
Care Unit, University Hospitals of Cleveland,
Cleveland, Ohio

NEUROLOGIC
Janet M. Delgado, RN, MN, CNRN, CCRN
Clinical Nurse Specialist and Adjunct Assistant
Professor, Department of Neurosurgery,
University of Miami, Miami, Florida

PULMONARY
Adele A. Large, RN, MSN, CCRN
Case Manager, Emergency Department,
University of Pittsburgh Medical Center,
Pittsburgh, Pennsylvania

RENAL
Suzanne S. Prevost, RN, PhD, CCRN, CNAA
Director, Outcomes Evaluation and Nursing
Education, Associate Professor, School of
Nursing, University of Texas Medical Branch,
Galveston, Texas

Quality care of the critically ill patient requires that the nurse be competent in critical care nursing practice and able to provide care by effectively using the nursing process. The American Association of Critical-Care Nurses (AACN) denotes competency in critical care nursing by means of its CCRN certification program. Certification in critical care nursing demands both a clinical practice requirement as well as successful completion of the CCRN examination, a written test on the cognitive elements that underlie critical care nursing practice. AACN's *Core Curriculum for Critical Care Nursing* defines the knowledge base for critical care nursing and its *Core Review for Critical Care Nursing* provides a means to verify acquisition of that knowledge basc.

In addition to its usefulness as a study guide, the *Core Review* is also designed to assist nurses who are preparing to take the CCRN certification examination. The *Core Review* attempts to achieve this object by blending the content of the *Core Curriculum* with the steps of the nursing process. The 600 test items in this book evaluate a nurse's ability to assess, diagnose, plan, implement, and evaluate nursing care for patients with life-threatening health problems. Achievement of these dual purposes necessitates retention of many aspects of the previous edition of this work as well as inauguration of some new features.

Some similarities with the previous edition include comprehensive coverage of topics contained in the most recent version of the *Core Curriculum*. This edition of the *Core Review* is based on the newly published (1998) fifth edition of the *Core Curriculum*. As with prior versions of the *Core Review*, items cover revised, continued, expanded, additional, and updated content from the most recent *Core Curriculum* and integrate psychosocial aspects of care. The test items still comprise four-option multiple-choice questions with provision of explanations for correct and incorrect answers. Case studies are again incorporated to ex-

emplify application of the nursing process. Grouping of items into three separate integrated tests of 200 questions each coincides with the number of items in the actual CCRN exam. The content areas included for each exam approximate their proportional coverage in the CCRN examination blueprint. Feedback on answers is again located at the end of each exam so that test completion and timing are not disrupted and item responses may more closely resemble completion of the actual CCRN examination. References for each answer and annotated bibliographies are again provided to assist readers in identifying relevant references for each content area in the CCRN exam blueprint.

Most of the new features of this edition of the *Core Review* have been introduced to more closely match the test content with the latest edition of the *Core Curriculum* as well as to more closely match the content and cognitive level distribution of the CCRN examination. Highlights of these new features include addition of the new *Core's* coverage of the multisystem content area, which added items related to the systemic inflammatory response syndrome (SIRS), the multiple organ dysfunction syndrome (MODS), drug and alcohol intoxication, poisoning, burns, hypothermia, and multisystem trauma to the tests. A second refinement with this edition of the *Core Review* is the matching of the distribution of cognitive levels (i.e., knowledge/comprehension, application/analysis, synthesis/evaluation) in each of the three tests to parallel their distribution in the CCRN examination. The area of legal/ethical aspects of critical care nursing has been deleted in this edition owing to its deletion from the current CCRN test blueprint.

Although these review tests are intended to simulate the CCRN examination, none of the test questions have been or will be actual CCRN exam items. Because changes in the CCRN exam occur from time to time, candidates preparing for this exam are encouraged to contact the AACN Certification

Corporation to obtain the exam blueprint that will be in effect for the date on which they plan to take the examination.

The contributors and reviewers for this book are experienced CCRN exam item writers. They have made every attempt to provide a study guide that is helpful in validating a nurse's ability to apply the content of the *Core Curriculum* to critical care nursing practice and in assisting nurses to prepare for the CCRN examination. We welcome your comments regarding how well we have achieved these objectives.

GRIF ALSPACH
Annapolis, Maryland

Publisher's Note: Although the previous edition of the *Core Review for Critical Care Nursing* was the second, we designate this edition as the fifth to align it with the corresponding edition of the *Core Curriculum for Critical Care Nursing*. The *Core Review* was not published in a third or fourth edition.

Instructions

Each of the three review tests in this book consists of 200 four-option multiple-choice questions. An answer sheet that can be used while taking these tests is provided on the following pages. Photocopy the answer sheet for use with each of the tests. Mark the number of the test on the line at the top of the first page of the answer sheet. To simulate taking a CCRN examination, mark your answer to each question on the answer sheet; allow a maximum of four hours to complete each test. After you have completed each test, compare your answers to those that appear in the answer key that follows that test.

A list of additional study references is provided for you in the annotated bibliographies for each content area of the CCRN examination. These bibliographies are located after the last of the three tests and are subdivided by topic area.

Core Review Test

Answer Sheet

1. ☐A ☐B ☐C ☐D	26. ☐A ☐B ☐C ☐D	51. ☐A ☐B ☐C ☐D
2. ☐A ☐B ☐C ☐D	27. ☐A ☐B ☐C ☐D	52. ☐A ☐B ☐C ☐D
3. ☐A ☐B ☐C ☐D	28. ☐A ☐B ☐C ☐D	53. ☐A ☐B ☐C ☐D
4. ☐A ☐B ☐C ☐D	29. ☐A ☐B ☐C ☐D	54. ☐A ☐B ☐C ☐D
5. ☐A ☐B ☐C ☐D	30. ☐A ☐B ☐C ☐D	55. ☐A ☐B ☐C ☐D
6. ☐A ☐B ☐C ☐D	31. ☐A ☐B ☐C ☐D	56. ☐A ☐B ☐C ☐D
7. ☐A ☐B ☐C ☐D	32. ☐A ☐B ☐C ☐D	57. ☐A ☐B ☐C ☐D
8. ☐A ☐B ☐C ☐D	33. ☐A ☐B ☐C ☐D	58. ☐A ☐B ☐C ☐D
9. ☐A ☐B ☐C ☐D	34. ☐A ☐B ☐C ☐D	59. ☐A ☐B ☐C ☐D
10. ☐A ☐B ☐C ☐D	35. ☐A ☐B ☐C ☐D	60. ☐A ☐B ☐C ☐D
11. ☐A ☐B ☐C ☐D	36. ☐A ☐B ☐C ☐D	61. ☐A ☐B ☐C ☐D
12. ☐A ☐B ☐C ☐D	37. ☐A ☐B ☐C ☐D	62. ☐A ☐B ☐C ☐D
13. ☐A ☐B ☐C ☐D	38. ☐A ☐B ☐C ☐D	63. ☐A ☐B ☐C ☐D
14. ☐A ☐B ☐C ☐D	39. ☐A ☐B ☐C ☐D	64. ☐A ☐B ☐C ☐D
15. ☐A ☐B ☐C ☐D	40. ☐A ☐B ☐C ☐D	65. ☐A ☐B ☐C ☐D
16. ☐A ☐B ☐C ☐D	41. ☐A ☐B ☐C ☐D	66. ☐A ☐B ☐C ☐D
17. ☐A ☐B ☐C ☐D	42. ☐A ☐B ☐C ☐D	67. ☐A ☐B ☐C ☐D
18. ☐A ☐B ☐C ☐D	43. ☐A ☐B ☐C ☐D	68. ☐A ☐B ☐C ☐D
19. ☐A ☐B ☐C ☐D	44. ☐A ☐B ☐C ☐D	69. ☐A ☐B ☐C ☐D
20. ☐A ☐B ☐C ☐D	45. ☐A ☐B ☐C ☐D	70. ☐A ☐B ☐C ☐D
21. ☐A ☐B ☐C ☐D	46. ☐A ☐B ☐C ☐D	71. ☐A ☐B ☐C ☐D
22. ☐A ☐B ☐C ☐D	47. ☐A ☐B ☐C ☐D	72. ☐A ☐B ☐C ☐D
23. ☐A ☐B ☐C ☐D	48. ☐A ☐B ☐C ☐D	73. ☐A ☐B ☐C ☐D
24. ☐A ☐B ☐C ☐D	49. ☐A ☐B ☐C ☐D	74. ☐A ☐B ☐C ☐D
25. ☐A ☐B ☐C ☐D	50. ☐A ☐B ☐C ☐D	75. ☐A ☐B ☐C ☐D

Core Review Test *(Continued)*

Answer Sheet

76. ☐A ☐B ☐C ☐D	101. ☐A ☐B ☐C ☐D	126. ☐A ☐B ☐C ☐D	
77. ☐A ☐B ☐C ☐D	102. ☐A ☐B ☐C ☐D	127. ☐A ☐B ☐C ☐D	
78. ☐A ☐B ☐C ☐D	103. ☐A ☐B ☐C ☐D	128. ☐A ☐B ☐C ☐D	
79. ☐A ☐B ☐C ☐D	104. ☐A ☐B ☐C ☐D	129. ☐A ☐B ☐C ☐D	
80. ☐A ☐B ☐C ☐D	105. ☐A ☐B ☐C ☐D	130. ☐A ☐B ☐C ☐D	
81. ☐A ☐B ☐C ☐D	106. ☐A ☐B ☐C ☐D	131. ☐A ☐B ☐C ☐D	
82. ☐A ☐B ☐C ☐D	107. ☐A ☐B ☐C ☐D	132. ☐A ☐B ☐C ☐D	
83. ☐A ☐B ☐C ☐D	108. ☐A ☐B ☐C ☐D	133. ☐A ☐B ☐C ☐D	
84. ☐A ☐B ☐C ☐D	109. ☐A ☐B ☐C ☐D	134. ☐A ☐B ☐C ☐D	
85. ☐A ☐B ☐C ☐D	110. ☐A ☐B ☐C ☐D	135. ☐A ☐B ☐C ☐D	
86. ☐A ☐B ☐C ☐D	111. ☐A ☐B ☐C ☐D	136. ☐A ☐B ☐C ☐D	
87. ☐A ☐B ☐C ☐D	112. ☐A ☐B ☐C ☐D	137. ☐A ☐B ☐C ☐D	
88. ☐A ☐B ☐C ☐D	113. ☐A ☐B ☐C ☐D	138. ☐A ☐B ☐C ☐D	
89. ☐A ☐B ☐C ☐D	114. ☐A ☐B ☐C ☐D	139. ☐A ☐B ☐C ☐D	
90. ☐A ☐B ☐C ☐D	115. ☐A ☐B ☐C ☐D	140. ☐A ☐B ☐C ☐D	
91. ☐A ☐B ☐C ☐D	116. ☐A ☐B ☐C ☐D	141. ☐A ☐B ☐C ☐D	
92. ☐A ☐B ☐C ☐D	117. ☐A ☐B ☐C ☐D	142. ☐A ☐B ☐C ☐D	
93. ☐A ☐B ☐C ☐D	118. ☐A ☐B ☐C ☐D	143. ☐A ☐B ☐C ☐D	
94. ☐A ☐B ☐C ☐D	119. ☐A ☐B ☐C ☐D	144. ☐A ☐B ☐C ☐D	
95. ☐A ☐B ☐C ☐D	120. ☐A ☐B ☐C ☐D	145. ☐A ☐B ☐C ☐D	
96. ☐A ☐B ☐C ☐D	121. ☐A ☐B ☐C ☐D	146. ☐A ☐B ☐C ☐D	
97. ☐A ☐B ☐C ☐D	122. ☐A ☐B ☐C ☐D	147. ☐A ☐B ☐C ☐D	
98. ☐A ☐B ☐C ☐D	123. ☐A ☐B ☐C ☐D	148. ☐A ☐B ☐C ☐D	
99. ☐A ☐B ☐C ☐D	124. ☐A ☐B ☐C ☐D	149. ☐A ☐B ☐C ☐D	
100. ☐A ☐B ☐C ☐D	125. ☐A ☐B ☐C ☐D	150. ☐A ☐B ☐C ☐D	

Core Review Test *(Continued)*

Answer Sheet

151. ☐A ☐B ☐C ☐D		176. ☐A ☐B ☐C ☐D	
152. ☐A ☐B ☐C ☐D		177. ☐A ☐B ☐C ☐D	
153. ☐A ☐B ☐C ☐D		178. ☐A ☐B ☐C ☐D	
154. ☐A ☐B ☐C ☐D		179. ☐A ☐B ☐C ☐D	
155. ☐A ☐B ☐C ☐D		180. ☐A ☐B ☐C ☐D	
156. ☐A ☐B ☐C ☐D		181. ☐A ☐B ☐C ☐D	
157. ☐A ☐B ☐C ☐D		182. ☐A ☐B ☐C ☐D	
158. ☐A ☐B ☐C ☐D		183. ☐A ☐B ☐C ☐D	
159. ☐A ☐B ☐C ☐D		184. ☐A ☐B ☐C ☐D	
160. ☐A ☐B ☐C ☐D		185. ☐A ☐B ☐C ☐D	
161. ☐A ☐B ☐C ☐D		186. ☐A ☐B ☐C ☐D	
162. ☐A ☐B ☐C ☐D		187. ☐A ☐B ☐C ☐D	
163. ☐A ☐B ☐C ☐D		188. ☐A ☐B ☐C ☐D	
164. ☐A ☐B ☐C ☐D		189. ☐A ☐B ☐C ☐D	
165. ☐A ☐B ☐C ☐D		190. ☐A ☐B ☐C ☐D	
166. ☐A ☐B ☐C ☐D		191. ☐A ☐B ☐C ☐D	
167. ☐A ☐B ☐C ☐D		192. ☐A ☐B ☐C ☐D	
168. ☐A ☐B ☐C ☐D		193. ☐A ☐B ☐C ☐D	
169. ☐A ☐B ☐C ☐D		194. ☐A ☐B ☐C ☐D	
170. ☐A ☐B ☐C ☐D		195. ☐A ☐B ☐C ☐D	
171. ☐A ☐B ☐C ☐D		196. ☐A ☐B ☐C ☐D	
172. ☐A ☐B ☐C ☐D		197. ☐A ☐B ☐C ☐D	
173. ☐A ☐B ☐C ☐D		198. ☐A ☐B ☐C ☐D	
174. ☐A ☐B ☐C ☐D		199. ☐A ☐B ☐C ☐D	
175. ☐A ☐B ☐C ☐D		200. ☐A ☐B ☐C ☐D	

Table of Contents

CORE REVIEW TEST

1–1. When assessing a transplant recipient, the critical care nurse is aware that a side effect common to both cyclosporine and tacrolimus but *not* to OKT3 is

A. Anorexia.
B. Nephrotoxicity.
C. Fever.
D. Pulmonary edema.

1–2. Q waves and ST segment elevation diagnostic for anterior wall myocardial infarction would be seen in which of the following leads?

A. I and aVL.
B. II, III, and aVF.
C. V_1 and V_6.
D. V_2, V_3, V_4, V_5, and V_6.

1–3. Which of the following is true of the initial ECG recorded after an acute myocardial infarction (MI)?

A. It always shows ST segment elevation and Q waves in acute MI.
B. It is normal in 25% to 50% of patients with acute MI.
C. It shows nonspecific changes in 90% of patients with acute MI.
D. It shows ST segment elevation and Q waves in only 25% of patients with acute MI.

Questions 1–4 through 1–6 relate to the following situation.

A 65-year-old man with a history of chronic obstructive pulmonary disease (COPD) is admitted to the ICU with a chief complaint of increasing dyspnea over the past several days. His chest radiograph in the emergency department shows bilateral fine infiltrates. His clinical presentation includes a respiratory rate of 32 breaths/min, barrel chest with accessory muscle use, and pursed-lip breathing.

1–4. What would this patient's arterial blood gas analysis be expected to show?

A. Acidosis, hypoxemia, and hypoventilation.
B. Acidosis, hyperemia, and hyperventilation.
C. Alkalosis, hypoxemia, and hypoventilation.
D. Alkalosis, hyperemia, and hyperventilation.

1–5. The patient's condition deteriorates and he is intubated and placed on a ventilator. The settings are tidal volume = 900 ml, respiratory rate = 20 breaths/min, PEEP = 5 cm H_2O, and FIO_2 = 30%. His arterial blood gas analysis results show pH = 7.55, $PaCO_2$ = 30 mm Hg, PaO_2 = 70 mm Hg, SaO_2 = 91%, and HCO_3^- = 35 mEq/L. What is the most likely cause of the acid-base disturbance?

A. Hypoxemia.
B. Lactic acidosis.
C. Nasogastric suction.
D. Overventilation.

1–6. What would be the most appropriate treatment to correct the acid-base imbalance?

A. Increase the respiratory rate.
B. Administer aluminum chloride.
C. Decrease the respiratory rate.
D. Increase the FIO_2.

1

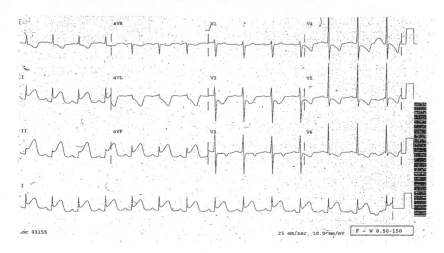

1–7. A 64-year-old man is admitted to the ICU with a history of ascending paralysis occurring over the past 36 hours. He also has a secondary diagnosis of chronic obstructive pulmonary disease and had his flu shot a week ago. A tentative diagnosis of Guillain-Barré syndrome is made. He has a respiratory rate of 30 breaths/min and spontaneous tidal volume of 200 ml. His arterial blood gas analysis results are pH = 7.32, $PaCO_2$ = 50 mm Hg, PaO_2 = 55 mm Hg, and SaO_2 = 88%. The physician orders oxygen at 35%. Which of the following oxygen delivery systems would be best for this patient?

A. Simple face mask.
B. Nasal cannula.
C. Partial rebreather mask.
D. Venturi mask.

1–8. The most common cause of chronic obstructive pulmonary disease (COPD) is

A. Smoking.
B. Pneumonia.
C. Allergies.
D. $Alpha_1$-antitrypsin deficiency.

1–9. Persistent ST segment elevation lasting weeks after an acute myocardial infarction may indicate

A. Extension of the infarct.
B. Hyperkinesis of the ventricle.
C. Ventricular aneurysm.
D. Nontransmural infarction.

1–10. The systemic inflammatory response syndrome (SIRS) refers to the systemic response to

A. Infection.
B. Anaphylaxis.
C. Bacteremia.
D. A variety of severe clinical insults.

1–11. The 12-lead ECG above indicates that this patient has an acute myocardial infarction (MI) of the

A. Anterior wall.
B. Anteroseptal wall.
C. Inferior wall.
D. Lateral wall.

1–12. Which of the following SjO_2 values is most likely indicative of global ischemia in the patient with a traumatic head injury?

A. 55%.
B. 65%.
C. 75%.
D. 85%.

1–13. Which of the following can lead to stress ulceration?

A. Tachycardia.
B. Vasodilative effect of norepinephrine.
C. Portal hypotension.
D. Local and systemic metabolic alkalosis.

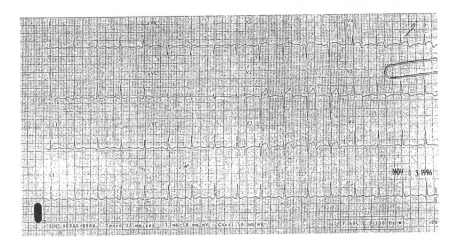

NOV 3 1996

1–14. The above 12-lead ECG indicates injury of the

A. Inferior wall.
B. Lateral wall.
C. Posterior wall.
D. Anteroseptal wall.

1–15. The care plan for a patient with an acute inferior wall myocardial infarction should indicate that the patient has an increased potential for which of the following?

I. Sinus bradycardia.
II. Sinus tachycardia.
III. Left-sided heart failure.
IV. Atrioventricular heart block.

A. I and II.
B. II and III.
C. III and IV.
D. I and IV.

1–16. The potential for intracranial hemorrhage in a patient receiving thrombolytic therapy is greatest in patients with which of the following characteristics?

A. Weight greater than 100 kg, age older than 65, and presence of hypertension.
B. Weight less than 70 kg, age older than 65, and presence of hypertension.
C. Weight greater than 100 kg, female sex, and postmenopausal.
D. Female sex, age older than 65, and presence of hypotension.

1–17. In developing the care plan for a patient with malignant vasovagal syncope who is undergoing percutaneous transluminal coronary angioplasty (PTCA) for coronary artery stenosis, the nurse would include which of the following?

I. Possible use of scopolamine patch during the procedure and sheath removal.
II. Administration of normal saline to maintain blood pressure.
III. Removal of femoral sheaths with patient in Trendelenburg position.
IV. Ingestion of a liberal salt diet.

A. I and III.
B. I, II, and III.
C. II, III, and IV.
D. I, II, III, and IV.

1–18. After a myocardial infarction an echocardiogram shows a left ventricular thrombus. Treatment of this condition would include

A. Anticoagulation with warfarin (Coumadin).
B. Administration of low-molecular-weight heparin.
C. Thrombectomy.
D. Streptokinase infusion.

1–19. Negative-pressure ventilation may be appropriate for a patient with

A. Guillain-Barré syndrome.
B. Pneumonia.
C. Pulmonary embolus.
D. Asthma.

1–20. The type of renal failure caused by a back-leak of glomerular filtrate is

A. Prerenal failure.
B. Postrenal failure.
C. Intrarenal failure.
D. Obstructive renal failure.

1–21. When the intracellular demand for oxygen exceeds the supply in the septic patient, the nurse would expect to find

A. An increase in carbon dioxide.
B. An increase in lactic acid.
C. A decrease in oxygen saturation.
D. A decrease in hydrogen ion concentration.

1–22. Patients who have had a myocardial infarction are placed on which of the following medications to prevent sympathetic increases in myocardial oxygen demand?

A. Aspirin.
B. Angiotensin converting enzyme (ACE) inhibitors.
C. Beta blockers.
D. Calcium channel blockers.

1–23. The goal of stress ulcer therapy is to

A. Inhibit bicarbonate secretion.
B. Control gastric pH.
C. Reduce endogenous prostaglandins.
D. Stimulate histamine release.

1–24. Which of the following is the most important intervention in managing intracranial pressure monitoring using an intraventricular cannula?

A. Maintaining the intracranial pressure at 20 mm Hg.
B. Zero-balancing the transducer only if erroneous readings are suspected.
C. Maintaining a closed system to prevent contamination.
D. Maintaining the transducer at the phlebostatic axis.

1–25. A patient is admitted to the ICU after neurosurgical removal of a pituitary tumor. A main priority in the postoperative care plan is

A. Strict restriction of fluids.
B. Accurate monitoring of intake and output.
C. Administration of hypertonic fluids.
D. Initiation of diuretic therapy.

1–26. A heart transplant recipient returns from the operating room after an endomyocardial biopsy. The biopsy specimen indicates severe rejection. The most appropriate treatment for this rejection would be

A. High doses of cyclosporine.
B. High doses of corticosteroids.
C. High doses of trimethoprim.
D. No treatment is necessary; this is a normal post-transplant finding.

Questions 1–27 through 1–29 relate to the following situation.

A 35-year-old woman with respiratory distress secondary to acute crack cocaine inhalation is intubated and on mechanical ventilation. Her settings are FIO_2 = 85%, PEEP = 22, tidal volume = 800 ml, respiratory rate = 26 breaths/min. Her hemodynamic values are

PaO_2	62 mm Hg
$P\bar{v}O_2$	33 mm Hg
SaO_2	89%
$S\bar{v}O_2$	65%
pH	7.33
$PaCO_2$	44 mm Hg
Mean PAP	28 mm Hg
PCWP	6 mm Hg
RAP	4 mm Hg
Cardiac output	5.2 L/min

1–27. She is placed on inverse I:E ratio ventilation. This mode of ventilation is used to

A. Increase time for expiration.
B. Increase time for inspiration.
C. Increase physiologic dead space.
D. Increase auto-PEEP.

1–28. Her arterial blood gas and hemodynamic values 15 minutes after implementing the inverse I:E ratio ventilation are

PaO_2	55 mm Hg
$P\bar{v}O_2$	28 mm Hg
SaO_2	83%
$S\bar{v}O_2$	58%
pH	7.27
$PaCO_2$	50 mm Hg
Mean PAP	30 mm Hg
PCWP	10 mm Hg
RAP	2 mm Hg
Cardiac output	2.5 L/min

The most likely reason for this change in her values is

A. Cardiogenic shock.
B. Hypovolemia.
C. Neurogenic shock.
D. Pulmonary embolus.

1–29. Appropriate therapy for this patient to maintain adequate hemodynamic and blood gas values while on inverse ratio ventilation (IRV) would consist of

A. Administering intravenous fluids.
B. Administering inotropic drugs.
C. Changing to volume ventilation.
D. Administering streptokinase therapy.

1–30. In a patient with sepsis the nurse would expect to find

A. Increased blood pressure (BP), decreased systemic vascular resistance (SVR), and decreased left ventricular (LV) ejection fraction.
B. Decreased BP, increased cardiac output (CO), and increased SVR.
C. Increased LV end-diastolic volume, increased heart rate, and increased CO.
D. Decreased LV end-diastolic volume, increased LV ejection fraction, and increased SVR.

1–31. Heparin is administered for the first 24 to 48 hours after acute myocardial infarction to maintain the

A. Prothrombin time (PT) between 10 and 14 seconds.
B. Activated clotting time (ACT) between 90 and 128 seconds.
C. Activated partial thromboplastin time (APTT) between 35 and 50 seconds.
D. Partial thromboplastin time (PTT) between 30 and 45 seconds.

1–32. The initial intervention for a patient with an acute myocardial infarction with a junctional rhythm at a rate of 60 beats/min and hypotension should be to

A. Place the patient in a supine position with legs elevated.
B. Administer a 250-ml bolus of lactated Ringer's solution.
C. Administer atropine, 0.5 mg IV.
D. Initiate transcutaneous pacing at a rate of 60 beats/min.

1–33. Ninety minutes after administration of streptokinase for acute myocardial infarction, the patient states he has chest pain. Rales are present at both bases, and ST segment elevation is increased. The patient is currently on a heparin drip at 1040 units/hr (15 units/kg/hr) and nitroglycerin at 90 μg/hr. Which of the following is the most appropriate treatment at this time?

A. Increase the heparin drip to 1200 units/hr.
B. Repeat streptokinase administration.
C. Administer tissue plasminogen activator (tPA).
D. Repeat administration of aspirin.

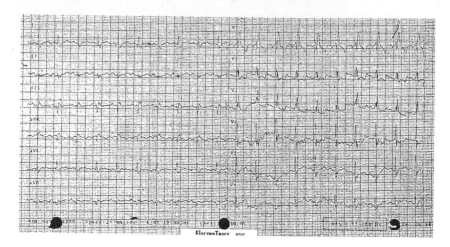

1-34. Inverse I:E ratio ventilation (IRV), which is the opposite of a normal ventilatory pattern, is used to allow a greater time for oxygen diffusion. An important patient care aspect related to IRV is that it

A. Requires a pulmonary artery catheter.
B. Requires that patients be kept sedated and paralyzed.
C. Can only be performed in select centers.
D. Requires 1:1 nursing care.

1-35. Endotracheal tube cuff pressures greater than 25 cm H_2O may result in

A. Mucosal ulceration.
B. Aspiration.
C. Self-extubation.
D. Infection.

1-36. An injury directly below the point of head trauma with a concomitant laceration at the opposite pole of impact is called a

A. Diffuse axonal injury.
B. Coup/contrecoup injury.
C. Hematoma.
D. Concussion.

1-37. Which of the following patient problems causes disruption of electrolyte absorption?

A. Curling's ulcers.
B. Stress ulcers.
C. Cushing's ulcers.
D. Chronic gastric ulcers.

1-38. The patient with the ECG above had an acute onset of chest pain and palpitations 1 hour before admission to the ICU. Blood pressure is 164/80 mm Hg. Relief of chest pain is best accomplished by administration of

A. Nitroglycerin spray.
B. Intravenous (IV) thrombolytic agents.
C. Morphine, 2 mg IV.
D. Atenolol, 5 mg IV.

1-39. A patient treated with thrombolytic therapy is in the CCU on a heparin drip at 600 units/hr, nitroglycerin at 60 μg/min, and lidocaine at 2 mg/min. The 12-lead ECG shows greatly decreased ST segment elevation when compared with the pre-thrombolytic ECG. The current activated partial thromboplastin time (APTT) is 45 seconds performed with a bedside APTT monitor. Appropriate treatment at this time is to

A. Administer morphine, 2 mg IV.
B. Increase the nitroglycerin drip to 80 μg/min.
C. Increase the heparin by 3 ml/hr.
D. Give a bolus with 1000 units of heparin and increase the drip by 3 ml/hr.

1–40. Which method of renal replacement therapy will be used to treat a patient who is moderately catabolic and hemodynamically unstable?

A. Continuous arteriovenous hemofiltration (CAVH).
B. Hemodialysis.
C. Slow continuous ultrafiltration (SCUF).
D. Peritoneal dialysis.

1–41. In planning care for a patient in early sepsis, the nurse will anticipate progression to septic shock in what percentage of cases?

A. 30%.
B. 40%.
C. 50%.
D. 60%.

1–42. A patient is admitted to the CCU after receiving streptokinase in the emergency department for ST segment elevation in leads II, III, and aVF. Which of the following best indicates reperfusion?

A. Reduction and relief of chest pain.
B. Presence of premature ventricular contractions.
C. Variable ST segment elevation and depression.
D. Nausea and diaphoresis.

1–43. Findings in a patient with unstable angina who is currently experiencing angina would typically include

A. Absence of ST segment and T wave changes.
B. ST segment elevation and Q waves.
C. ST segment depression.
D. ST segment elevation.

1–44. Which of the following describes the chest pain associated with unstable angina?

I. Pain similar to effort-induced angina but more intense.
II. Pain that radiates to additional sites.
III. Pain is "crushing" and lasts for more than 30 minutes.
IV. Nitroglycerin offers no relief of pain.

A. I and II.
B. I, II, and III.
C. II and III.
D. II, III, and IV.

Questions 1–45 through 1–47 relate to the following situation.

A 44-year-old man is admitted to the ICU after a farm accident in which he was trapped in an underground septic tank. He is unconscious secondary to sedation and chemical paralysis, intubated, and on a ventilator. He has fulminant pulmonary edema. The following arterial blood gas values are obtained on 100% oxygen:

pH	7.25
$Paco_2$	40 mm Hg
Pao_2	40 mm Hg
Sao_2	72%

1–45. What is the most likely cause of his hypoxemia?

A. Diffusion defect.
B. Hypoventilation.
C. Ventilation/perfusion ($\dot{V}/\dot{Q}$) imbalance.
D. Right-to-left shunt.

1–46. The following laboratory values are obtained:

WBC	2.5/mm³
Hgb/Hct	19.1 g/dl/52.9%
Lactic acid	8.2 mg/dl
K⁺	2.4 mEq/L
Sputum colloid osmolarity	19.0 mOsm/dl
Serum colloid osmolarity	14.9 mOsm/dl
Mean PAP	21 mm Hg
PCWP	4 mm Hg
RAP	5 mm Hg

The most likely cause of his pulmonary edema is

A. Respiratory distress syndrome.
B. Pulmonary embolus.
C. Cardiogenic shock.
D. Neurogenic shock.

1–47. What is the reason for this patient's hypokalemia?

A. Alkalosis.
B. Polycythemia.
C. Dehydration.
D. Lactic acidosis.

1–48. An 18-year-old patient is admitted to the ICU after sustaining closed-head trauma. The critical care nurse observes otorrhea. Which nursing intervention is appropriate at this time?

A. Apply pressure to the area.
B. Apply gentle suction.
C. Assess the drainage for the presence of glucose.
D. Pack the ear firmly with sterile dressings.

1–49. Which of the following principles should be considered in providing nursing care to a patient who has been admitted to the ICU after an acute gastrointestinal hemorrhage?

A. Minimize social stimuli during patient's customary awake time.
B. Monitor patient changes in terms of patient's expected biologic rhythms.
C. Reduce predictability of ICU routines.
D. Avoid direct communication of unfavorable prognoses.

1–50. The syndrome of inappropriate secretion of antidiuretic hormone (SIADH) is characterized by which of the following states in the plasma?

A. Hypotonicity and hypernatremia.
B. Hypertonicity and hyponatremia.
C. Hypotonicity and hyponatremia.
D. Hypertonicity and hypernatremia.

1–51. An adequate serum level of _____ is necessary for successful completion of the clotting cascade.

A. Sodium.
B. Calcium.
C. Phosphorus.
D. Potassium.

1–52. Broad-spectrum antibiotics in the septic patient are most effective at what period of time after administration?

A. 8–12 hours.
B. 12–24 hours.
C. 24–36 hours.
D. 48–72 hours.

1–53. To increase renal blood flow and increase cardiac perfusion in the septic patient, dopamine is infused at _____ µg/kg/min.

A. 2–4.
B. 6–8.
C. 10–12.
D. 14–16.

1–54. A patient with unstable angina and a documented 75% lesion of the left anterior descending artery should be monitored in which of the following leads to evaluate ECG changes?

A. MCL_1 in a three-lead system.
B. V_1 in a five-lead system.
C. Lead II in a three- or five-lead system.
D. V_2 or V_3 in a five-lead system.

1–55. The discharge plan for a patient with a diagnosis of unstable angina should include which of the following?

  I. Follow-up medical care.
  II. The role of aspirin.
  III. Identification of risk factors.
  IV. Nutrition counseling.

  A. I and II.
  B. I, II, and III.
  C. II, III, and IV.
  D. I, II, III, and IV.

1–56. A 28-year-old man is admitted to the ICU after a motor vehicle crash. He has a large, extended family who have been calling frequently, pulling the nurse away from patient care. Many have gathered in the small ICU waiting room so that there is little room for the other patient families. Family members frequently walk into the ICU without notification and have been very disruptive in the unit. What should be the nurse's first response?

  A. Establish a contract for each person visiting the patient.
  B. Hold a family conference.
  C. Have a social worker talk to the family about the problems with visiting.
  D. Identify one or two contact persons with whom staff can communicate.

1–57. Mechanisms to prevent a pneumothorax secondary to respiratory distress syndrome include all of the following *except*

  A. Increasing inspiratory time.
  B. Increasing end-expiratory alveolar pressure.
  C. Adding dead space.
  D. Increasing minute ventilation.

1–58. Which of the following is the most important consideration in the care plan for a patient with unstable angina on a nitroglycerin drip who develops a nitrate-induced headache?

  A. The headache will diminish with continued nitrate use.
  B. The headache is less problematic than the myocardial ischemia.
  C. The headache can be controlled with analgesics.
  D. Fear of headache may prevent appropriate patient self-medication.

Questions 1–59 and 1–60 refer to the following situation.

A patient arrives in the emergency department complaining of weakness, nausea, vomiting, and abdominal distention for 3 days. Vital signs are as follows: BP = 74/40 mm Hg, HR = 48 beats/min and irregular, RR = 12 breaths/min and shallow. The 12-lead ECG shows sinus bradycardia with prominent U waves. The patient's cardiac monitor shows sinus bradycardia with frequent premature ventricular contractions and intermittent (5 to 8 beat) runs of ventricular tachycardia. The patient's blood chemistry results are

Na^+	135 mEq/L
K^+	2.7 mEq/L
Cl^-	98 mEq/L
Mg^{2+}	0.9 mEq/L
Glucose	210 mg/dl
BUN	38 mg/dl
Ca^{2+}	8.5 mEq/L
Phosphate	4.6 mEq/L

1–59. What is the potential cause of this patient's ECG abnormalities?

  A. Hypokalemia.
  B. Hypocalcemia.
  C. Hyponatremia.
  D. Hypomagnesemia.

1–60. The physician orders the following:

Ringer's lactate at 150 ml/hr
KCl, 80 mEq IV, over 4 hours
Magnesium sulfate, 1 g IV soluset
over 1 hour × 4.

The nurse should

A. Administer the potassium before the magnesium.
B. Question the magnesium order as being too high.
C. Administer the magnesium before the potassium.
D. Refuse to administer such a high dose of potassium via the intravenous route.

1–61. An adult with regional enteritis is NPO and receiving multiple antimicrobial therapy. The patient's prothrombin time (PT) and partial thromboplastin time (PTT) are now grossly prolonged. The nurse suspects the patient has developed

A. Antibiotic allergy.
B. Uremia.
C. Vitamin K deficiency.
D. Thrombocytopenia.

Questions 1–62 through 1–64 relate to the following situation.

A 26-year-old man with decreased T-cell count secondary to known acquired immunodeficiency syndrome (AIDS) is admitted to the ICU with hypoxemia and respiratory distress. He is coughing and has chills, fever, and night sweats. His chest radiograph shows patchy areas of infiltration bilaterally.

1–62. What is the most likely causative agent of his pulmonary condition?

A. Pneumococcus.
B. *Legionella.*
C. *Pneumocystis.*
D. *Mycobacterium tuberculosis.*

1–63. The patient should be placed in a

A. Private room.
B. Regular isolation room.
C. Negative-pressure isolation room.
D. Two-bed room with a high-efficiency particulate air (HEPA) filter.

1–64. Sputum cultures times three for acid-fast bacilli are ordered. These should be collected

A. Each on a different day.
B. Thirty minutes apart.
C. By sputum induction.
D. Every 12 hours.

1–65. To prevent nitrate tolerance in patients with unstable angina

A. Transdermal nitroglycerin may be given instead of oral nitrates.
B. Oral isosorbide dinitrate is administered twice daily or three times a day instead of four times a day.
C. Oral nitrates are used instead of transdermal nitroglycerin.
D. Nitrates are administered only when a patient develops chest pain.

1–66. There is a difference in skin temperature in the legs of a patient 1 hour after he has returned from the cardiac catheterization laboratory. The side of the arterial puncture is cooler. The physician should be notified and which of the following performed?

A. Have the patient perform plantarflexion and extension exercises on the cooler side.
B. Apply heat to the warmer extremity to produce vasodilation in the cooler leg.
C. Apply heat to the cooler extremity to produce vasodilation.
D. Perform passive range of motion to the cooler extremity.

1-67. After percutaneous transluminal coronary angioplasty a patient is about to have the femoral sheath removed. Before removal of the femoral sheath the vital signs are BP = 134/80 mm Hg, heart rate = sinus rhythm at 80 beats/min, and respiratory rate = 20 breaths/min. As the sheath is being withdrawn, the heart rate decreases to 45 beats/min and the BP decreases to 90/50 mm Hg. The appropriate treatment is to

A. Administer 1 unit of packed cells.
B. Administer atropine, 0.5 mg IV.
C. Raise the legs above the level of the heart.
D. Apply firm direct pressure to the puncture site.

1-68. Which of the following indicates failure of therapy for unstable angina and the need for emergent coronary intervention?

A. A single anginal episode lasting 20 minutes on nonparenteral medication.
B. Recurrent 5-minute anginal episodes during a 24-hour period on nonparenteral medication.
C. Recurrent angina persisting for over 1 hour on parenteral medication.
D. Any recurrence of angina within 24 hours on parenteral therapy.

1-69. A patient intubated and on mechanical ventilation for 2 weeks is losing tidal volume with each breath, as air is escaping through his mouth. His cuff pressure is 20 cm H_2O. His saturation by pulse oximeter has decreased from 93% to 88%. What intervention should be instituted initially?

A. Reintubate with double-lumen endotracheal tube.
B. Use minimal-leak technique for cuff inflation.
C. Schedule for a tracheostomy.
D. Reintubate with a foam cuffed tube.

1-70. Sepsis-induced cardiogenic shock is treated by administration of

A. Dopamine and levarterenol.
B. Epinephrine and phenylephrine.
C. Atropine and dobutamine.
D. Dopamine and nitroprusside.

1-71. While the nurse is inspecting the groin site of a patient 2 hours after percutaneous transluminal coronary angioplasty (PTCA) sheath removal, the patient reports groin pain. The nurse notes a 4+ femoral pulse and 2+ popliteal and dorsalis pedis pulses. There is no active bleeding from the groin, but a firm, thick ecchymosis is noted around the puncture site. These findings suggest that

A. Hematoma formation is a common complication of PTCA and resolves without intervention.
B. Reapplication of a sand bag is necessary for 1 to 2 hours to resolve the hematoma.
C. Doppler ultrasonography may be necessary to evaluate the site for aneurysm or pseudoaneurysm.
D. Angiography may be necessary to evaluate structural wall defects in the femoral artery.

1-72. A 36-year-old patient is admitted following a gunshot wound to the head. Initial fluid orders include D5W to infuse at 50 ml/hr. The critical care nurse knows that the effects of this intravenous infusion include

A. Hyperosmolar solutions decrease brain water and thus decrease intracranial pressure.
B. Hyperosmolar solutions increase brain water and thus increase intracranial pressure.
C. Hypo-osmolar solutions reduce serum sodium and increase brain water and intracranial pressure.
D. Hypo-osmolar solutions decrease serum sodium and decrease brain water and intracranial pressure.

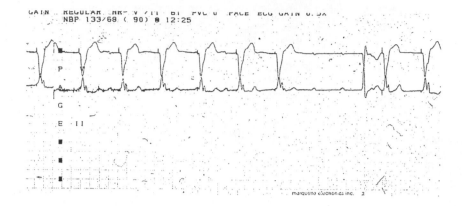

1–73. A 65-year-old patient is receiving magnesium-containing antacids every 2 hours via nasogastric tube. The patient is at risk for

A. Metabolic acidosis.
B. Aspiration.
C. Hyponatremia.
D. Constipation.

1–74. ECG characteristics of Wolff-Parkinson-White (WPW) syndrome include

A. Shortened PR interval and delta wave.
B. Prolonged PR interval and delta wave.
C. Prolonged QT interval and delta wave.
D. Prolonged QT interval and shortened PR interval.

1–75. Evaluate these laboratory results of a patient with diabetic ketoacidosis (DKA):

Magnesium   1.3 mEq/L
Phosphorus   2.3 mg/dl
Potassium   3.8 mEq/L
Calcium   8.4 mg/dl

Which electrolyte deficit should be corrected first?

A. Magnesium
B. Phosphorus
C. Potassium
D. Calcium

1–76. In planning the care of a patient with trifascicular block, the nurse should arrange to have which of the following at the bedside?

A. Defibrillator.
B. Transcutaneous pacemaker.
C. Adenosine.
D. Lidocaine.

1–77. The rhythm strip above (leads V_1 and II) belongs to a patient with a temporary ventricular demand pacemaker. The most appropriate treatment for the condition noted in this strip is to

A. Increase the sensitivity.
B. Decrease the sensitivity.
C. Increase the mA.
D. Decrease the mA.

Questions 1–78 and 1–79 refer to the following situation.

A 25-year-old man 3 days earlier was the victim of a motorcycle crash that resulted in fracture to his pelvis in three places. His fractures are unstable so he is placed on a low air loss bed with kinetic therapy to decrease his need for turning manually. He becomes progressively dyspneic, his pulse oximetry value decreases, his heart rate increases, his ECG remains normal, and he is confused and agitated. He also develops a petechial rash in his axillae and over his chest.

1–78. These findings suggest

A. Adult respiratory distress syndrome.
B. Fat embolism
C. Pneumothorax.
D. Pneumonia.

1–79. Appropriate management for this patient would likely include

A. Heparin.
B. Dextran.
C. Corticosteroids.
D. Tissue plasminogen activator.

1–80. A septic patient is receiving dopamine at an infusion rate of 20 µg/kg/min without evidence of sufficient tissue perfusion. The nurse should anticipate

A. Increasing the dopamine infusion rate to 30 µg/kg/min.
B. Starting levarterenol at a rate of 2 µg/min.
C. Initiating epinephrine to infuse at 20 µg/min.
D. Beginning phenylephrine to infuse at 8 µg/min.

1–81. During the onset phase of acute tubular necrosis (ATN), which of the following medications may be contraindicated?

A. Mannitol.
B. Nifedipine.
C. Indomethacin.
D. Furosemide.

1–82. In evaluating the care for a patient with a DDD pacemaker, which of the following supports the conclusion that potential problems of decreased cardiac output related to conduction defect and/or pacemaker failure are resolved?

A. Pacemaker rhythm strip demonstrates complete ventricular capture at a rate of 66 beats/min.
B. The patient's rhythm strip demonstrates regular sinus rhythm.
C. The patient's heart rate increases to 89 beats/min with activity.
D. ECG report states that during the treadmill test the patient had a Wenckebach response.

1–83. Pulsus alternans is a sign of

A. Severe left ventricular failure.
B. Severe right ventricular failure.
C. Hypovolemic shock.
D. Cor pulmonale.

1–84. A 42-year-old patient is admitted to the ICU with a diagnosis of cerebral aneurysm. During report the critical care nurse is told that the patient's aneurysm is a grade IV on the Hunt and Hess scale. In planning care for this patient the critical care nurse anticipates the patient will be

A. Awake with minimal neurologic deficit and have a mild to severe headache, nuchal rigidity, and no vasospasm.
B. Drowsy, be confused with mild focal neurologic deficit, and have no vasospasm.
C. Unresponsive, be hemiplegic, and may or may not have vasospasm.
D. Comatose with decerebrate (extensor) posture and will likely have vasospasm.

1–85. A 62-year-old patient with a history of "mild hepatitis" 25 years ago has developed cirrhotic changes and primary hepatic carcinoma. The hepatitis is classified as

A. Asymptomatic carrier.
B. Chronic persistent.
C. Acute fulminant.
D. Chronic active.

Questions 1–86 through 1–88 refer to the following situation.

A victim of a motor vehicle crash is admitted to the ICU. He has sustained blunt trauma to his chest from hitting the steering wheel. He was ejected from the vehicle and then it rolled over him. He is on a ventilator, and, after a couple hours, the peak inspiratory pressure alarm is activated. The patient is now agitated and restless, his pulse oximeter reading is dropping, and he has decreased breath sounds on the right side with dullness to percussion and a mediastinal shift to the left.

1-86. What intervention should the nurse anticipate?

A. Magnetic resonance imaging.
B. Computed tomography.
C. Surgery.
D. Chest tube placement.

1-87. Vigorous bubbling suddenly appearing in the water-seal chamber of a chest tube drainage system indicates the patient most likely has

A. Pulmonary edema.
B. A leak in the system.
C. Bronchopleural fistula.
D. Pulmonary contusion.

1-88. What intervention is the most appropriate in this situation?

A. Magnetic resonance imaging.
B. Thoracotomy.
C. Troubleshooting the chest tube drainage system.
D. Another chest tube placement.

1-89. At which of the following pulmonary capillary wedge pressures would the nurse expect to hear fine bibasilar rales?

A. 4-6 mm Hg.
B. 8-10 mm Hg.
C. 15-18 mm Hg.
D. 20-24 mm Hg.

1-90. The most reliable indicator for evaluating the adequacy of tissue perfusion during septic shock is related to

A. Oxygen consumption.
B. Renal function.
C. Hemodynamic status.
D. Respiratory status.

Questions 1-91 and 1-92 relate to the following situation.

An 85-year-old woman is admitted to the ICU from the emergency department. She lives with her son and daughter-in-law because she needs help with her activities of daily living. She has diabetes controlled by insulin, is blind from diabetic complications, and has renal failure requiring peritoneal dialysis at home. Her symptoms are shaking chills with temperature greater than 104°F, pleuritic chest pain, and racking cough productive of rusty sputum.

1-91. What is the most likely cause of her symptoms?

A. Pulmonary embolus.
B. Aspiration pneumonia.
C. *Mycoplasma* pneumonia.
D. Pneumococcal pneumonia.

1-92. In coordinating her care plan, in which order of importance should the following interventions be implemented?

A. Check blood glucose level, start antibiotic therapy, begin peritoneal dialysis.
B. Check blood glucose level, begin peritoneal dialysis, start antibiotic therapy.
C. Start antibiotic therapy, check blood glucose level, begin peritoneal dialysis.
D. Begin peritoneal dialysis, start antibiotic therapy, check blood glucose level.

1-93. A patient under treatment for acute heart failure complicated by atrial fibrillation is currently receiving digoxin, 0.25 mg/day; furosemide (Lasix), 40 mg/day; KCl, 30 mEq/day; and captopril, 50 mg twice daily. Fifteen minutes ago the patient was in sinus rhythm with a rate of 84 beats/min and respiratory rate was 24 breaths/min, with rales at both bases. Oxygen saturation is 96%. The potassium level is 4.6 mEq/L. The monitor currently shows the ECG tracing at the top of the facing page. Which of the following diagnostic tests is necessary to determine the cause of the rhythm change shown in the ECG tracing and to determine the appropriate treatment?

A. Serum digoxin level.
B. Serum potassium level.
C. Arterial blood gas analysis.
D. Serum blood urea nitrogen and creatinine levels.

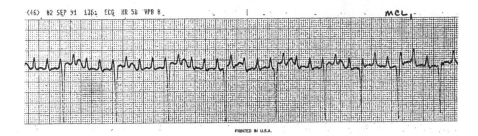

1–94. The care plan for a patient with a medical diagnosis of acute pulmonary edema due to diastolic dysfunction and a nursing diagnosis of fluid volume excess should include which of the following nursing interventions?

    I. Monitor intake and output.
    II. Weigh daily.
    III. Auscultate breath sounds.
    IV. Administer medication(s) to strengthen cardiac contraction.

    A. I and II.
    B. I, II, and III.
    C. I, II, and IV.
    D. I, II, III, and IV.

1–95. A major difference between a transient ischemic attack (TIA) and a reversible ischemic neurologic deficit (RIND) is

    A. A TIA results in a neurologic deficit that lasts longer than 24 hours and leaves little or no neurologic deficit.
    B. A RIND is a reversible short-lived neurologic deficit of less than 24 hours' duration.
    C. A RIND results in a neurologic deficit that lasts longer than 24 hours but leaves little or no neurologic deficit.
    D. A TIA is a reversible neurologic deficit that lasts no longer than a few minutes.

1–96. The critical care nurse anticipates which of the following interventions for a patient within the first 24 hours after a cerebral event caused by an embolus?

    A. Head of the bed flat.
    B. Anticoagulation therapy.
    C. Out of bed in chair 1 hour three times a day.
    D. Epidural catheter to monitor intracranial dynamics.

1–97. Which of the following is a sign of progressing hepatic failure?

    A. Hyperglycemia.
    B. Hyporeflexia.
    C. Hypernatremia.
    D. Hypokalemia.

1–98. The care plan for treatment of bleeding complications in a patient with a ventricular assist device (VAD) who is awaiting transplant for chronic left ventricular failure would include which of the following?

    A. Transfusions with packed cells to maintain hematocrit greater than 28%.
    B. Use of protamine sulfate to correct abnormal coagulation studies.
    C. Use of aminocaproic acid or aprotinin to minimize bleeding.
    D. Maintenance of VAD flow greater than 2 L/min.

1–99. The patient with systemic inflammatory response syndrome (SIRS) is noted to have an oxygen delivery of 800 ml/min and a urine output in the previous hour of 15 ml. The nurse would evaluate the patient for

A. Acute renal failure.
B. Hypothermia.
C. Insufficient hydration.
D. Vasoconstriction.

1–100. Drowsiness, lethargy, and headache during successful therapy for diabetic ketoacidosis may be indicative of

A. Cerebral edema.
B. Meningitis.
C. Acidosis.
D. Hypoxemia.

1–101. For a patient diagnosed with thrombotic thrombocytopenic purpura (TTP), the nurse should center care around the main goal to

A. Speed up platelet aggregation.
B. Prolong prothrombin and partial thromboplastin times.
C. Decrease tachycardia.
D. Inhibit platelet aggregation.

1–102. Which of the following is an abnormal muscle stretch reflex that may be seen in patients with acute spinal cord injury that would indicate diffuse cerebral dysfunction?

A. Grasp reflex.
B. Plantar reflex.
C. Achilles reflex.
D. Biceps reflex.

1–103. Angiotensin converting enzyme (ACE) inhibitors are used in the treatment of heart failure for which of their effects?

I. Decrease afterload.
II. Decrease preload.
III. Enhance diuresis.
IV. Improve cardiac output.

A. I, III, and IV.
B. I, II, and III.
C. I and II.
D. I, II, III, and IV.

1–104. Which of the following medications used in the treatment of heart failure and pulmonary edema reduces both preload and afterload, as well as sympathetic overdrive?

A. Digoxin.
B. Furosemide.
C. Morphine.
D. Captopril.

1–105. An 18-year-old man who sustained injuries from a motor vehicle crash a week ago is nasally intubated and on a ventilator at 70% FIO_2, CMV of 22 breaths/min, PEEP of 12 cm H_2O, and tidal volume of 800 ml. He is heavily sedated to reduce oxygen requirement and alleviate anxiety and agitation. When doing oral care, the nursing assistant notices a foul odor from his mouth and brown drainage from his nose and in the back of his mouth. What is the most likely explanation for this drainage?

A. Sinusitis.
B. Abscessed tooth.
C. Necrosis of oral tissue.
D. Tracheoesophageal fistula.

1–106. A 24-year-old man is admitted with an acute asthma attack. His blood gases are pH = 7.32, $PaCO_2$ = 50 mm Hg, PaO_2 = 65 mm Hg, and SaO_2 = 91% on 35% oxygen. Based on these results, the nurse would

A. Increase the oxygen percentage (FIO_2).
B. Give bronchodilator therapy.
C. Plan for intubation.
D. Give an intermittent positive-pressure breathing (IPPB) treatment.

1–107. In which order would treatment for mucus plugging in a patient with status asthmaticus be provided on a ventilator?

A. Humidification, hydration, postural drainage, bronchoscopy.
B. Hydration, postural drainage, bronchoscopy, humidification.
C. Bronchoscopy, hydration, postural drainage, humidification.
D. Postural drainage, bronchoscopy, hydration, humidification.

1–108. Treatment of heart failure caused by diastolic dysfunction includes which of the following mechanisms to treat or prevent myocardial ischemia?

    A. Digoxin to improve efficiency of myocardial contractility.
    B. Beta blockers to decrease heart rate and force of contraction.
    C. Dobutamine to improve cardiac output.
    D. Fluid boluses to maintain diastolic filling pressures.

1–109. An *early* laboratory finding characteristic of *acute* pancreatitis is

    A. Elevated serum calcium value.
    B. Decreased white blood cell count.
    C. Decreased blood glucose level.
    D. Elevated serum amylase value.

1–110. Laboratory data 24 to 48 hours after toxic ingestion of acetaminophen will likely demonstrate elevation of serum levels of

    A. Total bilirubin.
    B. Alkaline phosphatase.
    C. Amylase.
    D. Glucose.

1–111. A patient in acute pulmonary edema is intubated and placed on a ventilator. An arterial line and pulmonary artery catheter are inserted. Blood pressure is 130/80 mm Hg, mean arterial pressure (MAP) is 80 mm Hg, heart rate is 100 beats/min, pulmonary capillary wedge pressure (PCWP) is 15 mm Hg, right atrial pressure (RAP) is 12 mm Hg, and the cardiac output is 3.6 L/min. The patient has received 40 mg of furosemide (Lasix) and has diuresed 600 ml. Which of the following medications should be added?

    A. Nitroglycerin to improve coronary dilation.
    B. Dobutamine to improve contractility.
    C. Potassium, 10 mEq, to prevent hypokalemia.
    D. Nitroprusside to decrease preload and afterload.

1–112. A patient with left ventricular systolic dysfunction is being treated with spironolactone, enalapril, and isosorbide dinitrate. The current blood pressure is 94/64 mm Hg, heart rate is 110 beats/min, and respiratory rate is 28 breaths/min. There are rales at both lung bases. PaO_2 is 88%, and serum potassium concentration is 5.5 mEq/L. Current treatment should include

    A. Withhold enalapril and spironolactone.
    B. Withhold enalapril only.
    C. Withhold spironolactone only.
    D. Continue administration of spironolactone, enalapril, and isosorbide.

1–113. Altered gas exchange secondary to a pulmonary embolus is a result of

    A. Hypoventilation.
    B. Ventilation/perfusion mismatch.
    C. Diffusion impairment.
    D. Mucus plugging.

1–114. An immediate and serious consequence of remaining on bed rest would be

    A. Delayed hospital discharge.
    B. Ileus.
    C. Increased costs.
    D. Pulmonary embolus.

1–115. The effectiveness of treatment for a patient with right ventricular failure is best demonstrated by

    A. Clear breath sounds.
    B. Oxygen saturation greater than 96%.
    C. Pulmonary capillary wedge pressure 15 mm Hg.
    D. Jugular venous pulsations visible 2 cm above the angle of Louis.

1–116. The effectiveness of treatment for reduced left ventricular filling caused by diastolic dysfunction is demonstrated by

A. Decreased stroke volume and normal cardiac output.
B. Heart rate of 130 beats/min and cardiac output of 4.0 L/min.
C. Cardiac index of 3.0 L/min/m² and heart rate of 96 beats/min.
D. Normal heart size and ejection fraction.

1–117. A patient has been on relatively high doses of nitroprusside for 3 days to control his hypertension, despite attempts to wean using labetalol and nifedipine. On the previous shift the patient was alert, oriented, and cooperative, with a Glasgow Coma Scale score of 15. The patient is becoming increasingly confused and combative. Blood pressure is now 130/74 mm Hg with a heart rate of 110 beats/min that is attributed to agitation. The patient's skin is warm and pink with a capillary refill time of 1 second. Lungs are clear with an oxygen saturation of 96% on room air. Which of the following should be obtained?

A. A psychiatric consultation.
B. An arterial blood gas analysis.
C. A thiocyanate level.
D. A complete blood cell count.

1–118. Management of acute hydrocephalus from a ruptured cerebral aneurysm may include

A. Administration of dehydrating agents.
B. Administration of hypotonic intravenous fluids.
C. Surgical evacuation of stenotic scar tissue.
D. Surgical placement of a ventriculostomy.

1–119. Orogastric lavage is indicated for patients with life-threatening ingestions who receive medical attention within a maximum of _____ minutes.

A. 30.
B. 60.
C. 90.
D. 120.

1–120. During acute peritoneal dialysis, the rate of ultrafiltration is greatest during which phase of the peritoneal dialysis cycle?

A. The inflow phase.
B. The beginning of the dwell phase.
C. The end of the dwell phase.
D. The outflow phase.

1–121. In acute pancreatitis, the *first* priority is to

A. Administer nitroglycerin.
B. Titrate dietary protein intake.
C. Administer antibiotics.
D. Restore fluid volume.

1–122. A 22-year-old woman with cardiomyopathy after delivery of her second child is in the CCU awaiting a heart transplant. She is on bed rest to decrease her oxygen needs and intravenous antiarrhythmic agents to control her atrial fibrillation. Which of the following interventions would be the most important for her to prevent a pulmonary embolus?

A. Vena caval umbrella.
B. Low dose heparin.
C. Elastic stockings.
D. Ambulation.

1–123. Bowel loops in the thorax on chest radiograph indicate

A. Ileus.
B. Malposition of the patient.
C. Ascites.
D. Diaphragmatic rupture.

1–124. Differences in physical findings between hemothorax and simple pneumothorax include

A. Decreased vocal fremitus.
B. Percussion for dullness or hyperresonance.
C. Decreased breath sounds.
D. Unequal chest expansion.

1–125. In diabetic ketoacidosis, the key intervention aimed at resolving the acidosis is the administration of

A. Sodium bicarbonate.
B. Potassium.
C. Insulin.
D. Phosphorus.

1–126. A patient is diagnosed with thrombotic thrombocytopenic purpura (TTP). Based on the diagnosis, the most appropriate nursing measure would be to hold

A. Corticosteroids.
B. Aspirin.
C. Platelets.
D. Fresh frozen plasma.

1–127. In planning the care of a patient in hypertensive crisis being treated with a nitroprusside drip, which of the following nursing activities receives priority?

A. Monitoring for symptoms of thiocyanate toxicity.
B. Assisting the smooth transition from intravenous to oral antihypertensive agents.
C. Patient education regarding the complications of chronic hypertension.
D. Ensuring that blood pressure is lowered and maintained at prescribed levels.

1–128. Which of the following statements is true regarding the use of labetalol as an infusion to control blood pressure in hypertensive crisis? Labetalol is

A. Titrated to any dosage that achieves the desired effect.
B. Administered at 5 to 10 μg/kg/min.
C. Administered at 1 to 2 mg/min.
D. Given as bolus doses of 10 to 100 mg every 10 minutes until the desired effect is achieved or the heart rate decreases to less than 60 beats/min.

1–129. Which of the following indicates that initial interventions to reduce blood pressure (BP) in a patient with hypertensive crisis have been effective?

A. BP is 144/70 mm Hg; patient is confused.
B. BP is 150/90 mm Hg; patient is alert and cooperative.
C. BP is 110/60 mm Hg; patient is lethargic.
D. BP is 120/70 mm Hg; patient is oriented to person.

1–130. In an unconscious patient with an unknown ingestion history, suspected opioid overdose is treated with

A. Naloxone alone.
B. Flumazenil alone.
C. Naloxone and flumazenil.
D. Sodium bicarbonate.

1–131. During weaning of a patient from intra-aortic balloon counterpulsation, the patient exhibits the following:

Pulmonary capillary wedge pressure of 18 mm Hg
Cardiac index of 2.0 L/min/m^2
Clear breath sounds
Urine output > 30 ml/hr

These findings indicate
A. Adequate cardiac function to continue the weaning process.
B. Inadequate cardiac function to continue the weaning process.
C. Balloon pump dependence.
D. That the weaning attempt has been unsuccessful.

1–132. The critical care nurse is told that a patient with an intracranial hemorrhage is being admitted to the ICU. When planning for care of this patient, the nurse knows that the first priority will be to assess

A. Vital signs.
B. Pupillary response.
C. Motor and sensory ability.
D. Level of consciousness.

1–133. The patient's nasogastric tube is correctly placed and has drained a total of 1580 ml of clear green drainage during the past 24 hours. This volume most likely indicates

A. Normal secretion of gastric juice.
B. Acute pancreatitis.
C. Onset of gastric autodigestion.
D. Mesenteric ischemia.

1–134. The most common cause of postsurgical hypoxia is

A. Microatelectasis.
B. Pneumonia.
C. Pulmonary edema.
D. Pulmonary embolus.

1–135. A patient recovering from a myocardial infarction in the CCU collapses at dinnertime. Assessment reveals increased work of breathing with accessory muscle use, intercostal retractions, inspiratory stridor with minimal air exchange, wheezing on the right and left upper lobes, and absent breath sounds in the left base. The most likely explanation for these findings is

A. Pneumothorax.
B. Pulmonary embolus.
C. Cardiogenic shock.
D. Foreign body obstruction.

1–136. To improve peripheral circulation distal to the sheath insertion site of a patient with an intra-aortic balloon pump, how should the patient be positioned?

A. Elevate the head of the bed 45°.
B. Place the bed in Trendelenburg position.
C. Place the bed in reverse Trendelenburg.
D. Place the patient in semi-Fowler's position.

1–137. Which of the following medications causes the greatest increase in myocardial contractility?

A. Dobutamine.
B. Dopamine.
C. Epinephrine.
D. Norepinephrine.

1–138. Which of the following indicates migration of the intra-aortic balloon?

I. Decreased urine output.
II. Oozing around the insertion site.
III. Diminished pulse and temperature in the left arm.
IV. Diminished temperature of the insertion leg.

A. I and II.
B. I and III.
C. II and III.
D. III and IV.

1–139. After admission for cocaine overdose, the patient receives ascorbic acid 500 mg three or four times daily to

A. Restore cellular integrity.
B. Prevent muscle soreness.
C. Remove metabolites.
D. Maintain urinary pH.

1–140. While on hemodialysis, the patient becomes confused and agitated. He complains of nausea, weakness, and severe headache. Vital signs are BP = 186/110 mm Hg, heart rate = 110 beats/min, and respiratory rate = 32 breaths/min. The nurse administers nifedipine, 20 mg SL. After 15 minutes the patient's vital signs are BP = 212/114 mm Hg, heart rate = 125 beats/min, and respiratory rate = 36 breaths/min. The patient begins to vomit and then experiences a grand mal seizure. To best manage this acute crisis the nurse should expect to administer

A. Volume expanders.
B. Diuretics.
C. Antidysrhythmic agents.
D. Antihypertensive medication.

Questions 1–141 and 1–142 refer to the following situation.

A 75-year-old man is admitted with a closed-head injury after a motor vehicle crash. He is obtunded but responds to painful stimuli. Respirations are regular and deep. Arterial blood gases show pH = 7.47, $PaCO_2$ = 38 mm Hg, PaO_2 = 82 mm Hg, and SaO_2 = 95% on 30% oxygen.

1–141. The primary reason for his intubation would be to

A. Bypass an upper airway obstruction.
B. Manage secretions.
C. Protect the airway.
D. Provide mechanical ventilation.

1–142. During the intubation process, the most important nursing function is to continually monitor for hypoxemia and cardiac arrhythmias. Prevention measures for these potential complications include

A. Corticosteroid therapy.
B. Proper patient positioning.
C. Correct tube placement.
D. Strong suction available.

1–143. A 54-year-old man is admitted to the ICU after a fishing accident. He was in the water for 12 hours before being rescued. The patient is now lethargic, hypothermic, and disoriented. His arterial blood gases are pH 7.33, $PaCO_2$ = 38 mm Hg, PaO_2 = 65 mm Hg, and SaO_2 = 95% on room air.
What is the most important intervention needed at this point?

A. Provide oxygen.
B. Intubation.
C. Antibiotic therapy.
D. Rewarming.

1–144. Which of the following diagnostic tests would the critical care nurse anticipate for the patient with intracranial hemorrhage?

A. Lumbar puncture.
B. Cerebral angiography.
C. Computed tomography.
D. Myelography.

1–145. *Early* treatment of mesenteric ischemia will be directed at

A. Preventing metabolic alkalosis.
B. Correcting hypovolemia.
C. Administering vasoconstricting agents.
D. Providing potassium supplements.

1–146. Which of the following mixed venous oxygen saturation levels would indicate the left-to-right shunt typical of an atrial septal defect?

A. 60%.
B. 70%.
C. 85%.
D. 100%.

1–147. In the management of acute aortic regurgitation, which of the following medications decreases left ventricular wall stress and afterload and increases ejection fraction without slowing the heart rate?

A. Verapamil.
B. Diltiazem.
C. Propranolol.
D. Nifedipine.

1–148. The most frequent postoperative complication associated with thoracoabdominal aneurysm repair is

A. Pulmonary insufficiency.
B. Myocardial infarction.
C. Paralysis.
D. Cerebrovascular accident.

1–149. In patients with acetaminophen overdose, oral N-acetylcysteine (NAC) is administered

A. As long as the serum acetaminophen level remains elevated.
B. Until the serum acetaminophen level is reduced.
C. For 24 hours after the ingestion.
D. For an 18-dose course.

1–150. Given the following laboratory values, choose the best course of therapy.

	9 AM	10 AM
Serum glucose (mg/dl)	310	155
Urine ketones	+3	+3
Urine glucose	+3	+1

A. Discontinue insulin infusion and maintain saline infusion.
B. Continue insulin infusion and maintain saline infusion.
C. Discontinue insulin infusion and add dextrose to saline infusion.
D. Continue insulin infusion and add dextrose to saline infusion.

1–151. A patient has been on chronic warfarin (Coumadin) therapy for a mechanical heart valve. The admission International Normalized Ratio (INR) is 5.3. This ratio value would be interpreted as

A. Excessive anticoagulation.
B. Subtherapeutic anticoagulation.
C. Recommended range for prophylaxis of deep vein thrombosis.
D. Recommended range for patients with mechanical heart valves.

1–152. Which of the following methods of pulmonary toilet is appropriate for the patient who has had a repair of an aortic aneurysm?

A. Coughing and deep breathing exercises every 2 hours using pillow splinting.
B. Sitting the patient out of bed in a chair for 1 hour each shift to perform coughing and deep breathing exercises.
C. Rigorous suctioning via a nasal airway every 4 hours.
D. Sitting the patient in a chair for intermittent positive-pressure breathing treatments every 4 hours.

1–153. In hypovolemic shock, increased peripheral resistance causes which of the following effects on blood pressure?

A. Brachial blood pressure is equal to central aortic pressure.
B. Brachial blood pressure is generally lower than central aortic pressure.
C. Brachial blood pressure is generally higher than central aortic pressure.
D. Poorly palpable or faintly audible brachial blood pressure measurements are inaccurate.

1–154. Which of the following reflects the decrease in cardiac output seen in hypovolemic shock?

I. Urine output of 60 ml/hr.
II. Systemic vascular resistance of 1800 dynes/sec/cm⁵.
III. Increased urinary sodium.
IV. Blood pressure change from 120/80 to 120/100 mm Hg.

A. I and II.
B. II and III.
C. II and IV.
D. III and IV.

1-155. Protocols for correction of fluid loss suggest administering crystalloid in what proportion to each milliliter of actual or suspected blood loss?

A. 1 ml of crystalloid for each 5 ml of blood loss.
B. 2 ml of crystalloid for each 4 ml of blood loss.
C. 3 ml of crystalloid for each 1 ml of blood loss.
D. 5 ml of crystalloid for each 1 ml of blood loss.

1-156. During report, the critical care nurse is told that a patient with an intracranial hemorrhage has Glasgow Coma Scale values of 3–3–4. Evaluation of the patient's progress is based on the nurse's knowledge that this patient

A. Opens his eyes when spoken to.
B. Follows simple commands.
C. Makes no attempt to remove noxious stimuli.
D. Makes no attempt to vocalize.

1-157. Correction of fluid volume deficit should be anticipated in a patient with

A. Esophageal fistula.
B. Pulmonary edema.
C. Acute glomerulonephritis.
D. Hyperaldosteronism.

1-158. In the postoperative period after lower extremity vascular surgery, the patient has a blood pressure of 80/60 mm Hg and a hematocrit of 45%. Treatment to increase blood pressure should include

A. Infusion of packed cells.
B. Administration of crystalloid fluids.
C. Administration of vasopressors.
D. "Gatching" the bed so the legs are elevated.

1-159. A patient who exhibits an "ecchymotic mask" has most likely experienced

A. Traumatic asphyxia.
B. Near-drowning.
C. Carbon monoxide intoxication.
D. Airway obstruction.

1-160. Hyponatremia may be caused by all of the following except

A. Renal disease.
B. Cirrhosis.
C. Adrenal insufficiency.
D. Diabetes mellitus.

1-161. Clinical findings of a tension pneumothorax are

A. Neck vein distention and tracheal deviation away from the affected side.
B. Tracheal deviation toward the affected side and agitation.
C. Increased respiratory effort and decreased heart rate.
D. Increased cardiac output and cyanosis.

1-162. The murmur heard with right-sided infective endocarditis is best described as

A. Holosystolic at the apex.
B. Crescendo-descrescendo at the second intercostal space.
C. Holosystolic at the lower left sternal border.
D. Holosystolic at the right sternal border.

1-163. In a patient with endocarditis, blood samples for culture are drawn

I. Before antibiotic therapy and with temperature spikes.
II. From three separate sites over 1 hour.
III. From two separate sites concurrently.

A. I only.
B. I and II.
C. I and III.
D. II and III.

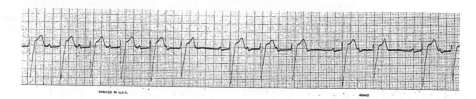

1–164. If the RR interval is constant, the heart rate can be determined most accurately by

A. Counting the number of QRS complexes in a 6-second strip.
B. Dividing the total number of large boxes between two consecutive R waves by 300.
C. Dividing the total number of small boxes between two consecutive R waves by 1500.
D. Using a precalculated table that uses the number of small squares between two R waves.

1–165. Which of the following indicates junctional rhythm with retrograde atrial conduction?

A. P waves are positive in leads II, III, and aVF.
B. P waves are negative in leads II, III, and aVF.
C. PR interval is greater than 0.40 second.
D. PR interval is less than 0.12 second.

1–166. The dysrhythmia indicated by the lead II ECG tracing above is

A. First-degree AV block.
B. Second-degree AV block Mobitz type I.
C. Second-degree AV block Mobitz type II.
D. Third-degree AV block.

1–167. One of the most difficult and individualized aspects of patient teaching for a patient with an implanted cardioverter/defibrillator (ICD) is

A. Instructing patients about changes in their medications.
B. Teaching patients about ICD sensing and shock delivery.
C. Assisting patients to make necessary life-style adjustments.
D. Convincing patients and families about the importance of learning cardiopulmonary resuscitation (CPR).

1–168. A 53-year-old patient is admitted to the ICU 3 weeks after a mild upper respiratory tract infection. The patient is diagnosed with Guillain-Barré syndrome (GBS). Which of the following interventions would the critical care nurse *not* anticipate?

A. Mechanical ventilation for paralysis of respiratory muscles.
B. Hemodynamic monitoring for assessing autonomic nervous system dysfunction.
C. Patient-controlled analgesia for acute pain.
D. Indwelling urinary catheter for bladder atony.

1–169. Two days after uncomplicated coronary artery bypass graft surgery, the patient complains of severe, cramping abdominal pain. The patient's white blood cell count is elevated. The abdomen is firm, and bowel sounds are absent. Which of the following therapies would be *discontinued* as soon as possible?

A. Vasoconstrictors.
B. Packed red blood cells.
C. Antibiotics.
D. Smooth muscle relaxants.

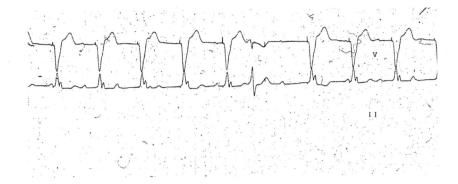

1-170. The most reliable indicator of the extent of carbon monoxide toxicity is

A. A carboxyhemoglobin level greater than 1%.
B. An oxygen saturation of hemoglobin higher than predicted.
C. An unexplained increase in anion gap metabolic acidosis.
D. A cherry-red skin color.

1-171. The nurse notices a nearly continuous air leak in the water-seal chamber of a patient with a tension pneumothorax. Measures to determine proper function of the chest tube include which of the following?

A. Stripping the chest tube.
B. Changing the water-seal system.
C. Quickly clamping the tube next to the insertion site.
D. Suctioning the chest tube.

1-172. On the basis of the rhythm strip above, the nurse plans to monitor for which potential problem?

A. Potential for ventricular tachycardia/fibrillation.
B. Potential for decreased cardiac output.
C. Potential for lead dislodgment.
D. Potential for cardiac tamponade.

1-173. The amount of energy recommended for the initial defibrillation attempt of a patient in ventricular fibrillation is _____ joules.

A. 100
B. 200
C. 300
D. 360

1-174. If administration of an initial 6-mg dose of adenosine (Adenocard) does not slow the ventricular response of a patient with Wolff-Parkinson-White syndrome, it is appropriate to administer

A. Another 6 mg of adenosine within 2 minutes.
B. A second dose of 12 mg of adenosine.
C. Verapamil, 5 mg.
D. Verapamil, 10 mg.

1-175. A patient is admitted to the ICU with a serum glucose value of 1172 mg/dl, hyperosmolality, hypokalemia, oliguria, tachycardia, and poor skin turgor. The first intervention in caring for this patient should be administration of

A. Insulin.
B. Normal saline.
C. Potassium.
D. Albumin.

1-176. A patient is admitted to rule out human immunodeficiency virus (HIV). Which of the following serum tests would be the most specific to make this evaluation?

A. Enzyme-linked immunosorbent assay (ELISA).
B. Western blot.
C. Coombs' test.
D. HIV antigen test.

1–177. Prophylactic irradiation of cellular blood components before transfusion is indicated for patients with

A. Kidney transplants.
B. Lung transplants.
C. Liver transplants.
D. Bone marrow transplants.

1–178. A brief sensory experience that occurs before the onset of some seizures is called a/an

A. Prodromal phase.
B. Aura.
C. Epileptic cry.
D. Ictus.

1–179. One of the measures to restore and maintain adequate oxygen delivery during the post-burn resuscitation period is to replace

A. Red blood cells to maintain hematocrit at more than 30%.
B. Serum albumin to maintain a level of 4 g/dl or greater.
C. Electrolytes associated with gastrointestinal losses.
D. Bicarbonate to lower lactic acid levels.

1–180. In planning the care of a patient receiving digoxin, assessment for which of the following electrolyte imbalances is essential?

A. Hyponatremia and hypermagnesemia.
B. Hyperkalemia and hyponatremia.
C. Hypocalcemia and hypomagnesemia.
D. Hypokalemia and hypercalcemia.

1–181. A 30-year-old patient is admitted through the emergency department after a motor vehicle crash with a liver laceration and possible splenic rupture. The patient is pale, anxious, tachycardic, and tachypneic. The blood pressure is 82/40 mm Hg. It is critical to assess this patient for signs of

A. Leukocytosis.
B. Ileus.
C. Hemorrhage.
D. Sepsis.

1–182. An 18-year-old man with adult respiratory distress syndrome has a tracheostomy and is on a ventilator at 90% FIo_2, CMV (controlled mandatory ventilation) of 28, PEEP of 20, and tidal volume of 850 ml. His peak inspiratory pressure is 75 with a plateau pressure of 68. During the initial assessment, the nurse notices subcutaneous bubbles with crackling on his chest and abdomen as well as scrotal and eyelid swelling. What would be the treatment of choice?

A. Suction out the air.
B. Make small cuts in the skin to release the air.
C. Do nothing.
D. Manually express out the air.

1–183. Immediate treatment of the dysrhythmia shown on the ECG tracing on the facing page is

A. Intravenous administration of 100 mg of lidocaine.
B. Intravenous administration of 6 mg of adenosine.
C. Synchronized cardioversion at 100 joules.
D. Direct-current countershock at 200 joules.

1–184. Which of the following best demonstrates that a therapeutic level of procainamide has been attained?

A. Serum N-acetyl procainamide (NAPA), 5 to 9 µg/ml.
B. Serum N-acetyl procainamide (NAPA) 10 to 20 µg/ml.
C. QRS complex width of 1.6 seconds.
D. Normal sinus rhythm on ECG.

1–185. Which of the following outcomes best demonstrates effective treatment of supraventricular tachycardia?

A. Improved cardiac output.
B. Decrease in heart rate.
C. Decrease in myocardial oxygen demand.
D. Return of atrial kick.

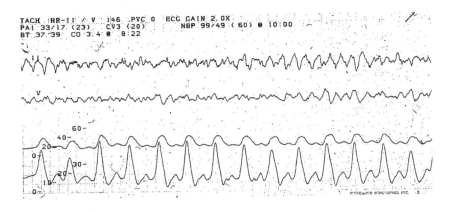

```
TACH  HR-II / V  146  PVC 0  ECG GAIN 2.0X
PAI 33/17 (23)  CV3 (20)      NBP 99/49 (60) @ 10:00
BT 37.39  CO 3.4 @ 8:22
```

1-186. A patient with hypertrophic cardiomyopathy has a pulmonary capillary wedge pressure (PCWP) of 24
mm Hg and cardiac output of 3.0
L/min. The respiratory rate is 30
breaths/min and labored, with
coarse rales throughout all lung
fields. Heart rate is 124 beats/min.
Which of the following medications
would the nurse anticipate administering?

   I. Dobutamine infusion.
  II. Propranolol.
 III. Diltiazem.

A. I only.
B. I and II.
C. II and III.
D. I, II, and III.

1-187. Treatment for septal rupture after
percutaneous laser myoplasty includes

A. Right-ventricular assist device.
B. Left-ventricular assist device.
C. Intra-aortic balloon counterpul-
sation and surgical intervention.
D. Open-heart repair with a Da-
cron patch.

1-188. A patient who was in a motor vehicle crash has a BP of 80/50 mm Hg,
heart rate of 126 beats/min, and respiratory rate of 28 breaths/min. The
12-lead ECG demonstrates sinus
tachycardia with atrial premature
contractions. Jugular veins are flat.
Heart tones are normal with no S_3
or S_4. Breath sounds are equal and
clear but shallow. Which of the following is the most likely cause of
the patient's hypotension?

A. Cardiac tamponade.
B. Hemothorax.
C. Pneumothorax.
D. Right ventricular contusion.

1-189. After repair of a ventricular stab
wound, a patient is having 6 to 10
premature ventricular contractions
per minute. Treatment should include

   I. Lidocaine bolus and infusion at
2 to 4 mg/min.
  II. Ventricular pacing.
 III. KCl, 10 mEq/hr prn for serum
potassium value less than 4.2
mEq/L.
 IV. Nitroglycerin, 50 mg/250 D5W,
to maintain systolic blood
pressure greater than 100 mm
Hg.

A. I and II.
B. II and III.
C. III and IV.
D. I and III.

1–190. A patient admitted to the ICU 5 days previously after sustaining a major electrical injury remains confused, restless, and agitated and exhibits severe short-term memory loss. The nurse implements

A. Seizure precaution measures.
B. Delirium tremens protocol.
C. Orientation to time and place protocol.
D. Sepsis work-up.

1–191. Three days after chest tube insertion for a tension pneumothorax, the nurse observes no bubbling or fluctuation in the water-seal chamber. This finding may indicate all of the following *except*

A. Bronchopleural fistula.
B. Tube obstruction.
C. Re-expansion of the lung.
D. Kinked tubing.

1–192. A 25-year-old patient in the ICU has a generalized tonic-clonic seizure. After the seizure has subsided, the critical care nurse expects the patient to exhibit which of the following as a characteristic behavior after a seizure?

A. Restlessness.
B. Lethargy.
C. Automatisms.
D. Incontinence.

1–193. A 19-year-old patient with multiple penetration injuries to the anterior trunk is admitted to the ICU. Which of the following are used to rapidly diagnose esophageal perforation?

A. Insertion of a chest tube and ingestion of methylene blue.
B. Peritoneal lavage and exploratory laparotomy.
C. Endotracheal intubation and suction.
D. Chest radiograph and contrast dye.

1–194. The classic symptom of aortoiliac occlusive disease is

A. Intermittent claudication.
B. Nonhealing leg ulcers.
C. A pulsatile mass over the iliac artery.
D. 2+ pulses noted at both the femoral and popliteal sites.

1–195. A patient with atherosclerotic heart disease and peripheral vascular disease was previously noted to have palpable bilateral dorsalis pedis and posterior tibialis pulses. In the initial assessment, the nurse notes the disappearance of the right dorsalis pedis pulse. Which of the following would be associated findings in an acute arterial occlusion?

I. Tenderness over the popliteal artery.
II. Severe, progressive pain in the toes and foot.
III. Positive blanching in mottled areas of the foot and calf.
IV. Nonblanching, mottled areas.

A. I and II.
B. II and IV.
C. II and III.
D. I, II, and III.

1–196. Which of the following medications is administered after peripheral arterial surgery to prevent vessel spasm?

A. Beta blockers.
B. Pyridamole.
C. Calcium channel blockers.
D. Prostaglandins.

1–197. A patient with chronic peripheral vascular disease has undergone revascularization surgery and has Ace wraps to the thigh. The patient reports intense pain in the calf that worsens when the foot is passively extended. The calf muscle is swollen and tender. Pedal pulses remain palpable at 1+. Capillary refill is 4 seconds, and compartment pressure is measured at 20 mm Hg. The nurse prepares for which corrective action?

A. Thrombectomy.
B. Administration of urokinase.
C. Removal and reapplication of Ace wraps.
D. Fasciotomy.

1–198. In evaluating the effectiveness of nutritional support during the post-resuscitation phase of burn injury, the most reliable indicator is

A. Indirect calorimetry.
B. Strict intake and output measurement.
C. Daily weight.
D. Nutrition formulas based on body and burn size.

1–199. A 25-year-old woman is admitted to the ICU after a motor vehicle crash. She has been unable to void, and the physician orders a Foley catheter to be inserted. Before catheter insertion, the nurse notes blood around the urinary meatus. The next action the nurse should take is to

A. Proceed with the Foley catheter insertion and inspect the urine.
B. Use a smaller straight catheter instead of a Foley catheter.
C. Cleanse the area and observe for continued bleeding.
D. Not insert the catheter and notify the physician immediately.

1–200. In a patient with suspected mild hypoglycemia, what is the first intervention the critical care nurse should implement?

A. Give intravenous glucose.
B. Obtain blood glucose level.
C. Determine last insulin dose and time.
D. Determine last oral intake.

1–1. (**B**) Nephrotoxicity is a side effect of both cyclosporine and tacrolimus but not OKT3. Anorexia, fever, chills, nausea, vomiting, diarrhea, weakness, and, less frequently, anaphylactic pulmonary edema, are side effects of OKT3.

Reference: Wahrenberger, A.: Differences in immunosuppressant agents. A.A.N.A.J. 19:566–567, 1992.

1–2. (**D**) The chest leads face the anterior wall of the left ventricle, specifically leads V_2 through V_6. Leads I and aVL face the lateral wall. Leads II, III, and aVF face the inferior wall.

Reference: Khan, M. G.: Heart Disease: Diagnosis and Therapy. Baltimore, Williams & Wilkins, 1996.

1–3. (**B**) Twenty-five to 50% of patients with acute MI have a normal initial ECG. Additional studies show that nondiagnostic changes account for 26% to 36% of patients admitted to rule out MI. ST segment elevation denotes injury on the 12-lead ECG and is considered indicative of pending MI. Q waves designate infarction.

Reference: Stack, L. B., Morgan, J. A., Hedges, J. R., Joseph, A. J.: Advances in the use of ancillary diagnostic testing in the emergency department evaluation of chest pain. Emerg. Med. Clin. North Am. 13:713–731, 1995.

1–4. (**A**) A patient with COPD normally has an increased $PaCO_2$ with normal pH and low normal oxygenation. In acute respiratory failure, ventilation is further impaired, leading to acidosis and hypoventilation, despite an increased respiratory rate and hypoxemia.

References: Alspach, J. G. (ed.): AACN Core Curriculum for Critical Care Nursing, 5th ed. Philadelphia, W. B. Saunders, 1998.
Kersten, L. D.: Comprehensive Respiratory Nursing: A Decision Making Approach. Philadelphia, W. B. Saunders, 1989.

1–5. (**D**) A patient with COPD normally has an elevated $PaCO_2$, compensated by retention of HCO_3^- leading to a normal pH. The arterial blood gas analysis results show that the ventilation supplied by the mechanical ventilation has blown off an excessive amount of CO_2. Because the kidneys have not had time to eliminate HCO_3^-, the pH becomes alkalotic. The arterial blood gases do not show hypoxemia or acidosis. Nasogastric suction would result in an alkalosis by removing gastric acid; however, there has not been sufficient time for this to occur.

References: Alspach, J. G. (ed.): AACN Core Curriculum for Critical Care Nursing, 5th ed. Philadelphia, W. B. Saunders, 1998.
Kersten, L. D.: Comprehensive Respiratory Nursing: A Decision Making Approach. Philadelphia, W. B. Saunders, 1989.

1–6. (**C**) The quickest way to correct the acute respiratory alkalosis would be to decrease the respiratory rate and allow the $PaCO_2$ to rise, thus correcting the pH to normal for this patient. This will also shorten weaning time because the HCO_3^- has already compensated for the patient's chronic respiratory acidosis. Ammonium chloride will also correct the disorder but usually is not used unless the patient's chloride is depleted or the respiratory rate cannot be decreased.

References: Alspach, J. G. (ed.): AACN Core Curriculum for Critical Care Nursing, 5th ed. Philadelphia, W. B. Saunders, 1998.
Kersten, L. D.: Comprehensive Respiratory Nursing: A Decision Making Approach. Philadelphia, W. B. Saunders, 1989.

1–7. (**D**) The nasal cannula, simple face mask, and partial rebreather mask are low-flow systems. Low-flow systems provide adequate gas flow partially by the system and partially by room air; and the FIO_2 varies depending on flow rate, ventilatory pattern, and anatomic dead space. This patient has an increased respiratory rate and decreased tidal volume (normal is around 500 ml), as well as hypoxemia and hypercarbia secondary to respiratory failure. A high-flow system is indicated to provide a consistent FIO_2 despite a low tidal volume. Either a Venturi mask or a heated nebulizer with face mask would be appropriate.

References: Alspach, J. G. (ed.): AACN Core Curriculum for Critical Care Nursing, 5th ed. Philadelphia, W. B. Saunders, 1998.
Kersten, L. D.: Comprehensive Respiratory Nursing: A Decision Making Approach. Philadelphia, W. B. Saunders, 1989.

1–8. (**A**) The most common cause of chronic bronchitis and emphysema is smoking. Alpha$_1$-antitrypsin deficiency is a genetic cause of emphysema. Patients with COPD are susceptible to pneumonia, which may then exacerbate COPD symptoms. Allergies may predispose a susceptible patient to asthma.

Reference: Alspach, J. G. (ed.): AACN Core Curriculum for Critical Care Nursing, 5th ed. Philadelphia, W. B. Saunders, 1998.

1–9. (**C**) Persistent ST segment elevation may indicate ventricular aneurysm. Ventricular aneurysms are an ischemic, noncontractile portion of the myocardium that expands during systole. New onset of ST segment elevation may represent extension of the area of infarct or a new infarction that is either transmural or nontransmural.

Reference: Kinney, M. R., Packa, D. R.: Andreoli's Comprehensive Cardiac Care, 8th ed. St. Louis, Mosby–Year Book, 1996.

1–10. (**D**) SIRS is the systemic response to any severe clinical incident. Extensive tissue damage is the result of a combination of maldistribution in blood flow leading to cell death and the effects of microorganisms or cellular by-products on cells. Anaphylaxis produces acute vasodilation, not inflammation. Infection is localized rather than systemic. Bacteremia refers to microorganisms in the circulation and is not a systemic response.

Reference: Clochesy, J. M.: Patients with systemic inflammatory response syndrome. *In* Clochesy, J. M., Breu, C., Cardin, S., et al. (eds.): Critical Care Nursing. Philadelphia, W. B. Saunders, 1996.

1–11. (**C**) Impressive ST segment elevation in the inferior leads (II, III, aVF) with reciprocal ST segment depression and T wave inversion in the anterolateral leads (I, aVL, and V_2 through V_4) indicate that this is an acute inferior wall MI. An acute anterior wall MI would have ST segment elevation in leads V_3 and V_4. An acute anteroseptal MI would have ST segment elevation in leads V_1 through V_4. An acute lateral wall MI would have ST changes in leads I and aVL and V_{5-6}.

Reference: Phalen, T.: The 12-Lead ECC in Acute Myocardial Infarction. St. Louis, Mosby–Year Book, 1996.

1–12. (**A**) Continuous jugular venous oxygen saturation (SjO_2) is an indirect measure of cerebral oxygenation. Transience of SjO_2 may indirectly reflect cerebral blood flow if measurements are made over a short period of time during which the cerebral metabolic rate for oxygen is assumed to remain unchanged. Arterial blood gases are simultaneously analyzed along with samples of venous blood withdrawn from the jugular catheter. Values derived are used to calculate the arteriovenous difference and, in conjunction with the cerebral blood flow measurements, determine the cerebral metabolic rate for oxygen. A normal SjO_2 value is approximately 65%; values below this are considered indicative of global ischemia.

References: Alspach, J. G. (ed.): AACN Core Curriculum for Critical Care Nursing, 5th ed. Philadelphia, W. B. Saunders, 1998.

Fortune, J. B., Feustal, P. J., Weigle, C. G., Popp, A. J. Continuous measurement of jugular venous oxygen saturation in response to transient elevations of blood pressure in head-injured patients. J. Neurosurg. 80:461–468, 1994.

1–13. (**A**) Ischemia of the gastrointestinal mucosa is a primary cause of stress ulcers. Elevated heart rate due to stress, fever, or other causes results in reduced gastrointestinal tract blood flow due to the vasoconstrictive effect of norepinephrine. Portal hypertension and local or systemic metabolic acidosis cause gastric mucosal ischemia. Hypovolemia, shock, occlusive diseases (emboli, thrombosis), and vascular spasm can also cause mucosal ischemia.

Reference: Prevost, S. S., Oberlie, A.: Stress ulceration in the critically ill patient. Crit. Care Nurs. Clin. North Am. 5:163–169, 1993.

1–14. (**D**) Leads V_2 through V_4 reflect the electrical activity of the anteroseptal wall. In this 12-lead ECG, ST segment elevation of 2 mm or greater is seen in leads V_2 and V_3, with slight ST segment elevation in leads V_1 and V_4. Inferior wall injury would be indicated by ST segment elevation in leads II, III, and aVF. Lateral wall injury would be indicated by ST segment elevation in leads I, aVL, V_5, and V_6. Posterior wall injury would be indicated by reciprocal ST segment depression in leads V_1 through V_4.

Reference: Thelan, L. A., Davie, J. K., Urden, L. D., Lough, M. E.: Critical Care Nursing, Diagnosis and Management, 2nd ed. St. Louis, Mosby–Year Book, 1994.

1–15. (**D**) Infarctions of the inferior wall are caused by occlusion of the right coronary artery, which supplies both the sinoatrial and atrioventricular nodes in most people. Patients with acute inferior wall myocardial infarction are therefore prone to heart blocks and bradyarrhythmias. Tachyarrhythmias and left-sided heart failure are associated with anterior wall myocardial infarction.

Reference: Thelan, L. A., Davie, J. K., Urden, L. D., Lough, M. E.: Critical Care Nursing: Diagnosis and Management, 2nd ed. St. Louis, Mosby–Year Book, 1994.

1–16. (**B**) Patients who are at higher risk of intracranial hemorrhage are thin, weighing less than 70 kg. Age older than 65 has been noted as a factor for increased risk of intracerebral bleeding. Hypertension has also been linked to intracerebral bleeding complications in patients receiving thrombolytic agents.

Reference: Braunwald, E. (ed.): Heart Disease: A Textbook of Cardiovascular Medicine. Philadelphia, W. B. Saunders, 1997.

1–17. (**D**) All of the therapies mentioned are used in malignant vasovagal syncope to prevent malignant syncopal reactions in the patient undergoing sheath removal. Sodium intake is encouraged to maintain preload. Trendelenburg position and normal saline infusion are used during sheath removal to prevent vagal hypotension. Scopolamine has atropine-like effects and prevents hypotension and bradycardia.

Reference: Barbiere, C.: Malignant vasovagal syncope after PTCA—a potential for disaster. Crit. Care Nurs. 14(2):90–93, 1994.

1–18. (**A**) The post–myocardial infarction patient with left ventricular thrombus is routinely placed on warfarin therapy for several weeks or months. Low-molecular-weight heparin is not approved for use in left ventricular thrombus therapy. Thrombectomy is not routinely performed because it is a high-risk open-heart procedure, and streptokinase administration is not used in this condition.

Reference: Kinney, M. R., Packa, D. R., Dunbar, S. B.: AACN's Clinical Reference for Critical Care Nursing, 3rd ed. St. Louis, Mosby–Year Book, 1993.

1–19. (**A**) Negative-pressure ventilation is provided externally and facilitates inspiration by pulling the chest outward, rather than pushing air in (e.g., iron lung, Cuirass ventilator). It is generally reserved for patients with respiratory failure who have normal lung parenchyma but concomitent ventilatory problems (e.g., neuromuscular disorders such as Guillain-Barré syndrome). Patients with lung disease such as pneumonia, pulmonary embolus, and asthma require more support than is generally able to be provided by the negative-pressure ventilator.

Reference: Alspach, J. G. (ed.): AACN Core Curriculum for Critical Care Nursing, 5th ed. Philadelphia, W. B. Saunders, 1998.

1–20. (**C**) Intrarenal or parenchymal renal failure is caused by primary or intrinsic damage to the nephrons, especially the tubular component, which results in a back-leak of glomerular filtrate. Prerenal failure is caused by decreased arterial blood flow to the kidneys. Postrenal or obstructive renal failure is caused by an obstruction of urine outflow.

Reference: Baer, C. L.: Acute renal failure. In Kinney, M. R., Packa, D. R., Dunbar, S. B. (ed.): AACN's Clinical Reference for Critical Care Nursing, 3rd ed. St. Louis, Mosby–Year Book, 1993.

1–21. (**B**) Maldistribution of blood flow occurs in septic shock, leading to inadequate tissue perfusion. As intracellular oxygen depletion occurs, lactic acid is produced. Lactic acid lowers the blood pH, producing a brain stem–mediated response that causes the patient to hyperventilate as carbon dioxide levels increase and pH levels decrease. Oxygen saturation is not decreased if the hemoglobin is fully saturated; rather, the deficit is between what is available (circulation) and what is required (metabolism).

Reference: Clochesy, J. M.: Patients with systemic inflammatory response syndrome. In Clochesy, J. M., Breu, C., Cardin, S., et al. (eds.): Critical Care Nursing. Philadelphia, W. B. Saunders, 1996.

1–22. (**C**) Beta blockers block sympathetic stimulation that causes increases in heart rate and, therefore, oxygen demand. Aspirin has no effect on the sympathetic or parasympathetic system. ACE inhibitors block angiotensin but not the systemic sympathetic response. Calcium channel blockers may stimulate the sympathetic response by vasodilation.

Reference: Kinney, M. R., Packa, D. R., Dunbar, S. B.: AACN's Clinical Reference for Critical Care Nursing, 3rd ed. St. Louis, Mosby–Year Book, 1993.

1–23. **(B)** The focus of stress ulcer prevention and treatment is usually directed toward gastric pH control. Inhibition of bicarbonate secretion would diminish the effectiveness of the gastric mucus. Endogenous prostaglandins are normally numerous in the gastric mucosa and provide a protective function by inhibiting gastric acid production, promoting mucus production, and promoting water and electrolyte absorption. H_2-receptor antagonists are used to block the histamine stimulation of gastric acid secretion.

Reference: Prevost, S. S., Oberlie, A.: Stress ulceration in the critically ill patient. Crit. Care Nurs. Clin. North Am. 5:163–169, 1993.

1–24. **(C)** The most important intervention in caring for a patient with an intraventricular cannula for intracranial pressure monitoring is to maintain a closed system to prevent contamination. Normal intracranial pressures should be less than 10 mm Hg: pressures between 10 and 20 mm Hg are considered mildly to moderately elevated. Although it may be necessary to open the system to zero-balance or to drain cerebrospinal fluid, care must be taken to avoid introduction of pathogens. The cannula is usually inserted into the lateral ventricle and connected by a stopcock to a transducer positioned at the level of the foramen of Monro using the middle of the ear as a reference point. It will be necessary to zero-balance the transducer if the patient's position is changed or if erroneous readings are suspected. The phlebostatic axis is used as a reference point for the transducer in intracardiac monitoring.

Reference: Alspach, J. G. (ed.): AACN Core Curriculum for Critical Care Nursing, 5th ed. Philadelphia, W. B. Saunders, 1998.

1–25. **(B)** The most common complication of pituitary tumor resection is diabetes insipidus, which results from hyposecretion of antidiuretic hormone (ADH) from the posterior lobe of the pituitary gland. Lack of ADH results in increased urine output due to inability to conserve water. Increased urine output is usually the first sign of diabetes insipidus. Management includes encouraging oral fluid intake and intravenous fluid replacement. Water losses result in hypernatremia. Hypertonic intravenous fluids, fluid restriction, and diuretics are all contraindicated.

Reference: Counsel, C. M., Gilbert, M., Snively, C.: Management of the patient with a pituitary tumor. Dimen. Crit. Care Nurs. 15(2):75–81, 1996.

1–26. **(B)** The gold standard for detecting cardiac rejection continues to be endomyocardial biopsy. Treatment of rejection is high-dose corticosteroids or monoclonal antibodies. Cyclosporine is indicated to prevent, not treat, rejection. Trimethoprim is used to prevent/treat *Pneumocystis* infection after transplantation.

References: Finkelmeier, B. A.: Cardiothoracic Surgical Nursing. Philadelphia, J. B. Lippincott, 1995.
Kobashigawa, J., Stevenson, L.: Managing complications in heart transplant recipients. J. Crit. Illness 8:678–689, 1993.
MacDonald, S. N.: Heart transplantation, Part I. *In* Sigardson-Poor, K. M., Haggerty, L. M.: Nursing Care of the Transplant Recipient. Philadelphia, W. B. Saunders, 1990.

1–27. **(B)** Normal inspiration to expiration time is 1:2. In severe respiratory distress syndrome, the stiff lungs do not expand sufficiently to allow adequate filling of the alveoli and diffusion of oxygen to the alveoli. Inverse I:E ratio ventilation increases lung volumes, which recruits (opens collapsed) alveoli without increasing the airway pressure. Expiratory time is shortened, and physiologic dead space may decrease. Auto-PEEP may occur and should be monitored, but that is not a reason to use inverse ratio ventilation.

Reference: Marini, J. J.: New options for the ventilatory management of acute lung injury. New Horizons 1:489–503, 1993.

1–28. (**B**) Her pulmonary wedge and right atrial pressures were decreased before instituting inverse I:E ratio ventilation. By prolonging the inspiratory time, venous return is impeded, leading to a hypovolemic picture in her hemodynamic values. Cardiogenic shock would show increased pulmonary capillary wedge and right atrial pressures. A pulmonary embolus large enough to affect the cardiac output would also increase the right atrial pressure.

Reference: Marini, J. J.: New options for the ventilatory management of acute lung injury. New Horizons 1:489–503, 1993.

1–29. (**A**) Because the change in blood gases and hemodynamics is due to hypovolemia, the treatment would be to administer intravenous fluids. Adequate intravascular volume is required before instituting inotropic therapy because the heart has to have an adequate filling volume to be able to contract effectively. If the blood gases and hemodynamics continue to deteriorate despite adequate intravenous fluid therapy and inotropic therapy, inverse I:E ratio ventilation should be discontinued. Streptokinase therapy is not indicated because a pulmonary embolus is not a factor.

Reference: Alspach, J. G. (ed.): AACN Core Curriculum for Critical Care Nursing, 5th ed. Philadelphia, W. B. Saunders, 1998.

1–30. (**C**) The cardiovascular response to sepsis produces a decrease in blood pressure, decrease in SVR, decrease in LV ejection fraction, an increase in LV end-diastolic volume, increased cardiac output, and increased heart rate. The response appears to be mediated by a substance secreted from macrophages, interleukin-1.

Reference: Clochesy, J. M.: Patients with systemic inflammatory response syndrome. *In* Clochesy, J. M., Breu, C., Cardin, S. et al. (eds.): Critical Care Nursing. Philadelphia, W. B. Saunders, 1996.

1–31. (**C**) The normal values for PT are 10 to 14 seconds; ACT, 90 to 128 seconds; and PTT, 30 to 45 seconds. For the first 24 to 48 hours after acute myocardial infarction, the APTT on heparin should be maintained at one and one-half to two times the control or normal value, which is 16 to 25 seconds. Therefore, an appropriate range for the APTT would be 35 to 50 seconds.

Reference: Ruppert, S. D., Kernicki, J. G., Dolan, J. T.: Dolan's Critical Care Nursing: Clinical Management Through the Nursing Process. Philadelphia, F. A. Davis, 1996.

1–32. (**A**) A priority in the care of patients with acute myocardial infarction is to prevent increased myocardial oxygen demands. Positioning the patient supine with the legs elevated should be performed as an initial intervention. This position increases blood return to the right ventricle, increases stroke volume, and thus improves blood pressure without increasing $M\bar{v}O_2$. If it fails to relieve the symptoms, the other methods may be attempted. If positioning restores blood pressure, a fluid challenge may be attempted. Transcutaneous pacing may be initiated at a higher rate if there is no improvement in blood pressure with positioning. Atropine is used when other methods fail to restore heart rate and blood pressure because the increases in heart rate are unpredictable and increase myocardial oxygen demand.

Reference: Braunwald, E. (ed.): Heart Disease: A Textbook of Cardiovascular Medicine. Philadelphia, W. B. Saunders, 1997.

1–33. **(C)** If reocclusion is suspected, tPA may be readministered or given after streptokinase. Streptokinase administration cannot be repeated because of the risk of anaphylaxis. Percutaneous transluminal coronary angioplasty or coronary artery bypass graft may also be performed. Aspirin should not be repeated, because the initial dose recommended by most protocols has already been administered. The heparin drip is at an appropriate rate for a patient who has received thrombolytic therapy.

Reference: Kinney, M. R., Packa, D. R., Dunbar, S. B.: AACN's Clinical Reference for Critical Care Nursing, 3rd ed. St. Louis, Mosby–Year Book, 1993.

1–34. **(B)** Because IRV reverses the normal I:E ventilatory pattern, it can be very anxiety producing for the patient. This change in ventilatory pattern does not feel normal and can produce a sensation of dyspnea. These patients can increase their oxygen needs or disrupt ventilation by being agitated, so they should be kept sedated and paralyzed. A pulmonary artery catheter may be helpful to assess hemodynamics but is not required. The patient may need 1:1 nursing care because of the complexity of care, but it is not required solely because of IRV. IRV can be used in any ICU with a ventilator capable of providing that mode of ventilation and with staff capable of caring for those patients.

Reference: Marini, J. J.: New options for the ventilatory management of acute lung injury. New Horizons 1:489–503, 1993.

1–35. **(A)** Increased endotracheal cuff pressures lead to high tracheal wall pressures, which then lead to mucosal ischemia. Mucosal ischemia leads to inflammation, hemorrhage, ulceration, and erosion. Too large an internal diameter may result in pulmonary aspiration and infection. Self-extubation has been associated with a decreased cuff volume.

Reference: Kersten, L. D.: Comprehensive Respiratory Nursing: A Decision Making Approach. Philadelphia, W. B. Saunders, 1989.

1–36. **(B)** Perivascular hemorrhages that surround small vessels around and directly beneath a point of impact along with a laceration that occurs on the opposite side of the brain as it strikes and rebounds on the skull is termed a *coup/contrecoup* injury. This mass movement of the intracranial contents causes bilateral and symmetric involvement. Diffuse axonal injuries, frequently called *shearing* injuries, differ based on their severity. A *hematoma* arises as a result of bleeding within the epidural or subdural space or as a clot within the brain tissue itself. *Concussion* is a clinical diagnosis that refers to transient neurogenic dysfunction after head trauma in which consciousness may or may not be lost; it results from a sudden release of acetylcholine.

Reference: Clochesy, J. M., Breu, C., Cardin, S., et al. (eds.): Critical Care Nursing, 2nd ed. Philadelphia, W. B. Saunders, 1996.

1–37. **(A)** Electrolyte absorption occurs most rapidly in the proximal portion of the small bowel. Disease processes that affect the duodenum are most likely to cause significant disruption of electrolyte absorption. Curling's ulcers are common in patients with severe burns and are usually located in the duodenum. Stress ulcers are usually located in the fundus of the stomach. Cushing's ulcers occur in patients with trauma, surgery, or central nervous system disease. They occur in the esophagus, stomach, and duodenum but are associated with hypersecretion of gastric acid and pepsin rather than with electrolyte imbalances. Chronic gastric ulcers are located in the stomach.

References: Prevost, S. S., Oberlie, A.: Stress ulceration in the critically ill patient. Crit. Care Nurs. Clin. North Am. 5:163–169, 1993.
Yamada, T. (ed.): Textbook of Gastroenterology, 2nd ed. Philadelphia, J. B. Lippincott, 1995.

Core Review Test 1 Answers 37

1–38. **(D)** Rapid heart rates increase the $M\bar{v}O_2$ and may precipitate chest pain. The rapid rate and right bundle-branch block indicate that the patient has rate-related problems, and rate reduction with atenolol should be attempted first. Nitroglycerin spray and morphine administration may increase the heart rate further as a result of vasodilation. Lack of ST segment elevation precludes the need for thrombolytic agents.

Reference: Kupersmith, J., Deedwania, P. C.: The Pharmacologic Management of Heart Disease. Baltimore, Williams & Wilkins, 1997.

1–39. **(D)** After thrombolytic therapy, the APTT is generally maintained at one and one-half to two times the control. Because nitroglycerin may decrease the activity of heparin many patients require higher doses of heparin. One of the primary reasons for reocclusion is inappropriately low heparinization after both revascularization and thrombolytic therapy. A bolus of heparin with an increase in the rate is the most appropriate intervention. Increasing the nitroglycerin or administering morphine is unnecessary because there is no chest pain or increase in ST segment elevation.

Reference: Crawford, M.: Current Diagnosis and Treatment in Cardiology. Norwalk, Conn., Appleton & Lange, 1995.

1–40. **(A)** CAVH/CAVHD is used for removal of waste products, as well as acids, electrolytes, and excess fluids in patients who are mildly to moderately catabolic and hemodynamically unstable. SCUF is used to rapidly remove excess fluid volume in hemodynamically unstable patients who are refractory to diuretics or in patients who are oliguric and require large volumes of fluid removed. Hemodialysis and peritoneal dialysis are used for removal of waste products, acids, electrolytes, and fluids in patients who are hemodynamically stable.

Reference: Baer, C. L.: Acute renal failure. *In* Kinney, M. R., Packa, D. R., Dunbar, S. B. (ed.): AACN's Clinical Reference for Critical Care Nursing, 3rd ed. St. Louis, Mosby–Year Book, 1993.

1–41. **(B)** Approximately 1 of 100 hospitalized patients develops sepsis, and 40% of these progress to septic shock.

Reference: Clochesy, J. M.: Patients with systemic inflammatory response syndrome. *In* Clochesy, J. M., Breu, C., Cardin, S., et al. (eds.): Critical Care Nursing. Philadelphia, W. B. Saunders, 1996.

1–42. **(A)** Reduction and relief of chest pain indicate reperfusion. Although premature ventricular contractions may indicate a reperfusion dysrhythmia, they are not specific to reperfusion and may indicate hypoxemia, potassium imbalances, or merely an irritable myocardium. Variable ST segment changes and nausea and diaphoresis may be symptoms of reinfarction.

Reference: Kinney, M. R., Packa, D. R.: Andreoli's Comprehensive Cardiac Care, 8th ed. St. Louis, Mosby–Year Book, 1996.

1–43. **(D)** ST segment elevation is typically found in patients with unstable angina during episodes of chest pain. They may have no ECG changes during pain-free periods. Q waves signify that infarction has taken place. ST segment depression is more commonly seen in chronic stable angina.

Reference: Crawford, M.: Current Diagnosis and Treatment in Cardiology. Norwalk, Conn., Appleton & Lange, 1995.

1–44. **(A)** The pain of unstable angina is described as similar to regular angina but more intense or as pain that radiates to different or additional sites. The pain may be described as pressure, squeezing, or heaviness. Pain of myocardial infarction lasts for more than 30 minutes or is unrelieved by nitroglycerin. Unstable anginal pain is reduced but generally not completely relieved by nitroglycerin.

Reference: Braunwald, E. (ed.): Heart Disease: A Textbook of Cardiovascular Medicine. Philadelphia, W. B. Saunders, 1997.

1–45. (**D**) Providing oxygen at 100% FIo_2 would correct for hypoxemia if it were due to diffusion defect, hypoventilation, or a $\dot{V}/\dot{Q}$ imbalance. Thus, the cause of his refractory hypoxemia is most likely a right-to-left shunt. When a right-to-left shunt occurs, venous blood passes unventilated alveoli and is not oxygenated. Providing 100% oxygen does not correct for the hypoxemia because oxygen cannot get to the capillaries through the unventilated alveoli and the collateral ventilation is not sufficient to overcome the deficiency.

References: Alspach, J. G. (ed.): AACN Core Curriculum for Critical Care Nursing, 5th ed. Philadelphia, W. B. Saunders, 1998.
Kersten, L. D.: Comprehensive Respiratory Nursing: A Decision Making Approach. Philadelphia, W. B. Saunders, 1989.

1–46. (**A**) Respiratory distress syndrome (RDS) is characterized by pulmonary edema from injury to the alveolar-capillary membrane. Unlike cardiogenic shock and pulmonary embolus, the right atrial and pulmonary wedge pressures are low to normal in RDS. Neurogenic pulmonary edema is due to a central nervous system problem. The telling information is that this patient's sputum colloid osmotic pressure is greater than his serum value, indicating that proteins are leaking into the alveoli.

Reference: West, J. B.: Pulmonary Pathophysiology, 4th ed. Baltimore, Williams & Wilkins, 1992.

1–47. (**D**) He is in lactic acidosis (8.2 mg/dl lactic acid level) secondary to the hypoxemia. In acidosis, the excess of hydrogen ions binds with carbon dioxide and potassium comes out of the cell. As the hypoxemia is corrected, potassium returns to the cell as hydrogen comes out of the cell to maintain electrical neutrality. Thus, the correction of hypoxemia is associated with hypokalemia.

Reference: West, J. B.: Pulmonary Pathophysiology, 4th ed. Baltimore, Williams & Wilkins, 1992.

1–48. (**C**) If otorrhea, the escape of fluid from the ear follows head injury, the fluid is likely cerebrospinal fluid (CSF). Because CSF contains glucose and lactate, it would be appropriate for the nurse to assess the drainage for the presence of these substances. In neurotrauma, pressure is never directly applied to the area of injury because possible compression of bone fragments into brain tissue may result. Meningitis, an infectious process, can result if microorganisms are introduced from packing the ear of a patient with drainage. Therefore, dressings are loosely applied to the external ear to allow for absorption of the drainage. Suction of the ear is not an appropriate nursing intervention because suction of cerebral contents can result.

Reference: Caine, R. M., Bufalino, P. M. (eds.): Nursing Care Planning Guides for Adults, 2nd ed. Baltimore, Williams & Wilkins, 1991.

1–49. (**B**) A newly admitted ICU patient will have endogenous biologic rhythms that are synchronized to his or her prehospital environment. Some of these internal rhythms include variations in heart rate, urine volume, and thermoregulation. Therefore, patient condition changes should be monitored in terms of normal variations in biologic rhythms. Sleep/wake cycles are promoted by increasing activity during customary wake time and reducing (or eliminating) activity during customary sleep time. Although hope is an important coping mechanism, unclear or unrealistic communication of expected outcomes disengages the caregiver(s) from the patient and family, adversely affecting care.

References: Chesla, C. A., Stannard, D.: Breakdown in the nursing care of families in the ICU. Am. J. Crit. Care 6(1):64–71, 1997.
Felver, L.: Patient-environment interactions in critical care. Crit. Care Nurs. Clin. North Am. 7:327–335, 1995.

1–50. (**C**) SIADH is characterized by plasma hypotonicity and hyponatremia that result from aberrant secretion of antidiuretic hormone due to failure of the negative feedback system. Water is retained relative to sodium, which results in dilute plasma with a low tonicity and a low sodium concentration.

Reference: Alspach, J. G. (ed.): AACN Core Curriculum for Critical Care Nursing, 5th ed. Philadelphia, W. B. Saunders, 1998.

1–51. (**B**) In the steps of the clotting cascade, reactions require calcium, coenzymes, or platelets to convert inactive proenzymes to active enzymes through proteolytic cleavage. Sodium, phosphorus, and potassium are not involved in the process of the clotting cascade.

Reference: Alspach, J. G. (ed.): AACN Core Curriculum for Critical Care Nursing, 5th ed. Philadelphia, W. B. Saunders, 1998.

1–52. (**D**) For the first 48 to 72 hours, broad-spectrum antibiotics may be ineffective because the drug may not be delivered to the affected tissues because of maldistribution of blood flow. As cardiovascular stability is restored, tissue perfusion increases and the drug is delivered to tissues.

Reference: Clochesy, J. M.: Patients with systemic inflammatory response syndrome. *In* Clochesy, J. M., Breu, C., Cardin, S., et al. (eds.): Critical Care Nursing. Philadelphia, W. B. Saunders, 1996.

1–53. (**A**) Low-dose dopamine (2 to 4 μg/kg/min) is administered to increase renal blood flow and cardiac perfusion. Heart rate and contractility increase with a moderate dose (5 to 10 μg/kg/min). High-dose dopamine (10 to 20 μg/kg/min) may strengthen myocardial contraction, heart rate, and cardiac output in patients not responding to lower dosages.

Reference: Roberts, S. L.: Multisystem deviations. *In* Critical Care Nursing: Assessment and Intervention. Stamford, Conn., Appleton & Lange, 1996.

1–54. (**D**) Lesions of the left anterior descending artery generally cause anterolateral ischemia, which is best viewed in leads V_2 through V_6.

Reference: Stiesmeyer, J. R.: Unstable angina associated with proximal left anterior descending coronary artery stenosis. Am. J. Crit. Care 2:48–53, 1993.

1–55. (**D**) The discharge plan for a patient with unstable angina should include medical follow-up, the use of aspirin, and risk factor modification. Identification of risk factors should occur as soon as the patient is stabilized, and the education plan for the patient should be tailored to the risk factors identified. Nutrition education may be identified as a component of risk factor modification.

Reference: Braunwald, E., Mark, D. B., Jones, R. H., et. al: Unstable Angina: Diagnosis and Management. Clinical Practice Guideline Number 10. ACHPR Publication No. 94–0602. Rockville, Md., Agency for Health Care Policy and Research and the National Heart, Lung and Blood Institute, Public Health Service, U.S. Department of Health and Human Services, March 1994.

1–56. (**D**) Large extended families can be very draining on ICU staff and the patient. One or two members of the family should be identified as spokes-persons to meet with the members of the team and update the rest of the family. This should decrease the number of calls because those calling would be directed to the spokespersons and may decrease the numbers and frequency of visitors because the information would be coming from someone they know and trust. If visiting continues to be an issue, a social worker could discuss visiting with them and assist in developing a visitation contract. Holding a family conference is usually hard in large families because it is difficult to bring everyone together at one time.

Reference: Kersten, L. D.: Comprehensive Respiratory Nursing: A Decision Making Approach. Philadelphia, W. B. Saunders, 1989.

1–57. (**C**) Adding dead space does not increase the mean airway pressure. Increasing the inspiratory time, end-expiratory alveolar pressure, and minute ventilation can all increase the mean airway pressure. Increasing the mean airway pressure equalizes the pressure between the alveolus and interstitium and thereby decreases the likelihood of a pneumothorax.

Reference: Marini, J. J.: New options for the ventilatory management of acute lung injury. New Horizons 1:489–503, 1993.

1–58. (**D**) Coronary vasodilation with nitroglycerin is the primary method to prevent angina and cardiac ischemia, which may lead to myocardial infarction. Nitrate headaches may prevent patients from appropriate self-medication. To help the patient become less fearful of the headache occurrence, the care plan for patients who develop nitrate headaches should include slow titration, analgesic medication, and encouragement that the headaches will diminish with increased use of nitrates.

Reference: Olson, H. G., Aronow, W. S.: Medical management of stable and unstable angina in the elderly with CAD. Clin. Geriatr. Med. 12:121–137, 1996.

1–59. (**A**) The presence of U waves on an ECG, along with bradycardia and ventricular ectopy, is associated with hypokalemia. ECG changes associated with hypocalcemia are lengthened QT intervals and dysrhythmias. Hyponatremia can cause tachycardia and orthostatic hypotension. ECG changes associated with hypomagnesemia include cardiac dysrhythmias, tachycardia, prolonged QT interval, and shortened ST segment.

Reference: Baer, C. L.: Fluid and electrolyte balance. *In* Kinney, M. R., Packa, D. R., Dunbar, S. B. (eds.): AACN's Clinical Reference for Critical Care Nursing, 3rd ed. St. Louis, Mosby–Year Book, 1993.

1–60. (**C**) Lack of magnesium causes calcium and potassium to move into the extracellular fluid where they are subsequently excreted. Therefore, low levels of magnesium can cause hypocalcemia and hypokalemia. If the hypomagnesemia is uncorrected, the patient will remain hypokalemic, despite potassium replacement.

Reference: Baer, C. L.: Fluid and electrolyte balance. *In* Kinney, M. R., Packa, D. R., Dunbar, S. B. (eds.): AACN's Clinical Reference for Critical Care Nursing, 3rd ed. St. Louis, Mosby–Year Book, 1993.

1–61. (**C**) Acquired coagulopathies are most commonly related to vitamin K deficiency, liver disease, and renal disease. The primary causes of vitamin K deficiency are gastrointestinal disorders (including regional enteritis, ulcerative colitis, and short bowel syndrome), medications (including broad-spectrum antibiotics, anticoagulants, and salicylates), and liver disease. Vitamin K deficiency is characterized by prolonged PT and PTT. Antibiotic allergy is demonstrated by symptoms of histamine release such as hives. Uremia can cause coagulopathy but is not apparent in this patient. Thrombocytopenia and other platelet abnormalities are characteristic of coagulopathies associated with renal disease.

Reference: Kimbrell, J. D.: Acquired coagulopathies. Crit. Care Nurs. Clin. North Am. 5:453–458, 1993.

1–62. (**D**) Tuberculosis is common in immunosuppressed individuals and may not present as the classic clinical and x-ray features because of the depressed immune system. The fever, chills, and night sweats should alert the nurse to the possibility of tuberculosis rather than infection with *Pneumocystis*. *Pneumocystis* pneumonia presents as tachypnea, dyspnea, and fever. Pneumococcal and *Legionella* pneumonias do not present as chills and night sweats but rather cough, fever, dyspnea, and chest pain.

Reference: Kinney, M. R., Packa, D. R., Dunbar, S. B. (eds.): AACN's Clinical Reference for Critical Care Nursing, 3rd ed. St. Louis, Mosby–Year Book, 1993.

1–63. (**C**) Any patient with suspected or known infectious tuberculosis should be placed in an isolation room with negative-pressure air flow that circulates from the hall to the patient room to prevent the aerosolized droplets from circulating and contaminating others. A private room, regular isolation room, and two-bed room would not have the negative air flow to prevent contamination of the area outside the room. A HEPA filter has no effect on aerosolized bacteria but filters pollens and other airborne particles.

Reference: Kinney, M. R., Packa, D. R., Dunbar, S. B. (eds.): AACN's Clinical Reference for Critical Care Nursing, 3rd ed. St. Louis, Mosby–Year Book, 1993.

1–64. (**A**) Smear and culture for acid-fast bacilli of three to five sputum specimens collected once daily, 24 hours apart, is the main diagnostic procedure for tuberculosis. Sputum induction by heated aerosol should not be necessary because sputum production is one of the identifying symptoms of tuberculosis.

Reference: Kinney, M. R., Packa, D. R., Dunbar, S. B. (eds.): AACN's Clinical Reference for Critical Care Nursing, 3rd ed. St. Louis, Mosby–Year Book, 1993.

1–65. (**B**) To prevent nitrate tolerance, free periods are incorporated into therapy. This may be accomplished by applying transdermal nitrates for only 12 of 24 hours or by administering isosorbide dinitrate twice or three times daily instead of four times a day.

Reference: Olson, H. G., Aronow, W. S.: Medical management of stable and unstable angina in the elderly with CAD. Clin. Geriatr. Med. 12:121–137, 1996.

1–66. (**B**) Application of heat to the warmer extremity will induce vasodilation of the other extremity owing to sympathetic action. If you apply heat to the cooler extremity you may further compromise oxygenation of the obstructed area of the affected extremity by increasing local metabolism. Increased activity of the extremity may loosen a thrombus that may be responsible for the decreased perfusion.

Reference: Ruppert, S. D., Kernicki, J. G., Dolan, J. T.: Dolan's Critical Care Nursing: Clinical Management Through the Nursing Process. Philadelphia, F. A. Davis, 1996.

1–67. (**B**) Vasovagal reactions during sheath removal are commonly treated with atropine, 0.5 mg IV. Atropine is a parasympatholytic medication that reverses vagal symptoms, thus increasing heart rate and blood pressure. Sheath removal would not cause immediate blood loss necessitating infusion of packed cells. Although manual pressure or a compression device is routinely applied after sheath removal, treatment of the vagal symptoms is necessary to increase heart rate and blood pressure. Raising the legs only would increase blood pressure but not restore the heart rate.

Reference: Ruppert, S. D., Kernicki, J. G., Dolan, J. T.: Dolan's Critical Care Nursing: Clinical Management Through the Nursing Process. Philadelphia, F. A. Davis, 1996.

1–68. (**C**) Angina lasting more than 1 hour on parenteral therapy indicates failure of the therapy and the need for more aggressive intervention. Recurrent angina on nonparenteral medications indicates the need for parenteral medication.

Reference: Braunwald, E., Mark, D. B., Jones, R. H., et al.: Unstable Angina: Diagnosis and Management. Clinical Practice Guideline Number 10. ACHPR Publication No. 94–0602. Rockville, Md.: Agency for Health Care Policy and Research and the National Heart, Lung and Blood Institute, Public Health Service, U.S. Department of Health and Human Services, March 1994.

1–69. (**B**) Minimal leak technique to inflate the cuff can be used initially to occlude the airway and maintain the tidal volume. Because this may necessitate higher cuff pressures than are desirable, the patient should be evaluated for weaning. If weaning is not possible, a foam-cuffed tube might be useful if high ventilator pressures or tidal volumes are not necessary. A tracheostomy may be appropriate if mechanical ventilation is going to be needed for a prolonged period of time. Use of a double-lumen endotracheal tube is unnecessary.

Reference: Kersten, L. D.: Comprehensive Respiratory Nursing: A Decision Making Approach. Philadelphia, W. B. Saunders, 1989.

1–70. (**D**) Sepsis-induced cardiogenic shock is treated with dopamine to increase strength of cardiac contractions and a vasodilator (nitroprusside) to decrease systemic vascular resistance to maintain mean arterial pressure, enhance myocardial contractility, and reduce afterload (systemic vascular resistance) and preload (pulmonary capillary wedge pressure). Levarterenol (Levophed), epinephrine, and phenylephrine (Neo-Synephrine) act systemically to produce peripheral vasoconstriction and would lead to decreased tissue perfusion. Atropine increases myocardial rate rather than improving contractility, which is the dysfunction associated with cardiogenic shock.

Reference: Roberts, S. L.: Multisystem deviations. *In* Critical Care Nursing: Assessment and Intervention. Stamford, Conn., Appleton & Lange, 1996.

1–71. (**C**) Pseudoaneurysm and aneurysm formation are indicated by the presence of a 4+ femoral pulse and firm, thick ecchymosis. Doppler ultrasonography would be used to evaluate these complications. A sandbag would not resolve the aneurysm or pseudoaneurysm. Although most hematomas do resolve without intervention, the presence of the 4+ pulse indicates aneurysm formation. Angiography is generally unnecessary because the defect relates to the puncture site.

Reference: Jones, C., Holcomb, E., Rohrer, T.: Femoral artery pseudoaneurysm after invasive procedures. Crit. Care Nurs. 15:47–51, 1995.

1–72. (**C**) Plasma osmolarity normally ranges between 280 and 295 mOsm/L. Intravenous fluid solutions that most closely match plasma osmolarity (e.g., 0.9% saline) are considered isotonic, those that exceed plasma osmolarity (e.g., D10W) are considered hypertonic (i.e., hyperosmolar), and those that have lower plasma osmolarities (e.g., D5W) are considered hypotonic (i.e., hypo-osmolar). Hypo-osmolar solutions, when administered to patients with traumatic brain injury, can be expected to reduce the serum sodium level and increase brain water and intracranial pressure. Hypertonic solutions can decrease brain water and intracranial pressure while temporarily increasing systolic blood pressure and cardiac output. Fluid restriction, as may occur in patients receiving 50 ml of intravenous fluids per hour, may not initially affect cerebral edema but may ultimately precipitate hypotension, which may increase intracranial pressure.

Reference: Zornow, M. H., Prough, D. S.: Fluid management in patients with traumatic brain injury. New Horizons 3:488–498, 1995.

1–73. (**B**) A nasogastric tube with frequent instillation of fluid antacids dramatically increases the potential for aspiration due to reflux through the penetrated gastric cardiac sphincter and a wick effect up the tubing. Other potential side effects of nasogastric antacids include metabolic alkalosis, hypernatremia, and diarrhea.

Reference: Prevost, S. S., Oberlie, A.: Stress ulceration in the critically ill patient. Crit. Care Nurs. Clin. North Am. 5:163–169, 1993.

1–74. (**A**) ECG characteristics of WPW syndrome include a shortened PR interval, a delta wave, and an abnormally wide QRS complex. In WPW there is an anomalous pathway connecting the atria and ventricles. This pathway bypasses the atrioventricular junction, which normally delays the impulse to the ventricle, causes the shortened PR interval, and may result in paroxysmal tachycardias.

Reference: Wright, J. E., Shelton, B. K.: Desk Reference for Critical Care Nursing, Boston, Jones & Bartlett, 1993.

1–75. (**C**) Potassium deficits are substantial in DKA. The extracellular fluid is hyperosmolar due to hyperglycemia, and fluid, along with potassium, shifts out of the cells. With acidosis, hydrogen ions shift into the cells, pushing potassium out, and a lack of insulin keeps potassium from entering the cells. The osmotic diuresis seen in DKA then causes excessive extracellular potassium to be excreted. If the serum potassium level measured is normal, there is still a deficit in the intracellular amount. If the measured serum potassium level is low, the deficit exists in both compartments, is more severe, and identifies patients at higher risk for morbidity and mortality. Aggressive potassium replacement in these patients is necessary because correction of volume deficits with saline and the concomitant administration of insulin both further lower the potassium concentration. The deficit of magnesium is seldom clinically important. Phosphorus deficiency is usually mild, and calcium deficiency occurs in less than 30% of patients.

Reference: Civetta, J. M., Taylor, R. W., Kirby, R. R. (eds.): Critical Care, 2nd ed. Philadelphia, J. B. Lippincott, 1992.

1–76. (**B**) Ventricular conduction is accomplished through three pathways or fascicles that exit the bundle of His. The right bundle is a single branch, and the left bundle divides into the anterior and posterior fascicles. When all three pathways are blocked, it is called trifascicular block. Because trifascicular block often progresses to complete heart block, a transcutaneous pacemaker should be at the bedside until a temporary or permanent pacemaker can be inserted. Trifascicular block does not cause ventricular fibrillation or tachyarrhythmias. Administration of adenosine would depress sinoatrial and atrioventricular node conduction, potentially worsening the block. Lidocaine depresses the myocardium and may inhibit ventricular escape beats if the patient becomes bradycardic.

Reference: Wright, J. E., Shelton, B. K.: Desk Reference for Critical Care Nursing. Boston, Jones & Bartlett, 1993.

1–77. (**B**) The pacemaker is sensing P waves as ventricular activity. The correct treatment is to decrease the sensitivity of the pacemaker to prevent further episodes of oversensing. Increasing the mA, or output, would change the energy level of the impulses delivered but would not cause the pacemaker to initiate paced beats.

Reference: Dossey, B. M., Guzzetta, C. E., Kenner, C. V.: Critical Care Nursing, Body—Mind—Spirit. Philadelphia, J. B. Lippincott, 1992.

1–78. (**B**) The clinical manifestations associated with fat embolism are often subtle with minimal changes evidenced. A definitive clue to this diagnosis is the petechial rash, which does not occur with adult respiratory distress syndrome, pneumothorax, or pneumonia. The petechial rash occurs from the fat molecules that accumulate in the capillaries.

Reference: Kinney, M. R., Packa, D. R., and Dunbar, S. B. (eds.): AACN's Clinical Reference for Critical Care Nursing, 3rd ed. St. Louis, Mosby–Year Book, 1993.

1–79. (**C**) Corticosteroids help to reduce the inflammation produced by the fat emulsions. Heparin and dextran are no longer used to treat fat emboli because they have not been found to be effective. Tissue plasminogen activator is not indicated because it is effective only on thrombi.

Reference: Kinney, M. R., Packa, D. R., Dunbar, S. B. (eds.): AACN's Clinical Reference for Critical Care Nursing, 3rd ed. St. Louis, Mosby–Year Book, 1993.

1–80. (**B**) Heart rate and contractility increase with dopamine infusions up to 20 μg/kg/min. If the response is not adequate, levarterenol (Levophed) can be administered at a rate of 2 to 8 μg/min. Epinephrine at a dose of 1 to 8 μg/min and phenylephrine (Neo-Synephrine) at a dose of 20 to 200 μg/min may be indicated to support arterial pressures unresponsive to the above.

Reference: Roberts, S. L.: Multisystem deviations. *In* Critical Care Nursing: Assessment and Intervention. Stamford, Conn., Appleton & Lange, 1996.

1–81. (**C**) Indomethacin, a prostaglandin inhibitor, may be contraindicated during the onset phase of ATN. Some prostaglandins act as vasodilator agents and may partially counteract the vasoconstrictive effects of sympathetic stimulation and angiotensin. Diuretics, such as furosemide or mannitol, can be effective in the early stages of ischemic-related ATN and in patients with toxic ATN by reducing oliguria and increasing solute excretion. Calcium channel blockers, such as nifedipine, lessen the degree of tubular necrosis by preventing the accumulation of toxic amounts of intracellular calcium.

Reference: Stark, J. L.: The renal system. *In* Alspach, J. G. (ed.): Core Curriculum for Critical Care Nursing, 5th ed. Philadelphia, W. B. Saunders, 1998.

1–82. (**D**) Appropriate function of the DDD pacemaker is demonstrated by the Wenckebach response to a rate faster than the preset pacemaker upper limit rate. Permanent pacemaker activity cannot be evaluated while the patient is in regular sinus rhythm. During complete capture ventricular pacing, pacemaker sensing of ventricular activity cannot be determined. An increase in patient heart rate to 89 beats/min with activity does not demonstrate pacemaker function.

Reference: Furman, S., Hayes, D., Holmes, D. R.: A Practice of Cardiac Pacing, 3rd ed. Mount Kisco, N.Y., Futura Publishing, 1993.

1–83. (**A**) Pulsus alternans reflects severe left ventricular failure. In left ventricular failure the systolic pressure may alternate by as much as 20 mm Hg as a result of the alternating contractility and stroke volume of the left ventricle. Hypovolemic shock and right ventricular failure both cause a general decrease in pulse pressure owing to decreased stroke volume. Cor pulmonale is a form of right ventricular failure caused by pulmonary hypertension.

Reference: Daily, E. K., Schroeder, J. S.: Techniques in Bedside Hemodynamic Monitoring, 5th ed. St. Louis, Mosby–Year Book, 1994.

1–84. (**C**) According to the Hunt and Hess aneurysm grading system, the following are the five grades of aneurysms: grade I—alert with no neurologic deficit, minimal headache, and slight nuchal rigidity; grade II—awake with minimal neurologic deficit, mild to severe headache, nuchal rigidity, and no vasospasm; grade III—drowsy, confused with mild focal neurologic deficit, and no vasospasm; grade IV—unresponsive, hemiplegic, and may or may not have vasospasm; and grade V—comatose with decerebrate (extensor) posture and will likely have vasospasm.

Reference: Alspach, J. G. (ed.): AACN Core Curriculum for Critical Care Nursing, 5th ed. Philadelphia, W. B. Saunders, 1998.

1–85. (**D**) Chronic active hepatitis is characterized by a long history of mild hepatitis with progressive liver damage, development of cirrhosis, and high risk of primary hepatocellular carcinoma. An asymptomatic carrier state is characterized by persistence of hepatitis antigen due to ineffective cellular immunity without liver damage but with a high risk of transmission to others. Chronic persistent hepatitis is associated with at least 6 months of chronic liver inflammation past the acute onset phase. Acute fulminant hepatitis is characterized by an acute onset of viral infection that is usually self-limiting.

Reference: Yamada, T. (ed.): Textbook of Gastroenterology, 2nd ed. Philadelphia, J. B. Lippincott, 1995.

1–86. (**D**) The patient's clinical presentation is consistent with a hemothorax that is clinically significant and should be drained immediately. The pressure in the chest from the hemothorax results in the dropping pulse oximeter reading from compression of the lungs, decreased breath sounds, and mediastinal shift. Magnetic resonance imaging and computed tomography are not necessary at this time because the chest tube should resolve the symptoms resulting from the hemothorax. Surgery is not indicated at this time, although it may be necessary at a later time if bleeding continues.

Reference: Kinney, M. R., Packa, D. R., Dunbar, S. B. (eds.): AACN's Clinical Reference for Critical Care Nursing, 3rd ed. St. Louis, Mosby–Year Book, 1993.

1–87. (**B**) Bubbling in the water-seal chamber indicates an air leak from the chest through the chest drainage system. A bronchopleural fistula develops from direct communication between the pleural space and tracheobroncheal tree and is identified by a near-continuous air leak through the water-seal system. Bronchopleural fistulas develop slowly over days, so that is not likely at this time. Pulmonary edema and contusion may produce an increase in secretions but not air in the system.

Reference: Kinney, M. R., Packa, D. R., Dunbar, S. B. (eds.): AACN's Clinical Reference for Critical Care Nursing, 3rd ed. St. Louis, Mosby–Year Book, 1993.

1–88. (**C**) Troubleshooting the chest drainage system is the first intervention to identify if there is a leak in the system. Differentiation between a leak in the system and a bronchopleural fistula can be determined by clamping the chest drainage system from the point of insertion into the chest and progressing toward the water-seal container. If at any point the leak stops, there is a leak in the system. Otherwise, the leak is in the chest or chest wall. Exploratory thoracotomy is not the first intervention to be considered. Magnetic resonance imaging or additional chest tube may be useful if the air is coming from the lung.

Reference: Kinney, M. R., Packa, D. R., Dunbar, S. B. (eds.): AACN's Clinical Reference for Critical Care Nursing, 3rd ed. St. Louis, Mosby–Year Book, 1993.

1–89. (**C**) The normal range of the pulmonary capillary wedge pressure is 4 to 12 mm Hg. Pulmonary capillary wedge pressures greater than 15 mm Hg signify the onset of pulmonary congestion. Pulmonary capillary wedge pressures of greater than 20 mm Hg indicate left ventricular failure and pulmonary edema. In pulmonary edema the nurse would hear coarse rales throughout lung fields.

Reference: Kinney, M. R., Packa, D. R., Dunbar, S. B. (eds.): AACN's Clinical Reference for Critical Care Nursing, 3rd ed. St. Louis, Mosby–Year Book, 1993.

1–90. (**A**) Sepsis results in cellular disruption and death. Oxygen consumption assesses oxygen transport and oxygen metabolism at the cellular level. Oxygen consumption is decreased in shock states but improves as tissue perfusion is restored. Although useful, the other choices are indirect measures that may not reflect the adequacy of tissue perfusion.

Reference: Shoemaker, W. C.: Diagnosis and treatment of the shock syndromes. *In* Shoemaker, W. C., Ayres, S. M., Grenvik, A., Holbrook, P. R. (eds.): Textbook of Critical Care, 3rd ed. Philadelphia, W. B. Saunders, 1995.

1–91. (**D**) The symptoms are classic for pneumoccocal pneumonia, which is a risk for the elderly and those with chronic underlying diseases. *Mycoplasma* pneumonia produces little sputum and a low-grade fever. The patient does not have risk factors for pulmonary embolus or aspiration.

Reference: Alspach, J. G. (ed.): AACN Core Curriculum for Critical Care Nursing, 5th ed. Philadelphia, W. B. Saunders, 1998.

1–92. (**C**) The most important intervention at this point is that antibiotics are administered as quickly as possible. Research has shown that the greatest impact on mortality is delay in antibiotic administration. Subsequently, assessment of the patient's blood glucose level can be quickly accomplished by a glucometer. Peritoneal dialysis can then be set up and administered.

References: Alspach, J. G. (ed.): AACN Core Curriculum for Critical Care Nursing, 5th ed. Philadelphia, W. B. Saunders, 1998.
American Thoracic Society: Guidelines for the initial management of adults with community-acquired pneumonia: Diagnosis, assessment of severity, and initial antimicrobial therapy. Am. Rev. Respir. Dis. 148:1418–1426, 1993.

1–93. (**A**) A serum digoxin level would be most helpful in determining the cause of atrial flutter in a patient on digoxin. Potassium administration in atrial flutter caused by elevated digoxin levels is controversial because potassium may further depress conduction. The serum potassium level is normal. Low potassium levels and hypoxemia are associated with ventricular, not atrial, irritability. The blood urea nitrogen/creatinine may be useful to determine the cause of the digoxin toxicity.

Reference: Khan, M. G.: Heart Disease: Diagnosis and Therapy. Baltimore, Williams & Wilkins, 1996.

1–94. (**B**) Accurate intake and output, daily weights, and breath sounds will provide information on the patient's fluid status. Weight loss and decreased pulmonary fluid evidenced by rales should correspond to the effects of diuretics and increased urinary output. Medications that are positive inotropes and strengthen myocardial contraction are contraindicated in heart failure patients with diastolic dysfunction because they increase cardiac work and therefore worsen the diastolic dysfunction.

Reference: Beattie, S., Pike, C.: Left ventricular diastolic dysfunction: A case report. Crit. Care Nurs. 16(2):37–52, 1996.

1–95. (**C**) A reversible ischemic neurologic deficit (RIND) is a neurologic deficit that lasts more than 24 hours but leaves little or no neurologic deficit. Transient ischemic attacks (TIAs) are ischemic events that result in reversible short-lived signs and symptoms of less than 24 hours' duration but may last only a few minutes. There may be neurologic deficits such as amaurosis fugax (loss of vision in one eye), dysarthria (impairment of speech muscles), numbness or weakness of a hand or leg, or aphasia. Lacunar TIAs generally result in a pure motor or pure sensory deficit lasting more than an hour.

Reference: Alspach, J. G. (ed.): AACN Core Curriculum for Critical Care Nursing, 5th ed. Philadelphia, W. B. Saunders, 1998.

1–96. (**B**) Anticoagulation therapy may be employed for stroke of embolic etiology. The head of the bed, in general, will be elevated 15° to 30° based on the patient's vital signs. Initially the patient with a cerebral embolus would be on bed rest to prevent dislodgment of the clot. Intracranial pressure monitoring is not a mainstay of treatment for this disorder.

Reference: Alspach, J. G.: AACN Core Curriculum for Critical Care Nursing, 5th ed. Philadelphia, W. B. Saunders, 1998.

1–97. (**D**) Hypokalemia occurs frequently in progressing hepatic failure. This is probably due to gastrointestinal potassium losses, hyperaldosteronism, or excessive renal losses secondary to alkalosis. Other signs of fulminating hepatic failure are hypoglycemia, hyperreflexia, and hyponatremia.

Reference: Kucharski, S. A.: Fulminant hepatic failure. Crit. Care. Nurs. Clin. North Am. 5:141–151, 1993.

1–98. (**C**) Aprotinin and aminocaproic acid are used to minimize bleeding, a common complication of VAD use. Aprotinin decreases antifibrinolytic activity and preserves platelet function. Aminocaproic acid reverses systemic fibrinolysis. Transfusions should be performed with leukocyte-poor blood, rather than with packed cells to prevent antibody development in a patient awaiting transplant. Protamine would reverse the effects of anticoagulation necessary to maintain flow. Low VAD flow rates (less than 2 L/min) would require more aggressive anticoagulation.

Reference: Braunwald, E. (ed.): Heart Disease: A Textbook of Cardiovascular Medicine. Philadelphia, W. B. Saunders, 1997.

1–99. **(C)** Administration of IV fluids sufficient to maintain adequate hydration is demonstrated by an oxygen delivery (Do_2) of 900 to 1200 ml/min or an oxygen delivery index (Do_2I) of 500 to 600 ml/min/m². Adequate hydration and tissue perfusion are demonstrated by a urine output of at least 20 to 30 ml/hr. Vasoconstriction increases tissue perfusion.

Reference: Roberts, S. L.: Multisystem deviations. *In* Critical Care Nursing: Assessment and Intervention. Stamford, Conn., Appleton & Lange, 1996.

1–100. **(A)** The development of headache and decreased level of consciousness during treatment of diabetic ketoacidosis (DKA) is ominous and suggests cerebral edema. Cerebral edema is theorized to occur secondary to the fluid shift that transpires as glucose levels drop in the serum and fluid moves back into the cells, including the cells of the central nervous system. A precipitous drop in glucose level could cause a rapid fluid shift and cellular edema, which readily leads to symptoms. Patients do not typically develop meningitis during successful treatment of DKA, but it is important to remember that infection is the major precipitating event of DKA. Acidosis is resolving during treatment, and hypoxemia is unusual in DKA, although the symptoms can be similar to those of cerebral edema, with restlessness and confusion usually occurring before profound deterioration of neurologic function.

References: Civetta, J. M., Taylor, R. W., Kirby, R. R. (eds.): Critical Care, 2nd ed. Philadelphia, J. B. Lippincott, 1992.
Clochesy, J. M., Breu, C., Cardin, S., et al. (eds.): Critical Care Nursing, 2nd ed. Philadelphia, W. B. Saunders, 1996.

1–101. **(D)** Because the formation of small platelet aggregates is responsible for the clinical manifestations of TTP, the main goal of therapies is to inhibit platelet aggregation, not speed it up.

Anticoagulants are not recommended in TTP, because platelet aggregation, not coagulation, is out of balance; therefore, PT and PTT are not altered. Although it is important to control tachycardia to maintain adequate cardiac output, this is not the main goal for treating TTP.

References: Alspach, J. G. (ed.): AACN Core Curriculum for Critical Care Nursing, 5th ed. Philadelphia, W. B. Saunders, 1998.
Kajs-Wyllie, M.: Thrombotic thrombocytopenic purpura: Pathology, treatment, and related nursing care. Crit. Care Nurs. 15(6):44–51, 1995.

1–102. **(A)** Diffuse cerebral dysfunction may be indicated by an abnormal grasp, snout, or glabellar reflex. Assessment of reflexes provides an indirect measure of motor ability and, more specifically, determination of spinal shock and differentiation between complete and incomplete spinal cord lesions. Percussion of a tendon with a reflex hammer (e.g., biceps, triceps, brachioradialis, quadriceps, and Achilles) causes stretch of a muscle with subsequent contraction of muscle fibers. Abnormal responses to reflex testing in this manner may indicate interruption of upper motor neuron pathways between the cerebrum and lower motor neurons. Absence of reflexes elicited in this manner is usually caused by lesions of lower motor neurons. Superficial reflexes (e.g., cremasteric, plantar) are generally tested by stroking the skin with a moderately sharp object. Abnormal or absent responses to this maneuver are generally found with upper motor neuron disorders.

Reference: Alspach, J. G. (ed.): AACN Core Curriculum for Critical Care Nursing, 5th ed. Philadelphia, W. B. Saunders, 1998.

1–103. (**D**) ACE inhibitors block angiotensin-converting enzyme, preventing the formation of angiotensin II and aldosterone. These actions reduce preload and afterload, cause mild diuresis, and improve cardiac output.

Reference: Kinney, M. R., Packa, D. R.: Andreoli's Comprehensive Cardiac Care, 8th ed. St. Louis, Mosby–Year Book, 1996.

1–104. (**C**) Morphine reduces anxiety, vasodilates to reduce both preload and afterload, and suppresses sympathetic overdrive. Furosemide decreases preload through its diuretic action. Digoxin has no direct effect on preload or afterload. Captopril decreases afterload through its effect on the renin angiotensin system and also has mild vasodilating properties. Furosemide, captopril, and digoxin have no effect on sympathetic overdrive.

Reference: Thelan, L. A., Davie, J. K., Urden, L. D., Lough, M. E.: Critical Care Nursing: Diagnosis and Management, 2nd ed. St. Louis, Mosby–Year Book, 1994.

1–105. (**A**) All endotracheal tubes, but especially nasotracheal tubes, can occlude sinus drainage and thereby foster growth of bacteria. An abscessed tooth would not produce drainage into the nasal passages. Ulceration and necrosis of oral tissue does not occur with a nasotracheal tube. A tracheoesophageal fistula is uncommon, especially with such a short time of intubation.

Reference: Stauffer, J. L.: Complications of translaryngeal intubation. In Tobin, M. J. (ed.): Principles and Practice of Mechanical Ventilation. New York, McGraw-Hill, 1994.

1–106. (**C**) The blood gas analysis results show a respiratory acidosis and hypoxemia. Asthma patients generally have a slight respiratory alkalosis (decreased $PaCO_2$) secondary to increased respiratory rate from "twitchy airways." When a patient with asthma retains CO_2, or even has a normal CO_2 value, it is a danger sign that he is tiring out. The increased work of breathing is due to increased resistance from the bronchoconstricted airways. Intubation should be planned for. Intermittent positive-pressure breathing may assist with breathing but also promotes air trapping. Bronchodilator therapy and increasing the FIO_2 may improve oxygenation but will not correct the hypercarbia.

Reference: Kersten, L. D.: Comprehensive Respiratory Nursing: A Decision Making Approach. Philadelphia, W. B. Saunders, 1989.

1–107. (**A**) Adequate humidification of the ventilator circuit is the most important first treatment to prevent mucus plugs from forming in the conducting airways. Adequate hydration is essential as a second step because dehydration can occur as a result of fluid loss from the tracheobronchial tree through increased respiratory rate during the preintubation phase. Postural drainage of lung lobes and segments can assist in moving thick secretions but may take time to be effective. Bronchoscopy may be indicated but only if lobes or segments were impacted with secretions.

Reference: Boggs, R. L., Wooldridge-King, M. (eds.): AACN Procedure Manual for Critical Care, 3rd ed. Philadelphia, W. B. Saunders, 1993.

1–108. (**B**) Beta blockers reduce the heart rate leading to more complete emptying of the left atrium, decrease myocardial oxygen demand, and decrease blood pressure. Digoxin and positive inotropes have the opposite effect in diastolic dysfunction, and often the deterioration they cause is the first clue to diastolic dysfunction instead of systolic dysfunction as the cause of heart failure.

Reference: Beattie, S., Pike, C.: Left ventricular diastolic dysfunction: A case report. Crit. Care Nurs. 16(2):37–52, 1996.

1–109. (**D**) In acute pancreatitis, the serum amylase level is dramatically elevated owing to the activation of proteolytic enzymes in the pancreas and pancreatic inflammation, leading to increased entry of amylase into the blood stream. In addition, the serum calcium level is decreased owing to binding with areas of fat necrosis, the white blood cell count is elevated owing to immune response, and the blood glucose level is elevated with the stress response and/or beta cell damage in the pancreas.

References: Krumberger, J. M.: Acute pancreatitis. Crit. Care. Nurs. Clin. North Am. 5:185–202, 1993. Urban, N., et al.: Guidelines for Critical Care Nursing. St. Louis, Mosby–Year Book, 1995.

1–110. (**A**) The clinical presentation of hepatotoxicity after acetaminophen ingestion occurs 24 to 48 hours after ingestion and results in elevation of total bilirubin and prothrombin time. Alkaline phosphatase and amylase levels remain near normal. Hypoglycemia may occur 3 to 4 days after ingestion as liver function abnormalities peak.

Reference: Clancy, C., Litovitz, T. L.: Poisoning. *In* Shoemaker, W. C., Ayres, S. M., Grenvik, A., Holbrook, P. R. (eds.): Textbook of Critical Care, 3rd ed. Philadelphia, W. B. Saunders, 1995.

1–111. (**D**) The systemic vascular resistance (SVR) in this patient is 1400 dynes/sec/cm^2, which is calculated by the formula [(mean arterial pressure − central venous pressure) ÷ cardiac output] × 80. Right atrial pressure is elevated (normal is 0 to 8 mm Hg). Therefore, the patient would benefit from both preload and afterload reduction from nitroprusside. Nitroglycerin is primarily an arterial vasodilator. Dobutamine is a positive inotropic medication that does not affect either preload or afterload. Potassium supplementation should be guided by serum potassium levels.

Reference: Braunwald, E. (ed.): Heart Disease: A Textbook of Cardiovascular Medicine. Philadelphia, W. B. Saunders, 1997.

1–112. (**A**) Angiotensin converting enzyme (ACE) inhibitors such as enalapril are contraindicated for use with potassium-sparing diuretics such as spironolactone because they increase serum potassium and may cause hyperkalemia. Side effects of ACE inhibitors include hypotension and increases in serum creatinine and potassium. Serum potassium concentration of 5.5 mEq/L is a contraindication to ACE inhibitor therapy unless the serum potassium concentration is reduced. The elevated serum potassium concentration warrants change to another diuretic than spironolactone. Isosorbide dinitrate should be continued to promote coronary and systemic vasodilation and lower blood pressure to decrease cardiac work. When enalapril is discontinued, the blood pressure will increase.

Reference: Konstam, M., Dracup, K., Baker, D., et al.: Heart Failure: Evaluation and Care of Patients with Left-Ventricular Systolic Dysfunction. Clinical Practice Guideline No. 11. ACHPR publication No. 94–0612. Rockville, Md.: Agency for Health Care Policy and Research, Public Health Service, U.S. Department of Health and Human Services, June 1994.

1–113. (**B**) In pulmonary embolism, blood flow is directed away from areas of obstruction; overperfusion of unobstructed areas of the lung results in low ventilation/perfusion ratios resulting in hyperventilation. Oxygen diffusion is not impaired in ventilated areas. Mucus plugging is not a relevant factor in this disorder.

Reference: Alspach, J. G. (ed.): AACN Core Curriculum for Critical Care Nursing, 5th ed. Philadelphia, W. B. Saunders, 1998.

1–114. (**D**) Although delayed discharge and increased costs may result from complications of immobilization, a more immediate concern and consequence to the patient's health is a pulmonary embolus. An ileus may occur as a result of bed rest, although it is not as serious a consequence as a pulmonary embolus.

Reference: Kersten, L. D.: Comprehensive Respiratory Nursing: A Decision Making Approach. Philadelphia, W. B. Saunders, 1989.

1–115. (**D**) Jugular venous pulsations greater than 5 cm above the angle of Louis are considered elevated and a sign of right ventricular failure. Clear breath sounds are normally found in right ventricular failure, which causes venous rather than pulmonary congestion. Pulmonary capillary wedge pressures may be low or normal in the patient with right ventricular failure, which causes symptoms of hypovolemia. Oxygen saturations remain normal in right ventricular failure unless there is coexisting lung disease.

Reference: Darovic, G. O.: Hemodynamic Monitoring: Invasive and Noninvasive Clinical Application, 2nd ed. Philadelphia, W. B. Saunders, 1995.

1–116. (**C**) In diastolic dysfunction, patients commonly have a normal heart size and ejection fraction; however, their stroke volume and cardiac output/index are decreased. Because heart size and ejection fraction are not generally affected in diastolic dysfunction, they are not reliable measures of the effectiveness of therapy. A heart rate of 130 beats/min with a normal cardiac output of 4.0 L/min indicates a decreased stroke volume. A cardiac index of 3.0 L/min with a normal heart rate of 96 beats/min indicates improved stroke volume.

Reference: Khan, M. G.: Heart Disease: Diagnosis and Therapy. Baltimore, Williams & Wilkins, 1996.

1–117. (**C**) Sodium nitroprusside is related to cyanide, and its metabolite is thiocyanate. Thiocyanate levels would indicate whether the patient's change in mental status was due to elevated levels of the metabolite. Thiocyanate toxicity is a potential complication of sodium nitroprusside therapy when it is delivered in high doses for several days. Signs and symptoms of toxicity include metabolic acidosis, blurred vision, psychosis, rash, seizures, and confusion.

Reference: Khan, M. G.: Heart Disease: Diagnosis and Therapy. Baltimore, Williams & Wilkins, 1996.

1–118. (**D**) Hydrocephalus in the adult is often the result of intracranial pathology that disrupts reabsorption of cerebrospinal fluid (CSF). Examples include intracranial tumors or hemorrhage that lead to an accumulation of CSF in the ventricles. This CSF is either not reabsorbed through the arachnoid villi (communicating—nonobstructive hydrocephalus) or its flow is obstructed (noncommunicating—obstructive). Normal-pressure hydrocephalus is usually reversible. Interventions for hydrocephalus include surgical placement of a ventriculostomy to shunt the excess CSF and administration of osmotic diuretics. Hypotonic intravenous fluids would be contraindicated in patients with hydrocephalus because they would reduce the serum sodium concentration, increase brain water, and increase intracranial pressure. Stenotic scar tissue does not generally occur with hydrocephalus.

References: Alspach, J. G. (ed.): AACN Core Curriculum for Critical Care Nursing, 5th ed. Philadelphia, W. B. Saunders, 1998.
Hickey, J. V.: The Clinical Practice of Neurological and Neurosurgical Nursing, 3rd ed. Philadelphia, J. B. Lippincott, 1992.

1–119. (**D**) Orogastric lavage is indicated in patients with life-threatening ingestions who reach medical attention within 2 hours after ingestion. Ingestion of substances associated with delayed gastric emptying such as anticholinergic agents may respond to even later treatment.

Reference: Clancy, C., Litovitz, T. L.: Poisoning. *In* Shoemaker, W. C., Ayres, S. M., Grenvik, A., Holbrook, P. R. (eds.): Textbook of Critical Care, 3rd ed. Philadelphia, W. B. Saunders, 1995.

1–120. (**B**) Peritoneal dialysis consists of three phases: inflow, dwell, and outflow. The dwell time allows for diffusion, osmosis, and ultrafiltration to occur. Ultrafiltration is greatest immediately after the infusion of fresh dialysate and decreases as the dwell phase progresses. Ultrafiltration is lowest during the outflow phase as the solution's osmolality equilibrates.

Reference: Carlson, K. K.: Acute peritoneal dialysis. *In* Urban, N. A., Krumberger, J. M., Winkelman, C. (eds.): Guidelines for Critical Care Nursing. St. Louis, Mosby–Year Book, 1995.

1–121. (**D**) Stabilization of fluid status is the first priority in all forms of acute pancreatitis. Nitroglycerin will reduce the abdominal pain caused by mesenteric ischemia. Protein intake is titrated in liver failure, whereas fat intake is titrated in pancreatitis. Antibiotics are indicated only for peritonitis associated with abdominal trauma.

References: Gupta, P. K., Al-Kawas, F. H.: Acute pancreatitis: Diagnosis and management. Am. Fam. Phys. 52:435–443, 1995.
Krumberger, J. M.: Acute pancreatitis. Crit. Care. Nurs. Clin. North Am. 5:185–202, 1993.

1–122. (**B**) Low-dose heparin is the main emphasis in prevention of pulmonary embolus. Although ambulation is generally used for prevention of a pulmonary embolus, this patient is not able to get out of bed at this time. An alternative may be range-of-motion or leg exercises that can be done in bed. Elastic stockings have not been shown to be effective in high-risk patients. Insertion of a vena caval umbrella is not indicated at this time.

Reference: Alspach, J. G. (ed.): AACN Core Curriculum for Critical Care Nursing, 5th ed. Philadelphia, W. B. Saunders, 1998.

1–123. (**D**) Bowel loops in the thorax on the chest radiograph indicate diaphragmatic rupture. Ascites and ileus would not generate sufficient pressure to push the bowel into the thorax. Malposition of the patient would not cause abdominal contents to penetrate the diaphragm.

Reference: Alspach, J. G. (ed.): AACN Core Curriculum for Critical Care Nursing, 5th ed. Philadelphia, W. B. Saunders, 1998.

1–124. (**B**) Hemothorax and pneumothorax both present as decreased vocal fremitus, decreased breath sounds, and unequal chest expansion. Blood in the thorax results in dullness on percussion, and air produces hyperresonance.

Reference: Alspach, J. G. (ed.): AACN Core Curriculum for Critical Care Nursing, 5th ed. Philadelphia, W. B. Saunders, 1998.

1-125. (**C**) Insulin is administered to treat diabetic ketoacidosis (DKA), which is a result of an insufficient or absent level of circulating insulin. In DKA, insulin-sensitive tissues (fat, liver, and muscle) alter their intermediary metabolism from a carbohydrate-metabolizing system to a fat-metabolizing system. The ketoacids formed are buffered by extracellular and cellular buffers, resulting in metabolic acidosis. Therefore, administration of insulin results in a decrease in acidosis because it enables normal carbohydrate metabolism.

Sodium bicarbonate therapy for acidosis is controversial; it has not been shown to improve outcomes or decrease the severity of acidosis.

Acidosis and hyperosmolality lead to water and potassium shifts out of the cells. Excessive urinary potassium losses secondary to osmotic diuresis are responsible for the development of potassium depletion. Correction of the loss is necessary, but this does not treat acidosis. Phosphorus shifts and is lost in a similar fashion to potassium in DKA. Correction of phosphorus loss is frequent during treatment, but this, too, does not treat the acidosis.

References: Alspach, J. G. (ed.): AACN Core Curriculum for Critical Care Nursing, 5th ed. Philadelphia, W. B. Saunders, 1998.
Kitabchi, A. E., Wall, B. M.: Diabetic ketoacidosis. Med. Clin. North Am. 79:9–37, 1995.

1-126. (**C**) Platelet transfusions are not usually indicated in TTP because the underlying problem is platelet consumption, not platelet production. Treatment of TTP includes corticosteroids, antiplatelet agents, plasmapheresis with administration of fresh frozen plasma to replace clotting factors, intravenous immunoglobulins to reduce platelet aggregation, and/or splenectomy.

Reference: Alspach, J. G. (ed.): AACN Core Curriculum for Critical Care Nursing, 5th ed. Philadelphia, W. B. Saunders, 1998.

1-127. (**D**) On admission, lowering and maintaining blood pressure within the prescribed parameters receives priority. Thiocyanate toxicity is a concern only after the patient has been on high levels of nitroprusside for several days. Patient education is inappropriate until the patient's condition has stabilized. The transition to oral antihypertensive medication takes place after the blood pressure is lowered to acceptable levels.

Reference: Khan, M. G.: Heart Disease: Diagnosis and Therapy. Baltimore, Williams & Wilkins, 1996.

1-128. (**C**) Labetalol is delivered at a rate of 1 to 2 mg/min as a continuous infusion.

Reference: Wright, J. E., Shelton, B. K.: Desk Reference for Critical Care Nursing, Boston, Jones & Bartlett, 1993.

1-129. (**B**) The goal for nursing management of this patient is to lower blood pressure gradually while maintaining cerebral perfusion and preventing complications. Lowering of blood pressure too rapidly can decrease cerebral perfusion causing lethargy, disorientation, confusion, or agitation. Control of blood pressure should be guided by maintenance of orientation to person, place, and time; absence of lethargy, agitation, and confusion; and the ability to follow commands and instructions.

Reference: Thelan, L. A., Davie, J. K., Urden, L. D., Lough, M. E.: Critical Care Nursing, Diagnosis and Management, 2nd ed. St. Louis, Mosby–Year Book, 1994.

1-130. (**C**) The administration of both naloxone, which reverses the effects of opiates, and flumazenil, which reverses the effects of benzodiazepine intoxication, is indicated because of the frequent occurrence of polysubstance abuse associated with opiate use. Activated charcoal is not administered to unconscious patients because of the risk of aspiration. Sodium bicarbonate is administered for cyclic antidepressant overdose.

Reference: Schnoll, S. H.: Drug abuse, overdose and withdrawal syndromes. In Shoemaker, W. C., Ayres, S. M., Grenvik, A., Holbrook, P. R. (eds): Textbook of Critical Care, 3rd ed. Philadelphia, W. B. Saunders, 1995.

1–131. (**A**) To initiate weaning from the intra-aortic balloon pump, patients should have a cardiac index of 2.0 L/min/m² or greater, a pulmonary capillary wedge pressure of 18 mm Hg or less, and evidence of renal perfusion. These findings demonstrate adequate cardiac function to proceed with the weaning process.

Reference: Ruppert, S. D., Kernicki, J. G., Dolan, J. T.: Dolan's Critical Care Nursing, 2nd ed. Philadelphia, F. A. Davis, 1996.

1–132. (**D**) Level of consciousness is always the essential component of any neurologic assessment because it is the earliest and most reliable indicator of cerebral perfusion. There are two components to level of consciousness: arousal and awareness. The Glasgow Coma Scale (GCS) is the most widely used assessment tool for determining level of consciousness. Pupillary response, motor and sensory abilities, and vital signs, although important components of the neurologic assessment, are not as singularly important as level of consciousness.

Reference: Barker, E. (ed.): Neuroscience Nursing, St. Louis, Mosby–Year Book, 1994.

1–133. (**A**) The stomach normally secretes 1500 to 3000 ml of clear, green gastric juice each day.

Reference: Yamada, T. (ed.): Textbook of Gastroenterology, 2nd ed. Philadelphia, J. B. Lippincott, 1995.

1–134. (**A**) Microatelectasis is the most common cause of hypoxia after surgery. Pulmonary embolus and pulmonary edema can cause hypoxia but are not specific to the postsurgical patient, nor do they develop shortly after a surgical procedure. Bacterial invasion of the lower airways or aspiration predisposes to pneumonia but does not necessarily result in postsurgical hypoxia.

References: Alspach, J. G. (ed.): AACN Core Curriculum for Critical Care Nursing, 5th ed. Philadelphia, W. B. Saunders, 1998.
Kersten, L. D.: Comprehensive Respiratory Nursing: A Decision Making Approach. Philadelphia, W. B. Saunders, 1989.

1–135. (**D**) The clinical presentation is suggestive of a foreign body obstruction on the left. Pneumothorax would present as absent breath sounds over a hemithorax rather than over a lobe. Pulmonary embolus would not present as wheezing and stridor. Cardiogenic shock would present as bilateral rales/crackles.

Reference: Alspach, J. G. (ed.): AACN Core Curriculum for Critical Care Nursing, 5th ed. Philadelphia, W. B. Saunders, 1998.

1–136. (**C**) Vascular position (reverse Trendelenburg) improves blood flow to the lower extremities. The sheath and balloon pump apparatus act as an obstruction and may diminish distal flow. The head of the bed in an IABP patient should not be elevated more than 30°. Trendelenburg positioning would decrease flow to the lower extremities. In semi-Fowler's position, in which both the head and legs are raised, flexion of the hips may cause balloon migration.

Reference: Ruppert, S. D., Kernicki, J. G., Dolan, J. T.: Dolan's Critical Care Nursing, 2nd ed. Philadelphia, F. A. Davis, 1996.

1–137. (**C**) Epinephrine is the strongest of the inotropes listed. All of these medications have positive inotropic effects but vary from strongest to weakest in inotropic activity: epinephrine, dobutamine, norepinephrine, and dopamine.

Reference: Khan, M. G.: Heart Disease: Diagnosis and Therapy. Baltimore, Williams & Wilkins, 1996.

1–138. (**B**) Migration of the intra-aortic balloon pump catheter caudad can cause occlusion of the subclavian artery, which supplies the left brachial artery causing decreased circulation to the left arm. Migration downward can cause occlusion of the renal artery, leading to decreased renal circulation and urinary output.

Reference: Ruppert, S. D., Kernicki, J. G., Dolan, J. T.: Dolan's Critical Care Nursing: Clinical Management Through the Nursing Process. Philadelphia, F. A. Davis, 1996.

1–139. (**C**) Ascorbic acid enhances secretion of amphetamine and its derivative by-products that accumulate after cocaine intoxication/overdose. Diuretics are administered when urinary pH is below 6.0. Cocaine overdose does not disrupt cellular integrity or cause muscle soreness.

Reference: Schnoll, S. H.: Drug abuse, overdose and withdrawal syndromes. *In* Shoemaker, W. C., Ayres, S. M., Grenvik, A., Holbrook, P. R. (eds.): Textbook of Critical Care, 3rd ed. Philadelphia, W. B. Saunders, 1995.

1–140. (**A**) Rapid osmolar shifts cause disequilibrium syndrome, which is characterized by hypertension, headache, confusion, nausea, vomiting, and seizures. Treatment is aimed at the reestablishment of normal osmolarity by the administration of volume expanders. The administration of diuretics may further aggravate the patient's hemodynamic state. Antihypertensives and antidysrhythmic medication will not correct the cause of the problem.

Reference: Carlson, K. K.: Acute hemodialysis. *In* Urban, N. A., Krumberger, J. M., Winkelman, C. (eds.): Guidelines for Critical Care Nursing. St. Louis, Mosby–Year Book, 1995.

1–141. (**C**) All options represent plausible reasons for intubation. In this patient situation, however, intubation is being used to protect the airway from aspiration. There is no indication of an upper airway obstruction or of excess secretions. His arterial blood gas analysis results do not indicate the need for mechanical ventilation.

Reference: Tobin, M. J. (ed.): Principles and Practice of Mechanical Ventilation. New York, McGraw-Hill, 1994.

1–142. (**D**) Strong suction should be available to prevent aspiration and quickly remove secretions should vomiting occur. Cardiac arrhythmias may occur during vomiting subsequent to stimulation of the vagus nerve. Hypoxemia and cardiac arrhythmias may also occur after vomiting and aspiration, which result in inflammation of the airway and decreased oxygen reaching the capillaries. Proper patient positioning and correct tube placement may not prevent vomiting. Corticosteroids may decrease the inflammatory response after aspiration has occurred but are not given routinely for prevention.

Reference: Boggs, R. L., Wooldridge-King, M. (eds.): AACN Procedure Manual for Critical Care, 3rd ed. Philadelphia, W. B. Saunders, 1993.

1–143. (**D**) Drowning frequently results in hypothermia. Rewarming should be done initially to reverse the effects of hypothermia. The hypothermia has shifted the oxygen dissociation curve to the left, inhibiting the release of oxygen from hemoglobin. This results in tissue hypoxia. His blood gases show a metabolic acidosis (lactic acidosis) from the tissue hypoxia. The saturation of 95% with a PaO_2 of 65 mm Hg indicates a stronger affinity of oxygen to hemoglobin than normal. Oxygen will improve tissue hypoxia although rewarming is the priority. Rewarming will shift the oxygen dissociation curve back toward normal, allowing release of oxygen from hemoglobin. Antibiotics and intubation are not indicated at this time.

Reference: Kinney, M. R., Packa, D. R., Dunbar, S. B. (eds.): AACN's Clinical Reference for Critical Care Nursing, 3rd ed. St. Louis, Mosby–Year Book, 1993.

1–144. (**C**) Computed tomography is a valuable diagnostic aid in almost all intracranial pathology and is particularly valuable in suspected intracranial hemorrhage. Lumbar puncture is generally contraindicated until intracranial pathology is ruled out because herniation may result. Likewise, cerebral angiography is associated with the risk of cerebrovascular accident resulting from a dislodged thrombus; therefore, intracranial hemorrhage is generally ruled out through use of computed tomography or magnetic resonance imaging before angiography. Myelography is typically used in patients with intervertebral disc disease or spinal cord injuries.

Reference: Alspach, J. G. (ed.): AACN Core Curriculum for Critical Care Nursing, 5th ed. Philadelphia, W. B. Saunders, 1998.

1–145. (**B**) Although the best treatment for acute mesenteric ischemia is prevention, early treatment is focused on correcting hypovolemia and acidemia. Vasoconstricting agents should be avoided. Hyperkalemia is likely if tissue death has occurred, so potassium supplementation would be inappropriate.

Reference: Quinn, A. D.: Acute mesenteric ischemia. Crit. Care Nurs. Clin. North Am. 5:171–175, 1993.

1–146. (**C**) The normal arterial oxygen saturation is 95% to 100%. Normal mixed venous oxygen saturation is 70% to 75%. A value of 85% would indicate a mixture of arterial with venous blood.

Reference: Kinney, M. R., Packa, D. R., Dunbar, S. B.: AACN's Clinical Reference for Critical Care Nursing, 3rd ed. St. Louis, Mosby–Year Book, 1993.

1–147. (**D**) In patients with aortic regurgitation, afterload reduction with nifedipine has significantly improved the survival rate of patients preoperatively as well as postoperatively. Verapamil, diltiazem, and propranolol are contraindicated because of their negative inotropic effects and bradycardia.

Reference: Khan, M. G.: Heart Disease: Diagnosis and Therapy. Baltimore, Williams & Wilkins, 1996.

1–148. (**A**) Pulmonary insufficiency is very common after thoracoabdominal aneurysm repair because the integrity of the diaphragm is disrupted by surgery and there are massive fluid shifts associated with cross-clamping the aorta and from abdominal manipulation. Meticulous attention to pulmonary toilet and gradual weaning from the ventilator are necessary to prevent pulmonary complications. Myocardial infarction, cerebrovascular accident, and paralysis are perioperative complications of this disorder.

Reference: Moore, W. S.: Vascular Surgery: A Comprehensive Review. Philadelphia, W. B. Saunders, 1993.

1–149. (**D**) If initially indicated, based on a nomogram of acetaminophen serum concentration hours after ingestion, oral NAC administration must be continued for the entire 18-dose course (loading dose and 17 maintenance doses) because the acetaminophen effects are prolonged and cannot be reversed without repeated administration of NAC over a prolonged period of time.

Reference: Clancy, C., Litovitz, T. L.: Poisoning. In Shoemaker, W. C., Ayres, S. M., Grenvik, A., Holbrook, P. R. (eds.): Textbook of Critical Care, 3rd ed. Philadelphia, W. B. Saunders, 1995.

1–150. (**D**) In a patient being treated for diabetic ketoacidosis, when the glucose concentration approaches 250 to 300 mg/dl, glucose should be incorporated into the parenteral fluids. Levels of glucose should not be reduced much more than this because of the increasing possibility of cerebral edema. The insulin dose should not be reduced to deal with the falling glucose concentration because the acidemia that has yet to be eliminated (as evidenced by ketones in the urine) will resolve more slowly.

Reference: Civetta, J. M., Taylor, R. W., Kirby, R. R. (eds.): Critical Care, 2nd ed. Philadelphia, J. B. Lippincott, 1992.

1–151. (**A**) The patient is at risk of increased and unnecessary bleeding. Optimal anticoagulation for mechanical heart valves is INR ratio of 2.5 to 3.5. The adoption of INR is recommended for the management of oral anticoagulant therapy because it is a value that is corrected for the variability in prothrombin time (PT) between laboratories. PT results between laboratories may vary owing to the variable sensitivities of thromboplastin reagents used by laboratories.

The INR is not a new laboratory test; it is a mathematical correction for variations in measurement of PT. The formula for calculating the INR = PTR^{ISI}, where PTR = prothrombin time ratio, which is the patient's PT (in seconds) divided by each laboratory's calculated mean PT, and ISI = International Sensitivity Index of each lot of thromboplastin reagent, as stated by the manufacturer.

References: Oertel, L. B.: International normalized ratio (INR): An improved way to monitor oral anticoagulant therapy. Nurse Pract. 20(9):15–22, 1995.
Hirsh, J.: Heparin: Mechanism of action, clinical effectiveness, and optimal therapeutic range. Chest Suppl. 108:231s–246s, 1995.

1–152. (**A**) Coughing and deep breathing with a pillow for splinting is preferred to the other methods of pulmonary toilet in the postoperative aortic aneurysm patient. The postoperative aortic surgery patient is not encouraged to sit in a regular chair because the bending applies pressure to the surgical sites. Rigorous suctioning is avoided because it may increase the blood pressure significantly.

Reference: Moore, W. S.: Vascular Surgery: A Comprehensive Review. Philadelphia, W. B. Saunders, 1993.

1–153. (**C**) The high peripheral resistance seen in hypovolemic shock causes amplification of the peripheral pressure that may exceed central aortic pressure. For patients in hypovolemic shock, one should assume that the aortic pressure is lower than radial or brachial artery pressures.

Reference: Daily, E. K., Schroeder, J. S.: Techniques in Bedside Hemodynamic Monitoring, 5th ed. St. Louis, Mosby–Year Book, 1994.

1–154. (**C**) In hypovolemic shock, as cardiac output falls, urine output decreases and sodium and water are retained. Vasoconstriction is demonstrated by increased systemic vascular resistance (SVR). Normal SVR is 800 to 1400 dynes/sec/cm^5. Decreased pulse pressure is related to decreased stroke volume and increased SVR and is reflected by the rise in diastolic pressure.

Reference: Ruppert, S. D., Kernicki, J. G., Dolan, J. T.: Dolan's Critical Care Nursing: Clinical Management Through the Nursing Process. Philadelphia, F. A. Davis, 1996.

1–155. (**C**) The 3:1 rule is used to replace blood losses with crystalloid because crystalloid remains in the intravascular space for a shorter period than colloid or blood. Three fourths of the crystalloid volume infused migrates to the extravascular compartment within approximately 20 minutes. Colloids remain in the intravascular space slightly longer because the size of the molecules is larger than in crystalloids.

Reference: Darovic, G. O.: Hemodynamic Monitoring: Invasive and Noninvasive Clinical Application, 2nd ed. Philadelphia, W. B. Saunders, 1995.

1–156. (**A**) The Glasgow Coma Scale (GCS) is an internationally recognized standardized assessment tool that evaluates level of consciousness, the most sensitive indicator of cerebral function. The patient's best responses in three areas—eye opening, motor response, and verbal response—are graded, and the scores are then summed. Scores range from a low of 3 to a high of 15, with 15 being normal. Glasgow Coma Scale values of 3–3–4 indicate that the patient opens his eyes when spoken to, is not able to follow commands but localizes pain and attempts to remove noxious stimuli when motor function is tested, and is able to vocalize but is confused (as determined by his inability to state his name, where he is, or the date). Medical and nursing care are based on a patient's improved or worsening of his or her summed score.

Reference: Clochesy, J. M., Breu, C., Cardin, S. (eds.): Critical Care Nursing, 2nd ed. Philadelphia, W. B. Saunders, 1996.

1–157. (**A**) Loss of gastrointestinal secretions through fistulas, vomiting, diarrhea, or suction predisposes a patient to fluid volume deficit. Pulmonary edema, acute glomerulonephritis, and hyperaldosteronism predispose a patient to fluid volume excess.

References: Doughty, D. B., Jackson, D. B.: Gastrointestinal Disorders. St. Louis, Mosby–Year Book, 1993.
Luckmann, J., Sorensen, K. C. (eds.): Medical Surgical Nursing, 4th ed. Philadelphia, W. B. Saunders, 1993.

1–158. (**B**) The hematocrit is normal so fluid is the treatment of choice. Had the hematocrit been below normal, transfusion of packed cells would have been indicated. Administration of vasopressors in the vascular patient with hypovolemia causes vasoconstriction and may impair limb perfusion. Elevating the legs of a patient who has had lower extremity surgery is contraindicated because this would decrease perfusion of the operative extremity.

Reference: Thelan, L. A., Davie, J. K., Urden, L. D., Lough, M. E.: Critical Care Nursing, Diagnosis and Management, 2nd ed. St. Louis, Mosby–Year Book, 1994.

1–159. (**A**) Sudden, severe crushing of the chest produces traumatic asphyxia, defined as asphyxia related to trauma that prevents respiratory movements. Associated findings, referred to as "ecchymotic mask," include subconjunctival hemorrhage plus petechiae, edema, and cyanosis of the head, neck, and upper extremities. The other options do not produce this effect.

Reference: Wilson, R. F.: Thoracic injuries. *In* Shoemaker, W. C., Ayres, S. M., Grenvik, A., Holbrook, P. R. (eds.): Textbook of Critical Care, 3rd ed. Philadelphia, W. B. Saunders, 1995.

1–160. (**D**) Hyperglycemia associated with diabetes can cause excessive fluid loss; this diuresis will decrease the extracellular fluid volume. Although there is a decrease in total body fluid, the quantity of body sodium remains constant, placing the patient at increased risk for the development of hypernatremia. Renal disease, cirrhosis, and adrenal insufficiency all cause hyponatremia.

Reference: Baer, C. L.: Fluid and electrolyte balance. *In* Kinney, M. R., Packa, D. R., Dunbar, S. B. (eds.): AACN's Clinical Reference for Critical Care Nursing, 3rd ed. St. Louis, Mosby–Year Book, 1993.

1–161. (**A**) Tension pneumothorax results from an injury to the pleura that allows air from the lung into the pleural space and traps it there. Atmospheric air may also enter the pleural space through an external wound that opens on inspiration and closes on expiration. The increasing air in the pleural space compresses the functional lung and surrounding area of the thorax. Clinical manifestations include neck vein distention, decreased cardiac output, decreased respiratory effort, agitation and restlessness, tracheal deviation away from the affected side, and cyanosis.

Reference: Kinney, M. R., Packa, D. R., Dunbar, S. B. (eds.): AACN's Clinical Reference for Critical Care Nursing, 3rd ed. New York, McGraw-Hill, 1993.

1–162. (**C**) Infective endocarditis is a common cause of tricuspid regurgitation. The murmur of a patient with right-sided endocarditis is heard best at the lower left sternal border and is holosystolic. Aortic stenosis is associated with crescendo-decrescendo murmur, heard best at the left second interspace. The murmur from mitral insufficiency is best heard as holosystolic at the apex.

Reference: Kinney, M. R., Packa, D. R.: Andreoli's Comprehensive Cardiac Care, 8th ed. St. Louis, Mosby–Year Book, 1996.

1–163. (**B**) For a patient with endocarditis, blood is drawn for culture from three separate sites over the course of 1 hour (20 minutes apart). This provides a greater chance that vegetations that may seed the endothelium may be obtained in the samples collected.

Reference: Khan, M. G.: Heart Disease: Diagnosis and Therapy. Baltimore, Williams & Wilkins, 1996.

1–164. (**D**) The most accurate method for calculating heart rate when the RR interval is constant takes into account the smallest number of boxes (0.04 second) via a precalculated table.

Reference: Kinney, M. R., Packa, D. R.: Andreoli's Comprehensive Cardiac Care, 8th ed. St. Louis, Mosby–Year Book, 1996.

1–165. (**B**) Retrograde P waves may be negative or biphasic in leads II, III, and aVF. Prolonged PR intervals indicate first-degree atrioventricular (AV) block. Shortened PR intervals indicate faster conduction through the AV node, usually owing to internodal or accessory tracts.

Reference: Kinney, M. R., Packa, D. R.: Andreoli's Comprehensive Cardiac Care, 8th ed. St. Louis, Mosby–Year Book, 1996.

1–166. (**B**) Criteria for second-degree AV block Mobitz type I are that the PR interval increases with each consecutively conducted P wave until a beat is dropped. Second-degree AV block Mobitz type II has intermittent nonconducted P waves with a constant PR interval. In third-degree AV block, P waves are independent of the QRS complex. In first-degree AV block, the PR interval is greater than 0.20 second, but the PR interval remains constant.

Reference: Thelan, L. A., Davie, J. K., Urden, L. D., Lough, M. E.: Critical Care Nursing, Diagnosis and Management, 2nd ed. St. Louis, Mosby–Year Book, 1994.

1–167. (**C**) Most patients will require adjustments in life style and activities related to ICD implant. Regular follow-up is necessary, and patients may have to alter their usual mode of dress so that waistbands and tight clothing are not worn over the device. The patient may not participate in contact sports and may be prohibited from using many electrical and magnetic devices. Some patients may be prohibited from driving. Medication changes are usually minor. Patients experience the shock delivered by the automatic ICD in the electrophysiology laboratory before discharge, so this will be familiar. Although teaching about sensing may be difficult, patients need only know basic elements. Many family members will readily accept the need to take CPR because the patient has probably needed emergency cardiac care in the past.

Reference: Sirovatka, B. M.: The implantable cardioverter defibrillator: Patient and family education. Dimen. Crit. Care Nurs. 12:328–334, 1993.

1–168. **(C)** Patients with Guillain-Barré syndrome (GBS) have an acquired inflammatory disorder that results in demyelinization of the peripheral nerves with a relative sparing of the axons. The patient usually presents several weeks after an upper respiratory tract infection with an ascending muscle weakness or total paralysis that is usually reversible. Many autonomic manifestations are present, including postural hypotension, heart block, and tachycardia; thus the patient will usually be monitored hemodynamically during the acute phase of the disorder. Bladder atony will require the use of an indwelling urinary catheter. Patients often have pain and tingling, experiencing various levels of pain. However, because of the paralysis associated with GBS, the patient will be unable to operate a patient-controlled analgesia system.

Reference: Barker, E. (ed.): Neuroscience Nursing. Mosby–Year Book, St. Louis, 1994.

1–169. **(A)** Severe, cramping abdominal pain, elevated white blood cell count, firm abdomen, and absent bowel sounds are classic symptoms of progressing mesenteric ischemia. Vasoconstrictive agents diminish gastrointestinal oxygen uptake, even when blood flow is normal. Packed red blood cells would improve oxygen-carrying capacity of the blood. Antibiotics would be given prophylactically in anticipation of gastrointestinal bacterial translocation. A smooth muscle relaxant such as papaverine dilates mesenteric arterioles.

Reference: Quinn, A. D.: Acute mesenteric ischemia. Crit. Care Nurs. Clin. North Am. 5:171–175, 1993.

1–170. **(C)** The most reliable indicator of carbon monoxide toxicity is the presence of an unexplained increase in anion gap metabolic acidosis. Carbon monoxide toxicity is identified by assessing the carboxyhemoglobin level (normal <5%). Because emergency responders are trained to treat suspected carbon monoxide toxicity by administering oxygen in the field, this value underestimates the magnitude of the problem in a patient who has received oxygen. The diagnosis may be based on a measured oxygen saturation of hemoglobin that is lower than predicted by the oxygen tension. Although carbon monoxide poisoning produces a cherry-red skin color, this only occurs in the presence of adequate tissue perfusion and is only detectable in light-skinned people; thus it is an unreliable indicator in patients in shock and in those with dark skin.

Reference: Demling, R. H.: Management of the burn patient. *In* Shoemaker, W. C., Ayres, S. M., Grenvik, A., Holbrook, P. R. (eds.): Textbook of Critical Care, 3rd ed. Philadelphia, W. B. Saunders, 1995.

1–171. **(C)** Briefly clamping the chest tube next to the insertion site will determine if there is a leak in the system or from the patient. A leak in the system will not be corrected by clamping the chest tube next to the insertion site; a leak from the patient will be stopped. If the leak is from the patient, a larger chest tube or increased suction may be necessary. If the leak is from the system, check for loose connections or a faulty/cracked system. Stripping the chest tube is to be avoided because it has been shown to generate high intrathoracic pressures and can damage pleural/lung tissue. The water-seal system only needs to be changed if it is cracked or full.

Reference: Boggs, R. L., Wooldridge-King, M. (eds.): AACN Procedure Manual for Critical Care, 3rd ed. Philadelphia, W. B. Saunders, 1993.

1–172. (**A**) The potential for ventricular tachycardia/fibrillation related to R on T phenomenon is demonstrated where a pacemaker spike is visible on the T wave. If a premature ventricular contraction or pacemaker spike occurs at this critical point, individual segments of myocardium can depolarize separately from each other resulting in ventricular tachycardia/fibrillation.

Reference: Thelan, L. A., Davie, J. K., Urden, L. D., Lough, M. E.: Critical Care Nursing, Diagnosis and Management, 2nd ed. St. Louis, Mosby–Year Book, 1994.

1–173. (**B**) The Advanced Cardiac Life Support (ACLS) guidelines call for an initial delivery of 200 joules.

Reference: Kinney, M. R., Packa, D. R.: Andreoli's Comprehensive Cardiac Care, 8th ed. St. Louis, Mosby–Year Book, 1996.

1–174. (**B**) If the administration of an initial 6-mg dose of adenosine is ineffective, a second dose of 12 mg may be attempted in 1 to 2 minutes. Adenosine is extremely short acting and has an immediate effect. Changing therapy to verapamil before therapeutic levels of adenosine have been reached is inappropriate.

Reference: Kinney, M. R., Packa, D. R.: Andreoli's Comprehensive Cardiac Care, 8th ed. St. Louis, Mosby–Year Book, 1996.

1–175. (**B**) These are the signs of a hyperglycemic hyperosmolar nonketotic state. The most important initial intervention is isotonic fluid administration because the patient is usually severely dehydrated and often hypotensive secondary to osmotic diuresis. Adequate fluid volume must be restored to maintain tissue perfusion. Colloids such as albumin can exacerbate vascular insufficiency and contribute to already elevated plasma viscosity. The large amount of glucose in the extracellular fluid preserves intravascular volume and organ perfusion despite a severe dehydration. If a patient is treated with insulin, extracellular glucose is decreased, water flows down the osmotic gradient into the cells, the extracellular and intravascular space contracts, and vascular collapse can occur. Potassium replacement should be considered as soon as adequate urine flow is established.

References: Alspach, J. G. (ed.): AACN Core Curriculum for Critical Care Nursing, 5th ed. Philadelphia, W. B. Saunders, 1998.
Lorber, D.: Nonketotic hypertonicity in diabetes mellitus. Med. Clin. North Am. 79:39–53, 1995.

1–176. (**B**) Western blot is the confirmatory test for HIV. ELISA is a test that is less expensive than Western blot and is used for HIV screening. The Coombs' test measures antigen-antibody complexes on the red blood cell membrane and is not used to test for HIV. HIV tests check for antibodies, not antigens.

Reference: Alspach, J. G. (ed.): AACN Core Curriculum for Critical Care Nursing, 5th ed. Philadelphia, W. B. Saunders, 1998.

1–177. (**D**) Patients who have undergone allogenic or autologous bone marrow transplantation are at high risk for graft-versus-host disease (GVHD). There is no evidence that patients receiving solid organ transplants have the same risk. Transfusion-associated graft-versus-host disease (TA-GVHD) is an immunologic reaction mediated by immunocompetent donor lymphocytes in cellular blood products that engraft in a transfused recipient, who is unable to recognize the transfused donor lymphocytes as foreign. (Engraftment is a process in which foreign lymphocytes invade a recipient's bone marrow and proliferate and mature. New blood cells can be found in the recipient's circulating blood. The process can be planned as in bone marrow transplantation or unplanned as in TA-GVHD.) Immunosuppression treatment for TA-GVHD has been disappointing. Thus, prophylactic irradiation of cellular blood components before transfusion is the only effective way to prevent TA-GVHD.

References: Gloe, D.: Common reactions to transfusions. Heart Lung 20:506–514, 1991.
Jeter, E., Spivey, M. A.: Noninfectious complications of blood transfusion. Hematol. Oncol. Clin. North Am. 9:187–204, 1995.

1–178. (**B**) An aura refers to a peculiar sensation that some patients with seizures experience immediately preceding the definite symptoms of a seizure. An aura may be visual, auditory, or gustatory, or it may consist of numbness or tingling of a body part. *Prodromal* is a term used to describe early symptoms of a disease. An *epileptic cry* is a sound sometimes produced by an individual during a seizure. *Ictus* refers to an acute seizure.

Reference: Hickey, J. V.: The Clinical Practice of Neurological and Neurosurgical Nursing, 3rd ed. Philadelphia, J. B. Lippincott, 1992.

1–179. (**A**) Hemodynamic support during this phase involves replenishing red blood cells to maintain a hematocrit at more than 30%, maintaining the serum albumin level at 2.5 g/dl or higher, and increasing oxygen delivery to decrease elevated lactic acid concentration. Electrolyte losses are corrected but do not directly affect oxygen delivery.

Reference: Demling, R. H.: Management of the burn patient. In Shoemaker, W. C., Ayres, S. M., Grenvik, A., Holbrook, P. R. (eds.): Textbook of Critical Care, 3rd ed. Philadelphia, W. B. Saunders, 1995.

1–180. (**D**) The development of hypokalemia, hypercalcemia, and/or hypomagnesemia may precipitate or aggravate digitalis toxicity. Hypokalemia and hypercalcemia may enhance the effects of digitalis to the point of toxicity.

Reference: Tucker, S. M., Canobbio, M. M., Paquette, E. V., Wells, M. F.: Patient Care Standards: Collaborative Practice Planning Guides, 6th ed. St. Louis, Mosby–Year Book, 1996.

1–181. (**C**) Liver laceration and splenic rupture injuries in trauma are known for causing large blood volume loss. If extensive blood loss occurs, low perfusion states are precipitated, leading to cellular hypoxia and anaerobic metabolism. Leukocytosis, ileus, and sepsis would indicate complications of bowel injury such as abscess, fistula, or obstruction, which are gradual in development and not acutely associated with abdominal trauma.

References: Aragon, D., Parson, R.: Multiple organ dysfunction syndrome in the trauma patient. Crit. Care Nurs. Clin. North Am. 6:873–881, 1994.
Lawrence, D. M.: Gastrointestinal trauma. Crit. Care Nurs. Clin. North Am. 5:127–140, 1993.

1–182. (**C**) Subcutaneous bubbles reflect air in planes of the tissues. Subcutaneous emphysema is not dangerous unless it occurs around the trachea and compresses tissues; it will eventually be reabsorbed. If the pressure is uncomfortable (scrotum) or disturbing to the patient or family (eyelids), small slits may be made in the skin to express the air out manually. Suctioning would not help and could traumatize tissue.

Reference: Kersten, L. D.: Comprehensive Respiratory Nursing: A Decision Making Approach. Philadelphia, W. B. Saunders, 1989.

1–183. (**D**) Immediate treatment of ventricular fibrillation is direct-current countershock at 200 to 400 joules, with the initial delivery at 200 joules.

Reference: Kinney, M. R., Packa, D. R.: Andreoli's Comprehensive Cardiac Care, 8th ed. St. Louis, Mosby–Year Book, 1996.

1–184. (**B**) The therapeutic range of procainamide is a serum N-acetyl procainamide (NAPA) level of 10 to 20 μg/ml. It is the most specific determination of therapeutic blood levels. QRS complex widening, greater than 0.12 second, is a symptom of procainamide toxicity. Procainamide is used to suppress ventricular ectopy, but the presence of normal sinus rhythm does not necessarily mean that therapeutic levels are present.

Reference: Kinney, M. R., Packa, D. R.: Andreoli's Comprehensive Cardiac Care, 8th ed. St. Louis, Mosby–Year Book, 1996.

1–185. (**A**) Improved cardiac output is the overall outcome that is sought in the treatment of supraventricular tachycardia. Decrease in heart rate is a component that aids in the improvement of cardiac output by allowing greater time for diastolic filling and decreasing myocardial oxygen demands. Return of atrial kick increases cardiac output by approximately 25%.

Reference: Ruppert, S. D., Kernicki, J. G., Dolan, J. T.: Dolan's Critical Care Nursing: Clinical Management Through the Nursing Process. Philadelphia, F. A. Davis, 1996.

1–186. (**C**) Beta blockers such as propranolol are used in hypertrophic cardiomyopathy to slow heart rate and decrease contractility. These actions decrease outflow obstruction and improve cardiac output. Calcium channel blockers such as diltiazem decrease cardiac work by slowing heart rate, and increasing diastolic relaxation and filling time. Positive inotropic medications such as dobutamine are not used in hypertrophic cardiomyopathy because they increase the obstruction of the outflow tract.

Reference: Thelan, L. A., Davie, J. K., Urden, L. D., Lough, M. E.: Critical Care Nursing, Diagnosis and Management, 2nd ed. St. Louis, Mosby–Year Book, 1994.

1–187. (**C**) Intra-aortic balloon therapy is used to decrease afterload and tension on the ruptured septum. The balloon pump is inserted before surgical repair of the rupture. A Dacron patch is not usually necessary for perforations because they are easily oversewn. Right- and left-ventricular assist devices are not utilized unless complications arise from the surgical repair of the rupture.

Reference: Enfanto, P. A., Pieczek, A. M., Kelley, K., et al.: Percutaneous laser myoplasty: Nursing care implications. Crit. Care Nurs. 14:94–101, 1994.

1–188. (**D**) The right ventricle is the most often affected with blunt trauma because of its anterior location and proximity to the sternum. Tamponade would cause increased neck vein distention, muffled heart tones, and pulsus paradoxus. Hemothorax and pneumothorax would cause decreased breath sounds over the affected lung.

Reference: Thelan, L. A., Davie, J. K., Urden, L. D., Lough, M. E.: Critical Care Nursing, Diagnosis and Management, 2nd ed. St. Louis, Mosby–Year Book, 1994.

1–189. (**D**) The myocardium is irritable from the edematous suture lines and defect. Lidocaine raises the threshold for ventricular premature contractions and decreases electrical instability. Potassium supplementation will decrease irritability.

Reference: Wright, J. E., Shelton, B. K.: Desk Reference for Critical Care Nursing, Boston, Jones & Bartlett, 1993.

1–190. (**C**) Severe short-term memory loss is a common sequela of major electrical injury and may persist for many weeks after electrical injury. There is no increased incidence of seizures after electrical injury. Delirium tremens occurs 48 to 72 hoursafter alcohol withdrawal. The mental status changes associated with sepsis do not persist for 5 days.

Reference: Kravitz, M.: Burn injuries. *In* Copstead, L. C.: Perspectives on Pathophysiology. Philadelphia, W. B. Saunders, 1995.

1–191. (**A**) A bronchopleural fistula would result in fairly continuous bubbling. Obstruction of the tube in the lung, kinked tubing, and re-expansion of the lung would produce minimal or no fluctuations in the water-seal chamber.

Reference: Kersten, L. D.: Comprehensive Respiratory Nursing: A Decision Making Approach. Philadelphia, W. B. Saunders, 1989.

1–192. (**B**) Typical postictal behavior includes confusion, lethargy, headache, and somnolence. The patient will usually sleep for an extended period of time after a seizure. Automatisms are repetitive, uncontrolled behaviors that are not characteristic after a seizure. Incontinence usually occurs during a seizure rather than after a seizure.

Reference: Clochesy, J. M., Breu, C., Cardin, S., et al. (eds.): Critical Care Nursing, 2nd ed. Philadelphia, W. B. Saunders, 1996.

1–193. (**A**) Esophageal rupture from penetration injury is diagnosed with insertion of a chest tube and ingestion of methylene blue. Chest drainage positive for methylene blue is confirmation of esophageal perforation. Exploratory laparotomy with peritoneal lavage confirms abdominal organ injury but not esophageal injury. Endotracheal intubation with suction and chest radiography with contrast medium enhancement are not diagnostic for esophageal injuries.

Reference: Lawrence, D. M.: Gastrointestinal trauma. Crit. Care Nurs. Clin. North Am. 5:127–140, 1993.

1–194. (**A**) Intermittent claudication is the classic symptom of aortoiliac occlusive disease with symptoms involving the muscles of the thigh, hip, buttocks, and calf. Symptoms of intermittent claudication occur typically during exercise. When metabolic demands of distal tissues exceed supply, pain occurs. Pulsatile masses are classic signs of aneurysms. Although diminished pulses may be a sign of occlusive disease, they may also be due to obesity, hypovolemia, or vasoconstriction. Palpable pulses are often found at rest because of collateral circulation.

Reference: Fahey, V.: Vascular Nursing, 2nd ed. Philadelphia, W. B. Saunders, 1994.

1–195. (**D**) A classic finding in acute occlusion of the popliteal artery is a painful, cool, pulseless foot that blanches to palpation. The area of occlusion is tender over the artery and proximal to it. As the occlusion becomes chronic, the skin and capillaries fail to blanch and pain decreases.

Reference: Moore, W. S.: Vascular Surgery: A Comprehensive Review. Philadelphia, W. B. Saunders, 1993.

1–196. **(C)** Calcium channel blockers are often used for their antispasmodic and vasodilation effects after peripheral arterial surgery. Prostaglandins cause arterial dilation but do not reduce spasm. Pyridamole is an antiplatelet agent. Beta blockers prevent sympathetic effects on the arterial wall but do not prevent spasm.

Reference: Thelan, L. A., Davie, J. K., Urden, L. D., Lough, M. E.: Critical Care Nursing, Diagnosis and Management, 2nd ed. St. Louis, Mosby–Year Book, 1994.

1–197. **(D)** Normal tissue pressure is zero. At pressures of 30 mm Hg, blood flow is severely impaired and compartment syndrome is present. Emergency treatment for compartment syndrome is fasciotomy. Loss of pulses would indicate thrombus as a potential source of the pain requiring thrombectomy or urokinase therapy. Reapplication of Ace wraps would not relieve the compartment syndrome.

Reference: Moore, W. S.: Vascular Surgery: A Comprehensive Review. Philadelphia, W. B. Saunders, 1993.

1–198. **(A)** Energy intake must equal the energy expended by the body's metabolism for optimal wound healing to occur. Energy expenditure is quantified using indirect calorimetry to measure metabolic status and thus determine whether the patient is in positive nutritional balance. Intake and outputs are difficult to measure accurately because of the inability to calculate fluids lost through the burn wound. Daily weights are not accurate assessments of nutritional status during the postresuscitation phase because of massive fluid shifts as edema resolves. The nutritional formulas are estimates, and individual patients may require substantially more or less nutritional support to meet actual energy expenditure.

Reference: Roberts, S. L.: Multisystem deviations. *In* Critical Care Nursing: Assessment and Intervention. Stamford, Conn., Appleton & Lange, 1996.

1–199. **(D)** Blood around the urinary meatus after renal trauma can indicate damage to the urethra. Insertion of a urinary catheter is contraindicated until urethral damage has been ruled out.

Reference: Smith, M. F.: Renal trauma: Adult and pediatric considerations. Crit. Care Nurs. Clin. North Am. 2:67–77, 1990.

1–200. **(B)** The symptoms of hypoglycemia are nonspecific. Initiation of treatment of autonomic symptoms such as tremors and diaphoresis should await confirmation of low blood glucose level because autonomic symptoms do not indicate a severely low glucose concentration. The time and type of the last insulin dose will tell when the peak effects should occur, indicating if the patient's symptoms are related to insulin therapy. The time and type of oral intake can also give information related to the cause of the hypoglycemic episode. Finding this information takes time and should follow measuring the patient's glucose level and treating the hypoglycemia, which can deteriorate if not treated. A patient with central nervous system manifestations such as disorientation or inability to respond is displaying symptoms of severe hypoglycemia, and immediate treatment would be the priority. Optimally, treatment would occur simultaneously with measurement of blood glucose concentration, so the exact glucose level is known.

Reference: Service, F. J.: Hypoglycemia. Med. Clin. North Am. 79:1–8, 1995.

CORE REVIEW TEST

2–1. Which of the following diagnostic studies would best contribute to the diagnosis of disseminated intravascular coagulation (DIC)?

A. Obtaining a chest radiograph.
B. Obtaining a serum sodium value.
C. Obtaining serum erythrocyte sedimentation rate.
D. Obtaining serum fibrin split products.

2–2. The nurse should use which of the following leads to distinguish right bundle branch block (RBBB) from left bundle branch block (LBBB)?

A. V_1 or V_2.
B. Lead I or lead II.
C. Lead II or lead III.
D. Lead III or lead I.

2–3. In addition to a crash cart, the nurse should arrange to have which of the following at the bedside of a patient with left bundle branch block (LBBB) during pulmonary artery catheter insertion?

A. A pacing defibrillator or transcutaneous pacemaker.
B. A pericardiocentesis tray.
C. A temporary transvenous pacemaker insertion tray.
D. A chest tube insertion tray.

Questions 2–4 through 2–6 relate to the following situation.

A 35-year-old man is admitted to the ICU after cholecystectomy. The patient is obese, is a diet-controlled diabetic, and has led a sedentary life style. His preoperative pulmonary function tests were marginal, which is explained by his smoking history of 30 pack-years. Extubation is performed in the recovery room, and the patient is sent to the ICU for observation overnight with oxygen at 3 L/min per nasal cannula.

2–4. In which order of importance should the following interventions be implemented?

A. Incentive spirometer, pain medication, cough and deep breathe.
B. Pain medication, incentive spirometer, cough and deep breathe.
C. Cough and deep breathe, pain medication, incentive spirometer.
D. Cough and deep breathe, incentive spirometer, pain medication.

2–5. The patient's oxygenation status remains tenuous. By the next morning, his oxygen saturation is 88%, he has a slightly productive cough and a slight fever and is splinting. What would be the most appropriate intervention?

A. Intermittent positive-pressure breathing (IPPB).
B. Antipyretics.
C. Early ambulation.
D. Patient-controlled analgesia pump.

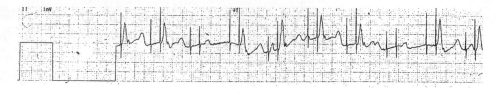

2–6. Which of this patient's risk factors has the most impact on his risk for developing atelectasis?

A. Abdominal surgery.
B. Smoking history.
C. Obesity.
D. Diabetes.

2–7. Which of the following is a possible cause for development of pneumonia?

A. Aspiration of gastric contents.
B. Organ transplant.
C. Immunosuppression.
D. Age.

2–8. *Pseudomonas* produces secretions that are thick, green, and foul smelling. This infection is usually

A. Community acquired.
B. Idiopathic.
C. Nosocomial.
D. The result of inappropriate antibiotic use.

2–9. The rhythm strip above (lead II) belongs to a patient with a temporary transvenous atrioventricular sequential pacemaker. The most appropriate treatment for the condition noted in this strip is to

A. Increase the sensitivity.
B. Decrease the sensitivity.
C. Increase the mA.
D. Decrease the mA.

2–10. In assessing a patient who has ingested lye, the nurse would expect to find the most tissue damage at the level of the

A. Mouth and lips.
B. Pharynx.
C. Esophagus.
D. Stomach.

2–11. For the nursing diagnosis Decreased Cardiac Output Related to Atrioventricular Block, which of the following findings indicates a need to revise the care plan?

A. The heart rate increases to 64 beats/min after withholding the ordered dose of digoxin.
B. The patient's heart rate decreases from 60 to 50 beats/min while having a bowel movement.
C. The patient maintains his blood pressure when placed supine during breakthrough tachycardia.
D. The patient's PR interval increases from 0.20 to 0.26 with isometric exercise.

2–12. When planning care for a patient with subarachnoid hemorrhage as a result of an arteriovenous malformation, the critical care nurse anticipates which of the following complications within the first 2 days after the initial rupture and hemorrhage?

A. Vasospasm.
B. Rebleeding.
C. Hydrocephalus.
D. Increased intracranial pressure.

2–13. A 50-year-old patient with fulminant hepatic failure presented yesterday with confusion, irritability, and sleep changes. This morning he is disoriented and somnolent. Essential assessment for this patient includes monitoring for

A. Impaired pupillary reflexes.
B. Hypotension.
C. Sinus tachycardia.
D. Hyperglycemia.

2–14. An elevated pulmonary capillary wedge pressure (PCWP) with high "v" waves is found in patients with

A. Hypovolemia.
B. Pulmonary edema.
C. Right ventricular failure.
D. Mitral regurgitation.

2–15. The chest radiograph of a patient with heart failure would show

A. Elevated hemidiaphragms.
B. Total whiteout of lung fields.
C. Small cardiac silhouette.
D. Cloudy lung fields.

2–16. A patient with chronic hypertension develops dyspnea. Data available include the following clinical findings:

BP = 180/96 mm Hg; heart rate = 120 beats/min; respiratory rate = 28 breaths/min.
12-lead ECG shows nonspecific ST changes and sinus tachycardia.
Chest radiograph shows interstitial and perivascular edema and a normal cardiac silhouette.
Doppler echocardiography demonstrates an ejection fraction of 50% with no evidence of aneurysm.

Which of the following is the probable cause of the patient's dyspnea?

A. Right ventricular failure.
B. Left ventricular systolic dysfunction.
C. Left ventricular diastolic dysfunction.
D. Myocardial contusion.

2–17. The care plan for patients with heart failure due to diastolic dysfunction should include education regarding

I. Symptoms of digoxin toxicity.
II. Achieving a balance of both exercise and rest.
III. Effects and actions of calcium channel blocking medications.
IV. Effects and actions of beta-blocking medications.

A. I and II.
B. II and III.
C. I, II, and III.
D. II, III, and IV.

2–18. For a patient with a ventricular-assist device for left ventricular failure, prevention of infection includes which of the following activities?

I. Meticulous cannula drive line care.
II. Removal of all invasive lines as soon as feasible.
III. High-dose triple-antibiotic prophylaxis.
IV. Use of masks and gloves for all patient contacts.

A. I and II.
B. II and III.
C. III and IV.
D. I and IV.

2–19. Which of the following places a patient at risk for pneumonia?

A. Mechanical ventilation.
B. Intravenous fluid therapy.
C. Intubation.
D. Percutaneous endogastric (PEG) tube.

2–20. Administration of which of the following medications will rapidly manage the cardiotoxic effects of hyperkalemia?

A. Calcium chloride.
B. Sodium bicarbonate.
C. Dextrose 50% and insulin.
D. Sodium polystyrene.

2–21. In an alert patient who has ingested diazepam, the first dose of activated charcoal is

A. 50 to 100 g given with a cathartic.
B. 50 to 100 g given without a cathartic.
C. 20 to 50 g given without a cathartic.
D. Contraindicated with diazepam ingestion.

2–22. Which of the following medications are used in heart failure to decrease renin-angiotensin activity?

 I. Furosemide.
 II. Captopril.
 III. Digoxin.
 IV. Bumetanide.

 A. II only.
 B. II and III.
 C. II and IV.
 D. II, III, and IV.

2–23. An initial sign of increasing cerebral edema in a patient with fulminant hepatic failure is

 A. Decreased muscle tone.
 B. Hypoventilation.
 C. Hypertension.
 D. Constricted pupils.

2–24. In a patient with Brown-Séquard syndrome, the critical care nurse would expect to find which one of the following on assessment?

 A. Contralateral sparing of vibration and touch.
 B. Contralateral loss of vibratory sensation.
 C. Ipsilateral loss of proprioception.
 D. Ipsilateral loss of pain and temperature sensation.

2–25. When the patient undergoing treatment for diabetic ketoacidosis develops ventricular dysrhythmias, the most probable cause is

 A. Myocardial infarction.
 B. Acidosis.
 C. Hypomagnesemia.
 D. Hypokalemia.

2–26. A critically ill patient develops prolonged bleeding without a previous history of bleeding. The nurse should plan care for a diagnosis of disseminated intravascular coagulation if which of the following predisposing signs are also present?

 A. Alkalosis and hypertension.
 B. Acidosis and hypertension.
 C. Alkalosis and hypotension.
 D. Acidosis and hypotension.

2–27. Protective mechanisms of the upper airway include all of the following *except*

 A. Cough reflex.
 B. Mucosal adherence.
 C. Filtration.
 D. Bacterial interference.

2–28. A major differentiation between the pulmonary function results for asthma and those for chronic obstructive pulmonary disease (COPD) is

 A. Responsiveness to bronchodilator.
 B. Reduced forced expiratory volume in 1 second (FEV_1).
 C. Decreased peak expiratory flow (PEF).
 D. Decreased forced vital capacity (FVC).

2–29. A patient with status asthmaticus is intubated and placed on a ventilator. He has a dry cough with minimal sputum production. What is he at greatest risk for?

 A. Pneumonia.
 B. Mucus plugging.
 C. Respiratory arrest.
 D. Barotrauma.

2–30. Cocaine overdose is initially treated with

 A. Naloxone.
 B. Flumazenil.
 C. Lorazepam.
 D. Haloperidol.

2–31. Which of the following are used in the treatment of heart failure to reduce preload?

 A. Furosemide, nitroglycerin, enalapril.
 B. Bemetamide, digoxin, captopril.
 C. Atenolol, minoxidil, nitroprusside.
 D. Sodium restriction, amiloride, dobutamine.

2–32. Therapy in heart failure directed to limit the effects of the renin-angiotensin-aldosterone system (RAAS) includes

A. Digoxin, diuretics, and potassium replacement.
B. Angiotensin converting enzyme (ACE) inhibitors, diuretics, and sodium restriction.
C. Beta blockers, calcium channel blockers, and diuretics.
D. Digitalis glycosides, calcium channel blockers, and ACE inhibitors.

2–33. A pulmonary artery catheter is inserted in a patient with left ventricular failure. While deflating the balloon after wedging, the nurse notes blood in the balloon catheter. These findings are documented. Which of the following is the most appropriate action?

A. Change the syringe to prevent infection.
B. Check to see if blood may be aspirated from the site.
C. Inject 1.5 ml of air to see if wedging is still possible.
D. Remove the syringe and close it with a dead end cap.

Questions 2–34 and 2–35 refer to the following situation.

An 85-year-old man had a closed reduction of the left femur after a motor vehicle–pedestrian accident. Three days later he experienced sharp pain in his chest and shortness of breath. His arterial blood gases were pH of 7.48; $PaCO_2$ of 30 mm Hg; PaO_2 of 55 mm Hg; and SaO_2 of 88%. He was transferred to the ICU and started on oxygen. Vital signs were blood pressure of 135/95 mm Hg, pulse of 110 beats/min, and respiratory rate of 23 breaths/min. A pulmonary embolus is suspected.

2–34. What tests would be most appropriate to order?

A. Spirometry.
B. Ventilation/perfusion scan.
C. Chest radiograph.
D. ECG.

2–35. The patient is diagnosed definitively as having had a pulmonary embolus. Which of the following therapies is the most appropriate to be implemented immediately?

A. Heparin.
B. Streptokinase.
C. Vena caval umbrella.
D. Tissue plasminogen activator.

2–36. After removal of a pituitary tumor, the critical care nurse knows that an intervention for postoperative headache is to

A. Administer narcotic analgesics.
B. Decrease fluid intake.
C. Elevate the head of the bed.
D. Keep patient stimulation to a minimum.

2–37. Severe, unrelenting left upper quadrant abdominal pain that is constant until treated is characteristic of

A. Angina.
B. Pulmonary emboli.
C. Acute pancreatitis.
D. Fulminant hepatitis.

2–38. A 70-year-old patient is admitted to the ICU in acute respiratory distress. Respiratory rate is 32 breaths/min, and heart rate is 124 beats/min. Chest radiograph shows right upper lobe infiltrates. PaO_2 is 70 mm Hg on 100% nonrebreather mask. Blood pressure is 142/92 mm Hg. There are crackles at both bases and decreased breath sounds in the right upper lobe. The 12-lead ECG shows Q waves in the anterior leads. There is a prominent systolic murmur. The patient is placed on a continuous positive airway pressure (CPAP) mask at 8 L and 5 cm H_2O. A pulmonary artery catheter is inserted and shows a pulmonary artery pressure of 78/40 mm Hg and a pulmonary capillary wedge pressure (PCWP) of 44 mm Hg. The patient would benefit from which of the following?

I. Digoxin loading dose of 0.25 mg every 4 hours for four doses.
II. Morphine sulfate, 2 to 4 mg IV.
III. Nitroprusside drip titrated to the PCWP.
IV. Furosemide, 40 mg IV.

A. I and II.
B. II and III.
C. III and IV.
D. II and IV.

2–39. Which of the following is used to confirm suspected pulmonary artery catheter knotting in a patient with left ventricular hypertrophy?

A. An overpenetrated chest radiograph.
B. The length of the catheter is noted to be 45 cm.
C. Inability to obtain a pulmonary capillary wedge waveform.
D. The waveform appears dampened and does not improve with flushing.

2–40. A patient is admitted to the ICU after a small bowel resection. Vital signs are BP = 94/62 mm Hg; heart rate = 128 beats/min; respiratory rate = 28 breaths/min. The patient's cardiac monitor shows sinus tachycardia with frequent premature ventricular contractions. The 12-lead ECG shows sinus tachycardia with prolonged QT interval and shortened ST segment. Chemistry results are as follows:

Na^+	132 mEq/L
K^+	2.4 mEq/L
Cl^-	95 mEq/L
Mg^{2+}	0.6 mEq/L
Glucose	165 mg/dl
BUN	28 mg/dl
Ca^{2+}	8.0 mEq/L
Phosphate	4.5 mg/dl

What is the potential cause of this patient's ECG abnormalities?

A. Hyponatremia.
B. Hyperchloremia.
C. Hypomagnesemia.
D. Hypercalcemia.

2–41. Ventricular arrhythmias associated with cocaine overdose are treated with

A. Beta blockers.
B. Calcium channel blockers.
C. Nitroglycerin.
D. Digoxin.

2–42. Which of the following indicates effective treatment for decreased cardiac output related to left ventricular failure?

A. MAP = 75 mm Hg, PCWP = 22 mm Hg, cardiac index = 2.0 L/min/m².
B. MAP = 60 mm Hg, PCWP = 4 mm Hg, cardiac index = 1.9 L/min/m².
C. MAP = 80 mm Hg, PCWP = 12 mm Hg, cardiac index = 2.5 L/min/m².
D. MAP = 80 mm Hg, PCWP = 25 mm Hg, cardiac index = 3.0 L/min/m².

2–43. In a patient being treated with vasodilators and diuretics for hypertensive crisis, assessment of tissue perfusion is focused on continuous
cardiac monitoring, continuous arterial pressure monitoring, and frequent assessment of

  A. Level of consciousness, urine
  specific gravity, and jugular venous pulsations.
  B. Level of consciousness, breath
  sounds, capillary refill, and
  urine output.
  C. Sensory and motor deficits, visual disturbances, and urinary
  protein.
  D. Skin temperature, jugular venous distention, intake and output, and urine specific gravity.

2–44. In the emergency department a patient with hypertensive crisis has
received two doses of nifedipine, 10
mg, 2 inches of nitropaste, and two
doses of labetalol, 20 mg IV. Blood
pressure is 160/100 mm Hg. Which
of the following would be anticipated for the care of this patient?

  I. A private, quiet room to
  decrease sensory stimuli.
  II. Infusion pumps to deliver
  fluids and antihypertensive
  medications.
  III. An automated blood pressure
  cuff to take frequent blood
  pressure readings.
  IV. Equipment for arterial line
  placement.

  A. I and II.
  B. II and III.
  C. I and IV.
  D. I, II, and IV.

2–45. The most frequent site of a pulmonary embolus is in the

  A. Lingula.
  B. Upper lobes.
  C. Middle lobe.
  D. Lower lobes.

**Questions 2–46 and 2–47 relate to the
following situation.**

A 45-year-old man is admitted to the ICU
with a presumptive diagnosis of primary
pulmonary hypertension. He has clinical
signs of cor pulmonale with no smoking history, and his pulmonary function test results are normal. A pulmonary artery catheter is placed, and initial measurements are

Mean PAP	50 mm Hg
PCWP	10 mm Hg
RAP	18 mm Hg
RVEDP	20 mm Hg
Cardiac output	2.8 L/min

2–46. What therapy might be implemented?

  A. Nitroglycerin patch.
  B. Prostacyclin.
  C. Nitroprusside.
  D. Diuresis.

2–47. A vasodilator drip is started and is
infusing directly into his lungs
through the infusion port of the pulmonary artery catheter. His pulmonary artery pressures slowly start
to decline. Suddenly, the patient
goes into ventricular fibrillation and
cardiac arrest. What is a likely
cause of his cardiac collapse?

  A. Hemodynamic collapse second-
  ary to saddle embolus.
  B. Right ventricular wall infarc-
  tion.
  C. Air embolus.
  D. Left ventricular wall infarction.

2–48. When assessing an elderly patient
with the following risk factors,
which places a patient at the greatest risk for a cerebrovascular accident?

  A. Previous stroke.
  B. Diabetes mellitus.
  C. Cardiac disease.
  D. Hypertension.

2–49. In a patient with acute pancreatitis, false elevation of serum amylase level may be caused by

A. Meperidine (Demerol).
B. Levorphanol tartrate (Levo-Dromoran).
C. Morphine.
D. Fentanyl.

2–50. Which set of laboratory values characterizes the usual presentation of diabetic ketoacidosis?

	A.	B.	C.	D.
Glucose (mg/dl)	1168	550	223	459
pH	7.23	7.15	7.39	7.18
Serum HCO_3^- (mEq/L)	19	13	17	26
Urine ketones	+2	+3	+4	−
Serum ketones	−	+	+	−
Serum osmolality	High	Variable	Low	Variable
Serum sodium (mEq/L)	155	135	130	140

2–51. Heparin is ordered for a patient with disseminated intravascular coagulation (DIC). To evaluate the appropriateness of this order, the nurse should know that the rationale for administration of heparin in DIC is to

A. Increase thrombin activity.
B. Enhance clot destruction.
C. Increase fibrin formation.
D. Slow the coagulation cycle.

2–52. The treatment for ethylene glycol ingestion is initiated on the basis of the patient's

A. History.
B. Anion gap acidosis.
C. Toxicology screen.
D. Osmolar gap.

2–53. The primary cause of death associated with drowning or near-drowning is related to

A. Respiratory failure.
B. Brain ischemia.
C. Hypoxia.
D. Multiple organ failure.

2–54. For a patient in hypertensive crisis with a suspected cerebrovascular accident (CVA), which of the following is an appropriate pharmacologic treatment?

A. Nifedipine, 10 mg sublingual PRN.
B. Sodium nitroprusside, 50 mg in 250 ml D5W titrated to maintain systolic blood pressure less than or equal to 150 mm Hg.
C. Diazoxide, 150 mg IV bolus.
D. Methyldopa, 250 mg IV every 4 to 6 hours for systolic blood pressure greater than 150 mm Hg.

2–55. Effective treatment for hypertensive crisis is indicated by return of blood pressure to normal range as well as which of the following clinical findings?

 I. Serum (venous) pH 7.45.
 II. Glasgow Coma Scale score 15.
III. Serum creatine kinase 140 U/L.
IV. Serum creatinine 1.8 mg/dl.

A. I and II.
B. II and III.
C. III and IV.
D. I and IV.

2–56. A flail chest is diagnosed by

A. Chest radiograph.
B. Paradoxical chest wall movement.
C. Patient history.
D. Arterial blood gas analysis.

2–57. The treatment of choice for diaphragmatic rupture is

A. Positive-pressure ventilation.
B. Surgical repair.
C. Phrenic nerve pacemaker.
D. Negative-pressure ventilation.

2–58. A patient has the following signs and symptoms:

Systolic BP of 80 mm Hg
PCWP of 20 mm Hg
Heart rate of 120 beats/min
Respiratory rate of 30 breaths/min
S_3, S_4
Urine output less than 30 ml/hr
Cool, clammy skin

What type of shock does this patient have?

A. Hypovolemic.
B. Cardiogenic.
C. Septic.
D. Anaphylactic.

Questions 2–59 and 2–60 refer to the following situation.

A patient is admitted to the ICU with a diagnosis of Small Bowel Obstruction, Rule Out Peritonitis. On review of the chemistry report the nurse notes a serum sodium concentration of 114 mEq/L.

2–59. The nurse should assess the patient for the following signs and symptoms:

A. Dehydration, flushed skin, and hypertension.
B. Hypotension, tachycardia, and oliguria.
C. Ileus, dysrhythmias, and a prolonged QT interval.
D. Hypertension, bradycardia, and slurred speech.

2–60. In planning the care of this patient, the nurse's priority intervention would be to

A. Institute seizure precautions.
B. Conserve the patient's energy by limiting activity.
C. Measure intake and output every 8 hours.
D. Promote patient comfort by controlling pain.

2–61. A patient with a history of ulcerative colitis was admitted yesterday with an acute myocardial infarction. The chest pain has been effectively controlled with morphine, but there is a persistent problem with hypokalemia. The patient suddenly begins to complain of severe abdominal pain. The abdomen is distended and tympanitic. This patient has most likely developed

A. Peptic ulcers.
B. Hepatic failure.
C. Toxic megacolon.
D. Costochondritis.

Questions 2–62 through 2–64 refer to the following situation.

An 18-year-old man is admitted to the ICU after a single car motor vehicle crash in which the car hit a tree. He was not wearing a seat belt. His initial chest radiograph shows several scattered pulmonary infiltrates. Six hours later, the patient is tachypneic and tachycardic, with crackles bilaterally and copious secretions. Arterial blood gas analysis results show hypoxemia and CO_2 retention.

2–62. What is the most likely cause of these findings?

A. Pneumothorax.
B. Hemothorax.
C. Adult respiratory distress syndrome.
D. Pulmonary contusion.

2–63. What would be the most appropriate treatment at this point?

A. Intubation and mechanical ventilation.
B. Chest tube.
C. Bronchoscopy.
D. Antibiotic therapy.

2–64. Three days later, his infiltrates on chest radiograph are resolving and weaning is attempted. Each time the patient is removed from the positive-pressure ventilation, he has paradoxical chest movements and he desaturates by pulse oximeter. What is the most likely cause of this deterioration?

A. Flail chest.
B. Adult respiratory distress syndrome.
C. Pain.
D. Diaphragmatic herniation.

2–65. Treatment of a patient in cardiogenic shock with a pulmonary capillary wedge pressure (PCWP) of 14 mm Hg would include

A. Dopamine.
B. Dobutamine.
C. Nitroglycerin.
D. Fluid administration.

2–66. In a patient with cardiogenic shock, which of the following is an appropriate treatment to improve cardiac contractility without increasing systemic vascular resistance?

A. Dobutamine, 10 μg/kg/hr.
B. Dopamine, 10 μg/kg/hr.
C. Norepinephrine, 10 μg/min.
D. Digoxin, 0.25 mg IV.

2–67. Which of the following indicates appropriate intra-aortic balloon pump (IABP) timing?

A. Inflation occurs at the end of ventricular diastole.
B. Deflation occurs just before ventricular systole.
C. Inflation occurs just before ventricular systole.
D. Deflation occurs at the beginning of ventricular diastole.

2–68. The severity of valvular aortic stenosis is demonstrated by

A. ST segment elevation in leads V_1 and V_2.
B. High-pressure gradients between the left ventricle and aorta on Doppler echocardiography.
C. Enlargement of the cardiac silhouette on chest radiograph.
D. Right-axis deviation of 90° to 150°.

2–69. The first step in treating the victim of a near-drowning is to

A. Determine serum alcohol and drug levels.
B. Establish an airway.
C. Rewarm the patient.
D. Remove water from the lungs.

2–70. In assessing a patient with burns, the nurse would expect the risk for potential airway obstruction to be higher in a patient with

A. Reddened oral mucosa in the absence of a facial burn.
B. Flame burns to both legs.
C. Scald burns to the entire trunk.
D. Carboxyhemoglobin levels of 10%.

2–71. Approximately 3 hours after coronary artery bypass graft surgery, the patient is mechanically ventilated with an oxygen saturation of 100%. Blood pressure is 90/60 mm Hg with a mean arterial pressure of 70 mm Hg. The heart rate is sinus rhythm at 66 beats/min and approximately 3 premature ventricular contractions per minute. Cardiac index is 2.2 L/min/m². Serum potassium concentration is 4.3 mEq/L. Which of the following therapies would best suppress dysrhythmias and increase the cardiac index?

A. Administer lidocaine, 100 mg IV bolus.
B. Initiate ventricular demand pacing at 70 beats/min.
C. Initiate atrioventricular sequential pacing at 80 beats/min.
D. Administer potassium, 10 mEq IV, over 1 hour.

2–72. A 72-year-old patient was admitted to the ICU after a cerebral embolic event. During report the critical care nurse is told that the patient has unilateral neglect, inattention to stimuli on the affected side, and homonymous hemianopsia and attempts to get out of bed without assistance. The critical care nurse knows that a nursing intervention necessary for patients with cerebral embolic events includes

A. Providing a safe environment by orienting this patient who has experienced a right-sided cerebral embolic event.
B. Providing a safe environment by orienting this patient who has experienced a left-sided cerebral embolic event.
C. Positioning objects in the affected visual field for this patient who has experienced a right-sided cerebral embolic event.
D. Positioning objects in the affected visual field for this patient who has experienced a left-sided cerebral embolic event.

2–73. A potential postoperative complication after surgical resection of a bowel infarction is

A. Infected pseudocyst.
B. Coagulopathy.
C. Necrosis of the anastomosis.
D. Metabolic alkalosis.

2–74. A blood pressure difference is noted between the right and left arms and a decrease in lower extremity pulses of a patient who was in a motor vehicle crash. These findings are associated with

A. Ruptured abdominal aortic aneurysm.
B. Ruptured ventricular aneurysm.
C. Aortic rupture.
D. Cardiac tamponade.

2–75. The first priority in management of patients with diabetic ketoacidosis is

A. Elimination of acidosis.
B. Decrease of serum glucose.
C. Restoration of fluid balance.
D. Replacement of electrolytes.

2–76. Which of the following is the most helpful to prevent pulmonary insufficiency after postoperative thoracoabdominal aneurysm repair?

A. Early extubation on the first postoperative day.
B. Frequent pulmonary toilet.
C. Serial arterial blood gas analysis.
D. Continuous oxygen saturation monitoring.

2–77. In addition to tachycardia, which of the following findings are associated with fluid volume losses of 750 to 1500 ml?

A. Narrowing of pulse pressure and respiratory alkalosis.
B. Widening of pulse pressure and metabolic acidosis.
C. Anuria and jugular venous distention.
D. Hypoxemia, metabolic acidosis, and oliguria.

Questions 2–78 and 2–79 relate to the following situation.

A 56-year-old homeless man is found unconscious under a freeway overpass. He is hypothermic and has a blood alcohol level of 0.23. He is admitted to the ICU and placed on a ventilator at FIO_2 of 40%, respiratory rate of 18 breaths/min, positive end-expiratory pressure of 8, and tidal volume of 800 ml. His arterial blood gas findings are pH = 7.32, $PaCO_2$ = 34 mm Hg, PaO_2 = 58 mm Hg, and SaO_2 = 89%.

2–78. The most likely explanation for his blood gas results is

A. Hypoventilation.
B. Alcoholic intoxication.
C. Aspiration.
D. Pulmonary embolus.

2–79. The most appropriate intervention for this patient initially would be

A. Antibiotic therapy.
B. Vigorous pulmonary hygiene.
C. Keep supine.
D. Corticosteroid therapy.

2–80. External heat sources are used to correct shivering in a burn patient to

A. Promote patient comfort.
B. Prevent shearing of skin grafts.
C. Lower metabolic rate.
D. Increase body temperature.

2–81. When educating the patient and family about the long-term effects of renal fracture secondary to trauma, the nurse must consider that

A. Peritoneal dialysis is the treatment method of choice.
B. Long-term dialysis may be required.
C. Renal transplant should be considered early on.
D. Short-term hemodialysis is usually sufficient.

2–82. Which of the following hemodynamic findings indicate hypovolemic shock related to blood loss?

A. Cardiac output of 3 L/min, PCWP of 3 mm Hg, heart rate of 120 beats/min.
B. Cardiac output of 6 L/min, PCWP of 10 mm Hg, heart rate of 120 beats/min.
C. Cardiac output of 5 L/min, PCWP of 5 mm Hg, heart rate of 120 beats/min.
D. Cardiac output of 4.5 L/min, PCWP of 8 mm Hg, heart rate of 100 beats/min.

2–83. Which of the following should be performed for a patient with hypovolemic shock who is to receive multiple consecutive blood transfusions?

A. Administer calcium chloride, 100 mg, with each transfusion.
B. Use pressure cuffs to ensure rapid transfusion.
C. Use a blood warmer for high-rate intravenous fluids and transfusions.
D. Obtain the blood sample for a complete blood cell count within 15 minutes after the transfusion.

2–84. A 64-year-old patient underwent thrombolytic therapy in the emergency department 12 hours after symptoms of a stroke began. Which of the following is correct with regard to thrombolytic therapy for stroke?

A. The principal clot-specific therapeutic agent is streptokinase.
B. The principal action of thrombolytic therapy is to convert plasmin to plasminogen.
C. The half-life of the major clot-specific agent is 30 minutes.
D. The use of thrombolytic agents for stroke poses an increased risk of intracranial hemorrhage after 6 hours.

2–85. An alert, stable patient has been admitted to the ICU with an acute perforated viscus. Which of the following body positions is most appropriate for this patient?

A. Semi-Fowler's.
B. Prone.
C. Supine.
D. Sims'.

2–86. Which interventions differentiate "wet" and "dry" near-drowning?

    A. Mask continuous positive airway pressure (CPAP).
    B. Mechanical ventilation.
    C. Positive end-expiratory pressure (PEEP).
    D. Rewarming.

Questions 2–87 and 2–88 refer to the following situation.

A 32-year-old man with cystic fibrosis has been intubated for 8 days for hypoxemia secondary to mucus plugging, which then progressed to adult respiratory distress syndrome. He requires high peak pressures with a returned tidal volume of 600 ml. He suddenly loses consciousness and his eyes roll back. He becomes tachycardic and hypotensive, his peak pressure increases, and the ventilator alarm sounds. Within a few minutes, the patient's blood pressure stabilizes, his heart rate returns to normal, his ventilator stops sounding an alarm, and he becomes alert.

2–87. The critical care nurse should

    A. Draw blood for arterial blood gas analysis.
    B. Obtain an ECG.
    C. Set up for a chest tube.
    D. Plan for a ventilation/perfusion scan.

2–88. The patient is at risk for a bronchopleural fistula because of his pre-existing disease that has scarred his lung parenchyma and weakened areas of lung that are prone to rupture. Therefore, he is more susceptible to pneumothoraces and bronchopleural fistula. The nurse may implement all the following measures in this patient to reduce the likelihood of an air leak *except*

    A. Change ventilation mode to intermittent mandatory ventilation.
    B. Decrease the inspiratory time.
    C. Avoid using an expiratory retard.
    D. Employing the lowest level suction on the water seal that maintains lung inflation.

2–89. A patient with intestinal obstruction has a blood pressure of 84/66 mm Hg, hematocrit of 47%, and serum potassium value of 5.2 mEq/L. Which of the following should be administered?

    A. Normal saline, 500-ml bolus.
    B. Lactated Ringer's solution, 500-ml bolus.
    C. One unit of fresh frozen plasma.
    D. One unit of packed red blood cells.

2–90. A patient 10 days after severe burn injury was extubated 7 days earlier and underwent a successful skin grafting procedure 5 days ago. The patient's electrolytes for the past 12 hours are as follows:

	Sodium	*Potassium*
6:00 AM	140 mEq/L	3.5 mEq/L
Noon	135 mEq/L	3.8 mEq/L
6:00 PM	128 mEq/L	4.2 mEq/L

The most important nursing action to take now is to

    A. Check gastric secretions for blood.
    B. Anticipate starting colloid intravenous fluids.
    C. Check the patient's hematocrit.
    D. Assess for signs of sepsis.

Questions 2–91 and 2–92 refer to the following situation.

A 72-year-old man with chronic obstructive pulmonary disease (COPD) is admitted to the ICU with dyspnea, tracheal deviation to the left, minimal to absent breath sounds on the right, tachycardia, and hypotension. Arterial blood gases show pH of 7.28, $PaCO_2$ of 50 mm Hg, PaO_2 of 54 mm Hg, and SaO_2 of 87% on room air. He is intubated and placed on a ventilator at 35% FIO_2, synchronized intermittent mandatory ventilation (SIMV) of 10 breaths/min, and tidal volume of 700 ml.

2–91. What is the most likely reason for his clinical presentation?

    A. Pneumonia.
    B. COPD exacerbation.
    C. Pulmonary embolus.
    D. Spontaneous pneumothorax.

2–92. The nurse observes continuous bubbling in the water-seal chamber of the chest tube drainage system. This most likely indicates

A. Plugged chest tube lumen.
B. Chest tube pulled out of the chest wall.
C. Bronchopleural fistula.
D. Kinked tubing.

2–93. Which of the following diagnostic findings would best diagnose pericarditis?

A. Chest radiograph with normal heart size.
B. ECG with ST segment depression.
C. Echocardiography confirming pericardial fluid.
D. Chest pain increasing on inspiration.

2–94. On the first day after an acute myocardial infarction, a patient develops pericarditis. Which of the following pharmacologic therapies would be prescribed?

A. Indomethacin.
B. Ibuprofen.
C. Anticoagulants.
D. Corticosteroids.

Questions 2–95 and 2–96 refer to the following situation.

A 43-year-old patient admitted several days ago after an automobile accident has multiple fractures including a right femur fracture, lacerations, and an acute subdural hematoma. The patient underwent surgery to evacuate the hematoma. Vital signs and laboratory data are

Vital Signs
Blood pressure	92/64 mm Hg
Heart rate	108 beats/min
Respiratory rate	26 breaths/min

Laboratory Values
Hemoglobin	15.5 g/dl
Hematocrit	59%
Serum Na^+	145 mEq/L
Serum K^+	4 mEq/L
Serum osmolarity	305 mOsm/L
Urine osmolality	280 mOsm/L
Urine specific gravity	1.001

Intake & Output
24-hour fluid intake	1600 ml
24-hour urine output	4800 ml

2–95. The above laboratory values are consistent with

A. Hypotension and hypernatremia related to syndrome of inappropriate secretion of antidiuretic hormone (SIADH).
B. Hyperosmolarity and polyuria related to SIADH.
C. Hypo-osmolarity and polyuria related to diabetes insipidus.
D. Hypernatremia and polyuria consistent related to diabetes insipidus.

2–96. Based on the data provided, which of the following treatment modalities would the critical care nurse expect to implement?

A. Hypertensive hypervolemic therapy and administration of antidiuretic hormone (ADH).
B. Calcium channel blockers and diuretics.
C. Infusion of 0.9% normal saline and ADH.
D. Fluid restriction and calcium channel blockers.

2–97. An ICU patient 24 hours after abdominal aortic aneurysm repair develops severe periumbilical pain, elevated serum amylase level, decreased breath sounds, hypotension, metabolic acidosis, and blood-tinged, foul-smelling stools. Which of the following diagnostic procedures should the nurse expect?

A. Radiography.
B. Endoscopy.
C. Laparoscopy.
D. Angiography.

2–98. As the heart rate increases, the QT interval

A. Remains constant.
B. Decreases.
C. Increases.
D. Varies by approximately 0.2 second.

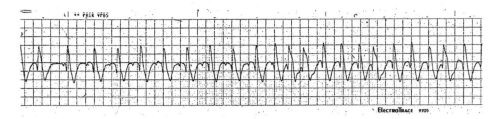

2–99. During the postresuscitation phase of burn care, the effectiveness of interventions related to altered peripheral tissue perfusion is indicated by

A. Decreased oxygen consumption.
B. Restoration of gastric motility.
C. Reduced dependent edema formation.
D. Maintenance of a normal hemoglobin concentration.

2–100. A patient with diabetic ketoacidosis has the following set of laboratory values

	5 PM	6 PM
Serum glucose (mg/dL)	256	145
Bicarbonate (mEq/L)	18	21
Serum ketones	+	−
Urine ketones	+	−

The nurse's plan of care should include

A. Discontinue IV insulin; add dextrose to fluids.
B. Discontinue IV insulin; begin subcutaneous insulin regimen.
C. Maintain IV insulin until blood glucose level falls below 140 mg/dl.
D. Maintain IV insulin; add dextrose to IV fluids.

2–101. Which of the following laboratory values usually remains normal in patients diagnosed with thrombotic thrombocytopenic purpura (TTP)?

A. Partial thromboplastin time.
B. Fibrin split products.
C. Hematocrit.
D. Lactic dehydrogenase.

2–102. A 29-year-old patient is admitted with severe headache, photophobia, nuchal rigidity, a fever of 103°F, and positive Kernig and Brudzinski signs. The admitting diagnosis is "Suspicious of Meningitis." The critical care nurse anticipates which one of the following interventions?

A. Immediate tracheostomy.
B. Lumbar puncture.
C. Magnetic resonance image of the spinal cord.
D. Electroencephalogram.

2–103. A patient has the following clinical findings:

ECG: rhythm regular, P rate 110/min, QRS rate 110/min.
P waves precede each QRS complex.
Neck veins show constant cannon "a" waves.

These findings support a diagnosis of

A. Atrial flutter.
B. Atrioventricular (AV) junctional rhythm.
C. Wolff-Parkinson-White reciprocating tachycardia.
D. Nonparoxysmal AV junctional tachycardia.

2–104. Carotid massage is being applied during the initial 3 seconds of the above lead II rhythm strip. The rhythm strip represents

A. Ventricular tachycardia.
B. Accelerated idioventricular tachycardia.
C. Nonparoxysmal atrioventricular (AV) junctional tachycardia.
D. Supraventricular tachycardia.

2–105. The major pathophysiologic mechanisms that can cause acute respiratory failure include all of the following *except*

A. Hyperventilation.
B. Ventilation/perfusion mismatch.
C. Shunt.
D. Diffusion impairment.

Questions 2–106 and 2–107 relate to the following situation.

A 42-year-old woman is admitted to the ICU with a chief complaint of a 3-month history of increasing shortness of breath that has limited her activities of daily living. A presumptive diagnosis of emphysema is made. She has a 12-pack-year history of smoking, is still smoking, and uses marijuana socially. Her father and an uncle died of chronic obstructive pulmonary disease in their 60s and had long smoking histories. She is scheduled for bedside pulmonary function tests.

2–106. What blood test would be important in supporting a diagnosis of emphysema?

A. Carboxyhemoglobin.
B. Theophylline level.
C. Alpha₁-antitrypsin level.
D. Methemoglobin.

2–107. What would be important to plan for regarding administration of medications before performing pulmonary function tests?

A. Hold bronchodilators.
B. Administer anxiolytics.
C. Hold oxygen.
D. Keep NPO.

2–108. The critical care nurse's primary responsibility in caring for a patient with second-degree heart block, Mobitz type I, is to

A. Administer atropine, 0.5 mg IV, for heart rates less than 60 beats/min.
B. Initiate transcutaneous pacing if the heart block progresses to type II.
C. Monitor the patient for progression of heart block or symptoms of low blood pressure.
D. Limit activities that require increases in heart rate to prevent syncope.

2–109. An 18-year-old is admitted to the emergency department after a high-speed car crash into a tree. The patient was wearing a two-point fixation lap belt. Which type of injury is suspected?

A. Rupture of abdominal solid viscera.
B. Hollow viscus injury.
C. Large vessel laceration.
D. A cavitation wound.

2–110. In the early stages of septic shock, the patient's skin may appear

A. Cold and clammy.
B. Cyanotic.
C. Hot and sweaty.
D. Flushed.

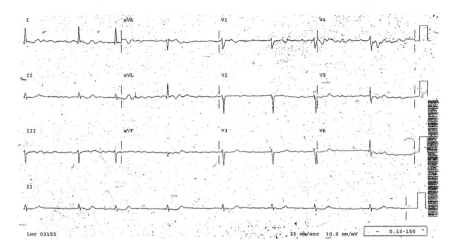

Loc 03155   25 mm/sec   10.0 mm/mV   0.15-150

2–111. The care plan for a patient with the above 12-lead ECG would include the potential for which of the following?

A. VVI or VVIR pacemaker implant.
B. DDD pacemaker implant.
C. Administration of a beta blocker.
D. Insertion of a temporary pacemaker for rapid atrial pacing.

2–112. Which of the following is the appropriate method to administer intravenous amiodarone?

A. Administer 1 mg/kg as a rapid infusion followed by a continuous infusion of 1 mg/min.
B. Administer 5 mg/kg as a bolus over 30 minutes followed by a continuous infusion of 1 g/day.
C. Administer 50 mg/kg over 1 hour followed by a continuous infusion of 1 mg/min.
D. Administer bolus doses of 1 to 3 mg/kg over 30 minutes as needed for breakthrough dysrhythmias during continuous infusion at 0.5 mg/min.

2–113. Mechanical ventilation is provided for patients with inability to sustain spontaneous ventilation to

A. Hyperinflate the lungs.
B. Decrease lung volumes.
C. Prevent pneumonia.
D. Reduce the work of breathing.

2–114. A 52-year-old man with a past history of hypertension is admitted with a presumptive diagnosis of cerebrovascular disease. His respiratory rate starts to decrease over the next 2 hours from 28 to 12 breaths/min, and he is intubated and placed on a ventilator. His nursing diagnosis is "Inability to Sustain Spontaneous Ventilation." Which of the following is the most appropriate mode of ventilation for him?

A. Pressure support.
B. Continuous positive airway pressure (CPAP).
C. Synchronized intermittent mandatory ventilation (SIMV).
D. Inverse ratio ventilation (IRV).

2–115. Treatment for a wide-complex tachycardia of undetermined origin would include which of the following?

I. Verapamil, 10 mg IV.
II. Lidocaine, 1 mg/kg IV.
III. Synchronized cardioversion.
IV. Adenosine, 6 mg IV.

A. I, II, and III.
B. II, III, and IV.
C. I, II, and IV.
D. I, III, and IV.

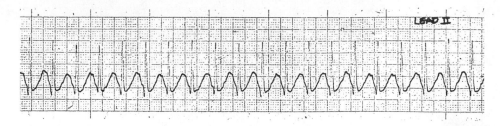

2–116. The patient with the rhythm noted above has a blood pressure of 118/60 mm Hg, respiratory rate of 28 breaths/min, and temperature of 38°C. Oxygen saturation by pulse oximeter is 96%. Coarse rhonchi are present in all lung fields, and chest radiograph shows right lower lobe consolidation. Reduction of heart rate is best accomplished by administration of

A. Acetaminophen and chest physiotherapy.
B. Propranolol and oxygen at 2 L by nasal prongs.
C. Verapamil, 10 mg, by mouth and oxygen at 2 L by nasal prongs.
D. Oxygen at 2 L by nasal prongs and chest physiotherapy.

2–117. The function of a newly implanted automatic implantable cardioverter-defibrillator (AICD) pacemaker is usually tested

A. At the bedside.
B. During treadmill stress-testing.
C. In the electrophysiology laboratory.
D. During postdischarge follow-up.

2–118. A 19-year-old patient is admitted with generalized seizures and is receiving phenytoin (Dilantin) and phenobarbital. Phenytoin levels are monitored. The critical care nurse knows that which of the following laboratory values for phenytoin is within the therapeutic level?

A. 15 μg/ml.
B. 31 μg/ml.
C. 51 mg/ml.
D. 71 mg/ml.

2–119. Shortly after receiving an intravenous infusion of antibiotic, the patient expresses a sense of "impending doom." The nurse should assess the patient for

A. Delirium tremens.
B. Seizure.
C. Anaphylaxis.
D. Anxiety.

2–120. Intrarenal acute renal failure is characterized by a blood urea nitrogen (BUN):creatinine ratio of

A. 10:1.
B. 20:1.
C. 30:1.
D. 40:1.

2–121. The most important nursing interventions for a patient with large bowel traumatic injuries are those that

A. Prevent malabsorption.
B. Treat hemorrhage.
C. Monitor for biliary fistula.
D. Prevent sepsis.

Questions 2–122 through 2–124 relate to the following situation.

A 58-year-old woman was admitted to the ICU 3 weeks previously after a motor vehicle crash. She has had two tension pneumothoraces secondary to increased inspiratory pressures and high oxygen levels required for adequate ventilation and oxygenation. Weaning has been attempted several times but has been unsuccessful because of hypercarbia and hypoxemia. Her chest radiograph shows a fibrotic appearance and prominent pulmonary arteries. Her lung compliance remains low.

2–122. What is the most likely reason for her inability to be weaned?

A. Pneumonia.
B. Diaphragm fatigue.
C. Chronic respiratory distress syndrome.
D. Pneumothorax.

2–123. A tracheostomy is being considered. What would be the reason for a tracheostomy in this patient's situation?

A. Improve oxygenation.
B. Bypass airway obstruction.
C. Facilitate secretion removal.
D. Decrease dead space.

2–124. Six days after the tracheostomy, she is weaned to an FIo_2 of 40% and continuous positive airway pressure of 10. She is unable to write because of a fractured wrist on one arm and fractured fingers on the other. She tries to talk, but the staff and family have difficulty reading her lips and she becomes very agitated when she is not understood. What should the nurse consider using?

A. Sedation.
B. A Passey-Muir speaking valve.
C. An alphabet board.
D. An artificial larynx.

2–125. In a hyperglycemic hyperosmolar nonketotic (HHNK) state, vigorous treatment with insulin in the presence of inadequate fluid replacement increases the risk of

A. Cerebral edema.
B. Vascular thrombosis.
C. Hypoglycemia.
D. Hypokalemia.

2–126. A 45-year-old man is admitted to ICU with dyspnea, nonproductive cough, cyanosis, and respiratory alkalosis. Which of the following findings would best support the nurse to implement an immunosuppressive care protocol?

A. Leukocytosis.
B. Delayed response to skin testing.
C. Hypersensitivity to skin testing.
D. Pneumonia.

2–127. Which of the following is used to evaluate permanent pacemaker capture when a patient's intrinsic rate is faster than the pacemaker lower limit rate?

   I. Application of the pacemaker magnet to the generator site.
  II. Patient performance of isometric exercise.
 III. Chest wall stimulation.
  IV. Carotid massage or patient performance of Valsalva maneuvers.

A. I and II.
B. II and III.
C. III and IV.
D. I and IV.

2–128. For a patient admitted with hypertrophic cardiomyopathy, which of the following medications would the nurse plan to use in the treatment of dysrhythmias?

A. Amiodarone.
B. Adenosine.
C. Digoxin.
D. Lidocaine.

2–129. Vasodilators are used in treatment of cardiomyopathy because they

   I. Relieve symptoms of heart failure.
  II. Improve survival.
 III. Improve cardiac contractility.
  IV. Improve cardiac ejection fraction.

A. I and II.
B. I, II, and III.
C. I, II, and IV.
D. I, II, III, and IV.

2–130. In reviewing factors contributing to sepsis related to microbial translocation, the nurse will assess the patient's

A. Level of consciousness.
B. Nutritional status.
C. Renal function.
D. Source of infection.

2–131. A patient who has had multiple stab wounds to the thorax has the following clinical findings:

Blood pressure is 70/60 mm Hg.

Heart rate is 136 beats/min, sinus tachycardia with frequent premature ventricular contractions.

Radial pulses are 1+ palpable with pulsus paradoxus.

Respiratory rate is 36 breaths/min with clear breath sounds, decreased at both bases.

Neck veins are flat.

The most likely cause of the patient's hypotension is

A. Pneumothorax.
B. Hemothorax.
C. Cardiac tamponade.
D. Aortic transection.

2–132. When planning to administer a loading dose of phenytoin (Dilantin), the critical care nurse knows that the correct method of administration is

A. 1 g intravenously over 60 minutes.
B. 5 mg intramuscularly.
C. 75 mg intravenously over 1 minute.
D. 75 mg intramuscularly.

2–133. The patient with acute gastrointestinal hemorrhage has a pulse of 146 beats/min, urine output of 5 ml/hr, and blood pressure of 68/36 mm Hg. What is the patient's estimated total blood volume loss?

A. Less than 15%.
B. 15% to 30%.
C. 31% to 40%.
D. Greater than 40%.

2–134. Acute respiratory failure is associated with which of the following arterial blood gas alterations?

A. $\uparrow Paco_2$, $\uparrow Pao_2$
B. $\downarrow Paco_2$, $\uparrow Pao_2$
C. $\uparrow Paco_2$, $\downarrow Pao_2$
D. $\downarrow Paco_2$, $\downarrow Pao_2$

2–135. Hallmarks of respiratory distress syndrome include all of the following except

A. An increased right-to-left shunt.
B. Decreased dead space.
C. Decreased pulmonary compliance.
D. Increased pulmonary vascular resistance.

2–136. Shortly after a ventricular stab wound repair, a patient has the following clinical data:

Heart rate	120 beats/min
Hematocrit	32%
Pulmonary capillary wedge pressure	4 mm Hg
Systemic vascular resistance	1600 dynes/sec/cm^5
Cardiac index	2 L/min/m^2

Which of the following is appropriate at this time?

A. Increase dopamine drip from 5 to 10 µg/kg/min.
B. Administer a normal saline bolus of 500 ml.
C. Administer 50 ml of salt-poor albumin.
D. Transfuse 2 units of packed red blood cells.

2–137. Segmental Doppler pressures in a patient with aortoiliac occlusive disease typically show a

I. Normal ankle-brachial index at rest.
II. Near-normal resting ankle pressure.
III. Fall in ankle pressure immediately after exercise.
IV. Increased ankle-brachial index after exercise.

A. I and II.
B. II and III.
C. I, II, and III.
D. I, II, and IV.

2–138. A postoperative aortofemoral by-pass patient's blood pressure has remained stable at 94 to 120 mm Hg systolic without the use of nitroprusside. Femoral pulses are 2 +. Urinary output has been 80 ml, 60 ml, and 30 ml, respectively for the last 3 hours. Which of the following should be included in a focused assessment of the patient?

A. Temperature and pulse.
B. Urine specific gravity and review of current blood urea nitrogen and creatinine values.
C. Glasgow Coma Scale score.
D. Doppler assessment of the lower extremities.

2–139. The purpose of administering a high dose of dopamine along with crystalloids during resuscitation for shock is to

A. Reduce capillary leak.
B. Increase tissue perfusion.
C. Increase serum osmolality.
D. Decrease oxygen consumption.

2–140. The most common reason for beginning dialysis in the patient with acute renal failure is

A. Fluid overload.
B. Hyponatremia.
C. Hyperkalemia.
D. Metabolic acidosis.

Questions 2–141 through 2–143 refer to the following situation.

A 21-year-old woman is admitted with pneumococcal pneumonia that rapidly progressed into septic syndrome. She then developed respiratory distress syndrome that became chronic, requiring continuous mandatory ventilation of 28, FIO_2 of 90%, positive end-expiratory pressure (PEEP) of 18 cm H_2O, and tidal volume of 850 ml. Her oxygenation is marginal (PaO_2, 58 mm Hg; $P\bar{v}O_2$, 33 mm Hg), and she requires inotropic medication and fluids to maintain an adequate cardiac output. She is sedated and chemically paralyzed.

2–141. What alternatives to conventional mechanical ventilation would be appropriate to consider initially?

A. Intravenous oxygenator (IVOX).
B. Extracorporeal membrane CO_2 removal (ECCO$_2$R).
C. Extracorporeal membrane oxygenation (ECMO).
D. High-frequency ventilation.

2–142. Her arterial blood gases after 40 minutes on a ventilatory rate of 120 beats/min and tidal volume of 90 ml, FIO_2 of 90% and PEEP of 12 are pH, 7.37; $PaCO_2$, 38 mm Hg; PaO_2, 68 mm Hg; SaO_2, 93%; $P\bar{v}O_2$, 38 mm Hg, and $S\bar{v}O_2$, 69%. The reason for the improvement in her oxygenation is

A. Increased lung compliance.
B. Decreased oxygen needs.
C. Decreased respiratory effort.
D. Improved regional distribution of oxygen.

2–143. Her pulmonary capillary wedge pressure (PCWP) has been 18 to 20 mm Hg with a mean pulmonary artery pressure (PAP) of 30 mm Hg. Her wedge is now 12 mm Hg although her mean PAP remains stable. What is the most likely explanation for the change in PCWP?

A. Bubble in the system.
B. Leak in the system.
C. Decreased intrathoracic pressure.
D. Catheter cuff leak.

2–144. Increased intracranial pressure as a result of metabolic encephalopathy may be monitored best by determining which one of the following?

A. Blood urea nitrogen.
B. Serum glucose.
C. Serum osmolarity.
D. Serum ammonia.

2–145. The priority in care of the patient with an acute gastric hemorrhage is to

A. Administer prostaglandins.
B. Reduce portal hypotension.
C. Reverse enzyme stimulation.
D. Achieve hemostasis at the bleeding site.

2–146. Which of the following is administered to prevent thrombosis and improve blood flow after peripheral arterial surgery?

A. Low-molecular-weight dextran.
B. Aspirin.
C. Atenolol.
D. Nitroglycerin.

2–147. A patient who has had vascular surgery is receiving an infusion of low-molecular-weight dextran at 100 ml/hr, nitroglycerin at 66 μg/min, and 0.45 normal saline with 100 mEq/L of sodium bicarbonate at 75 ml/hr. The patient's skin is warm and pink. Blood pressure is 100/58 mm Hg, and heart rate is sinus rhythm at 100 beats/min. Abruptly, the blood pressure decreases and the patient develops audible wheezes. Skin temperature remains warm but is a deeper pink. Which of the following interventions should be performed?

  I. Decrease the rate of nitroglycerin infusion.
 II. Discontinue the dextran infusion.
III. Increase the bicarbonate and saline infusion to 250 ml/hr.

A. I only.
B. I and II.
C. I and III.
D. I, II, and III.

2–148. Myocardial ischemia is demonstrated on the electrocardiogram by

A. T wave inversion.
B. ST segment elevation.
C. Q waves.
D. Q waves and ST segment depression.

2–149. In planning care for a septic patient with a D-dimer level greater than 2.0 mg/ml, the nurse would

A. Support nutritional status.
B. Prevent urinary tract infection.
C. Protect the skin from bruising.
D. Improve respiratory status.

2–150. Which of the following medications can interfere with exhibition of the symptoms of mild hypoglycemia?

A. Diltiazem (Cardizem).
B. Lidocaine.
C. Metoprolol (Lopressor).
D. Nitroglycerin.

2–151. A patient is in the ICU 2 hours after admission following a liver transplantation. His blood type is A+. There is an order to administer 2 units of packed red blood cells. To prevent an anaphylactic reaction, which of the following statements is true for safe blood administration to this patient?

A. The patient cannot receive blood until therapeutic immunosuppression is achieved 24 to 48 hours postoperatively.
B. The patient should receive type B blood, because blood compatibility reverses after liver transplantation.
C. The patient should receive type A blood, because blood compatibility remains the same after liver transplantation.
D. The patient should receive type AB blood, because patients after liver transplantation are universal recipients.

2–152. Optimal electrode placement for continuous ST segment monitoring in a patient with documented left anterior descending coronary artery occlusion would be

A. The standard five leads with the chest lead at V_6
B. MCL_6.
C. Lead III.
D. The standard five leads with the chest lead at V_2.

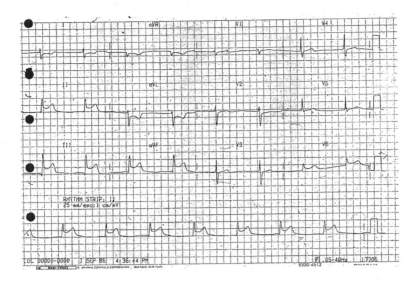

2-153. Early reperfusion after thrombolytic therapy for acute myocardial infarction is demonstrated by

A. ST segment elevation resolving rapidly and accelerated development and resolution of Q waves.
B. ST segments elevating rapidly but Q waves never appearing.
C. The development of ST segment elevation and Q waves that do not resolve.
D. The development of ST segment elevation and T wave inversion.

2-154. The above 12-lead ECG indicates an acute myocardial infarction (MI) of the _____ wall.

A. Anterior
B. Lateral
C. Inferior
D. Posterior

2-155. Acute pulmonary edema and symptoms of shock develop abruptly in a patient with an inferior wall myocardial infarction (MI). The nurse would also expect to find which of the following?

A. Holosystolic murmur.
B. ST segment elevation in leads facing the anterior wall.
C. Muffled heart tones.
D. ST segment elevation in leads V_3R and V_4R.

2-156. Which one of the following has been shown to control increased intracranial pressure (ICP) in a patient who has not responded to other methods to control ICP?

A. Hyperventilation.
B. Sedation.
C. Loop diuretics.
D. Barbiturate therapy.

2-157. Synthetic prostaglandin therapy is particularly useful for ulcers associated with

A. Nonsteroidal anti-inflammatory drugs (NSAIDs).
B. Lidocaine.
C. Calcium channel blockers.
D. Warfarin.

2-158. The care plan for a patient with an acute right ventricular wall myocardial infarction (MI) should indicate that the patient has an increased potential for which of the following?

I. Pulmonary edema.
II. Hypotension.
III. Bradycardia.
IV. Papillary muscle rupture.

A. I and II.
B. II and III.
C. II and IV.
D. I and IV.

2–159. The primary reason why patients with sepsis who progress to septic shock receive fresh frozen plasma (FFP) is to

A. Expand circulating volume.
B. Restore host defenses.
C. Increase serum albumin.
D. Correct coagulation disorders.

2–160. Which diuretic is frequently used to prevent acute renal failure?

A. Mannitol.
B. Furosemide.
C. Spironolactone.
D. Bumetanide.

2–161. In the acute phase of respiratory distress syndrome, corticosteroids

A. Are effective when sepsis is the cause.
B. Have not been proven to be efficacious.
C. Prevent the chronic phase of respiratory distress syndrome.
D. Have not been researched.

2–162. For a patient with right ventricular infarction, which of the following should be included in the care plan?

A. Titrate nitroglycerin to maintain systolic blood pressure greater than 90 mm Hg.
B. Titrate intravenous fluids to maintain pulmonary capillary wedge pressure between 16 and 18 mm Hg.
C. Titrate dopamine to maintain systolic blood pressure greater than 90 mm Hg.
D. Administer angiotensin converting enzyme (ACE) inhibitors to promote gentle diuresis and decrease afterload.

2–163. The most appropriate placement for the V or chest lead in a patient with evolving inferior wall myocardial infarction (MI) is at the

A. Fourth intercostal space, right sternal border.
B. Fifth intercostal space, right midclavicular line.
C. Fifth intercostal space, left anterior axillary line.
D. Fifth intercostal space, left midaxillary line.

2–164. Which of the following thrombolytic regimens is appropriate for a patient who has received streptokinase for a previous myocardial infarction?

A. Systemic urokinase.
B. Systemic streptokinase (SSK).
C. Recombinant tissue plasminogen activator (rt-PA).
D. Intracoronary streptokinase.

2–165. A patient in coronary care awaiting a single-vessel percutaneous transluminal coronary angioplasty (PTCA) informs his nurse that he is extremely fearful of needing open-heart surgery and that he might lose his job if he is unable to return to work within 2 weeks. Which of the following responses is the most appropriate?

A. Your cardiologist has done thousands of PTCAs and you need to trust that your PTCA will be successful.
B. Because you only have one diseased vessel, you won't need emergency open heart surgery.
C. You need to talk to your physician about return to work plans after you have your PTCA.
D. Although there are no guarantees, many PTCA patients return to work within 1 to 2 weeks.

2–166. For a patient with myocardial infarction, which of the following would necessitate withholding propranolol and notification of the physician?

I. Pulmonary capillary wedge pressure greater than or equal to 20 mm Hg.
II. Rales to one third of lung fields.
III. PR interval of 0.24 second.
IV. Wheezes on auscultation.

A. I, II, and III.
B. II, III, and IV.
C. I, III, and IV.
D. I, II, III, and IV.

2–167. Three hours after percutaneous transluminal coronary angioplasty (PTCA), the patient complains of chest pain. Sheaths are in place. A 12-lead ECG demonstrates ST segment elevation. The patient is currently on a heparin drip at 1000 units/hr and the activated partial thromboplastin time (APTT) is two times control. The physician is notified and is unable to return the patient to the catheterization laboratory for 2 hours. The most appropriate immediate intervention for this patient is to

A. Increase the heparin drip to 1200 units/hr.
B. Initiate a nitroglycerin drip and titrate to pain and blood pressure.
C. Discontinue the heparin drip in preparation for emergency surgery.
D. Notify the family of the patient's change in condition.

2–168. After head trauma, which of the following subjective complaints would likely indicate to the critical care nurse that a patient had sustained an anterior fossa basilar skull fracture?

A. Liquid in the ear.
B. Double vision.
C. Paresthesias.
D. Salty or sweet taste in the mouth.

2–169. The normal inflation pressure range for esophageal balloon tamponade is

A. Less than 10 mm Hg.
B. 10 to 15 mm Hg.
C. 20 to 45 mm Hg.
D. Greater than 50 mm Hg.

2–170. As the patient in early sepsis begins to receive dopamine, the nurse informs the patient of possible side effects, which may include

A. Headache and vomiting.
B. Drowsiness.
C. Diarrhea.
D. Dry mouth.

2–171. Patients with respiratory distress syndrome are placed on a mechanical ventilator with positive end-expiratory pressure. This results in increased airway pressures. A potential complication that can result from increased airway pressure is

A. Pneumonia.
B. Decreased cardiac output.
C. Volutrauma.
D. Oxygen toxicity.

2–172. Which of the following medications is used for patients during and after percutaneous transluminal coronary angioplasty (PTCA) to prevent vasoconstriction and vasospasm?

A. Nitroglycerin.
B. Beta blockers.
C. Angiotensin converting enzyme (ACE) inhibitors.
D. Calcium channel blockers.

2–173. Two hours after returning from the cardiac catheterization laboratory for percutaneous transluminal coronary angioplasty (PTCA) the patient complains of low back pain. When he is logrolled to a side-lying position, he complains of increased pain radiating to his abdomen and the sensation of urinary urgency. The physician is notified and orders an abdominal CT scan. Which of the following interventions would the nurse perform first?

A. Administer furosemide, 40 mg IV.
B. Administer morphine, 5 mg IV.
C. Discontinue the heparin drip.
D. Initiate a nitroglycerin drip.

2–174. A patient is readmitted to the CCU 5 days after percutaneous transluminal coronary angioplasty (PTCA) with placement of three overlapping intracoronary stents. The patient has been on maintenance warfarin (Coumadin) therapy for 1 month. The 12-lead ECG demonstrates ST segment elevation in the inferior leads. Which of the following would be considered appropriate interventions?

   I. Emergent PTCA.
  II. Administration of systemic thrombolytic agents.
 III. Heparin bolus and infusion.
 IV. Emergent transluminal extraction catheter atherectomy.

A. I and II.
B. II and III.
C. I, II, and III.
D. I, II, III, and IV.

2–175. In the care plan for the patient with diabetes insipidus, the ICU nurse should prioritize the monitoring of which parameters?

A. Urine specific gravity and serum osmolality.
B. Central venous pressure and urine osmolality.
C. Urine electrolytes and serum electrolytes.
D. Serum glucose and urine output.

Questions 2–176 and 2–177 refer to the following situation.

A 45-year-old man 2 weeks status post-allogeneic bone marrow transplantation (BMT) is admitted with increased bilirubin, increased ammonia, and decreased clotting factors.

2–176. These findings are most likely due to

A. Infection.
B. Renal failure.
C. Veno-occlusive disease.
D. Cyclosporine therapy.

2–177. Which of the following would be the most appropriate therapy for these findings?

A. Administer albumin intravenously.
B. Administer granulocyte colony-stimulating factor.
C. Total-body irradiation.
D. Administer normal saline.

2–178. Which of the following interventions has the highest priority for the patient who has sustained a traumatic brain injury?

A. Take the patient's vital signs.
B. Assess the patient's pupils for a consensual response.
C. Assess the patient's motor strength.
D. Determine the patient's level of consciousness.

2–179. When starting an infusion of epinephrine to treat refractory septic shock, the nurse will

A. Infuse medication through the proximal pulmonary artery catheter port.
B. Expect the medication to be brown after the mixture is prepared.
C. Expect a decrease in diastolic blood pressure.
D. Prepare a 1-mg ampule of 1:1000 solution in 250 ml for a 16-µg/ml concentration.

2–180. A contraindication to the use of continuous arteriovenous hemofiltration (CAVH) to treat acute renal failure is a

A. Hemoglobin of 10.2 g/dl.
B. Mean arterial pressure of 90 mm Hg.
C. Systolic blood pressure of 85 mm Hg.
D. Hematocrit of 48%.

2–181. The patient's esophageal balloon tamponade has been present for 48 hours. The patient now complains of substernal pain that increases with inspiration and expiration. The nurse suspects

A. Pharyngeal obstruction.
B. Esophageal perforation.
C. Gastric wall erosion.
D. Bowel obstruction.

2–182. Corticosteroid therapy has been suggested as being useful in the treatment of

A. Pneumonia.
B. Thrombotic pulmonary embolus.
C. Sepsis.
D. Chronic respiratory distress syndrome.

2–183. Which of the following provides the best information on coronary blood flow?

A. Multiple gated acquisition (MUGA) blood pool imaging.
B. M-mode echocardiography.
C. Coronary angiography.
D. Exercise stress testing.

2–184. Common ECG findings in unstable angina include

A. Transient ST depression or elevation, usually with T wave inversion.
B. ST segment depression and T wave inversion that persist for more than 12 hours before beginning to resolve.
C. Transient Q waves.
D. Transient ST segment elevation and Q waves that resolve within 12 hours.

2–185. A patient has percutaneous balloon angioplasty for unstable angina. Immediately after sheath removal and application of a compression device, nursing assessment should include

A. Palpation of the insertion site for hematoma formation.
B. Palpation of pedal pulses in the affected leg.
C. Assessment of heart tones for symptoms of tamponade.
D. Assessment of heart tones for signs of coronary dissection.

2–186. Which of the following angiographic findings are consistent with a diagnosis of unstable angina?

A. Up to 75% occlusion of a coronary artery.
B. Lesions of greater than 75% occlusion of a coronary artery.
C. Twenty percent multivessel occlusion.
D. Ischemic symptoms with near-normal coronary arteries.

2–187. Immediate treatment goals for the care of patients with unstable angina include

I. Evaluation of the cause of the symptoms.
II. Relief of pain.
III. Prevention of ischemia/ infarction.
IV. Reduction of risk factors.

A. I and II.
B. II and III.
C. III and IV.
D. I, II, III, and IV.

2–188. Which is the highest priority for a patient with unstable angina?

A. Patient education in risk factor modification.
B. Evaluation of chest pain and prevention of myocardial ischemia.
C. Obtaining the patient history and identification of risk factors.
D. Identification of patient knowledge deficits related to coronary artery disease.

2–189. Which of the following calcium channel blockers has been shown to increase the risk of myocardial infarction in unstable angina?

A. Verapamil (Isoptin, Calan).
B. Nifedipine (Procardia, Adalat).
C. Felodipine (Plendil).
D. Diltiazem (Cardizem).

2–190. After starting infusions of dopamine and nitroprusside in a patient in sepsis-induced cardiogenic shock, desired outcomes include

A. Increased systemic vascular resistance (SVR), increased pulmonary capillary wedge pressure (PCWP), mean arterial pressure (MAP) greater than 60 mm Hg.
B. Decreased SVR, decreased PCWP, MAP greater than 60 mm Hg.
C. Increased cardiac output (CO), increased SVR, decreased PCWP.
D. Increased CO, increased SVR, increased PCWP.

2–191. When one is drawing a sample for mixed venous blood gas analysis to assess overall oxygenation status, the blood sample must be drawn

A. At a rate of 1 ml/min.
B. From a wedged pulmonary artery catheter.
C. From the right atrial port of the pulmonary artery catheter.
D. From the ventricular infusion port of the pulmonary artery catheter.

2–192. When evaluating the initial treatment of the patient with intracranial hypertension after traumatic brain injury, which of the following does the critical care nurse know to be the most appropriate position?

A. Head of the bed elevated to 30°.
B. Side-lying.
C. Prone.
D. Head of the bed flat.

2–193. Which of the following is a complication of vasopressin therapy in a woman with esophageal varices?

A. Hypotension.
B. Angina.
C. Dehydration.
D. Uterine cramping.

2–194. The most effective method to stop bleeding around the insertion site in a patient with sheaths in place after percutaneous transluminal coronary angioplasty is to

A. Apply ice to the site.
B. Apply direct pressure to the insertion site.
C. Discontinue heparin infusion.
D. Apply manual pressure 1 inch above the insertion site.

2–195. A patient with a diagnosis of unstable angina is currently on a nitroglycerin drip at 66 μg/min and receives 100 mg of atenolol and 1 mg of amlodipine daily. The patient develops a headache, and blood pressure decreases to 90/50 mm Hg. The most appropriate action would be to

A. Hold the daily amlodipine and atenolol but maintain the nitroglycerin at 66 μg/min.
B. Administer the atenolol and hold the amlodipine while decreasing the nitroglycerin drip to 60 μg/min.
C. Administer the amlodipine and hold the atenolol while decreasing the nitroglycerin drip to 60 μg/min.
D. Decrease the nitroglycerin drip to 40 μg/min and administer the amlodipine and atenolol.

2–196. Effectiveness of the plan for preventing activity intolerance in a patient with unstable angina is best demonstrated by the patient who

A. Is observed taking his pulse while ambulating.
B. Ambulates around the CCU after eating lunch.
C. Has a heart rate of 124 beats/min during ambulation.
D. Is able to sit in a chair for 30 minutes.

2–197. A patient admitted with a diagnosis of unstable angina is treated with aspirin, heparin, and nitroglycerin. The nurse notes that the CK2 value has increased in the second set of creatinine kinase isoforms drawn. This finding signifies that therapy

A. Has been appropriate to the condition of the patient and the plan needs no alteration.
B. With the nitroglycerin drip should be increased.
C. With the heparin drip should be increased.
D. Requires modification to include treatment for myocardial ischemia/infarction.

2–198. In dealing with the family of an ICU patient, the most critical need the nurse must provide is

A. Comfort.
B. Information.
C. Proximity.
D. Assurance.

2–199. A patient is admitted to the ICU with a diagnosis of acute renal failure (ARF). Which type of ARF is associated with the following results: specific gravity, 1.004; creatinine clearance, 72 ml/min; urine osmolality, 310 mOsm/L, and urine sodium, 47 mEq/L?

A. Prerenal.
B. Obstructive.
C. Intrarenal.
D. Postrenal.

2–200. Select the set of laboratory values that characterize the syndrome of inappropriate secretion of antidiuretic hormone (SIADH).

	Serum Sodium (mEq/L)	Serum Osmolality (mOsm/L)
A.	127	264
B.	138	296
C.	115	289
D.	152	254

2–1. (**D**) Fibrin split products are increased in DIC owing to increased fibrin degradation production. Radiologic examinations are usually noncontributory to the diagnosis of DIC. The erythrocyte sedimentation rate is best used to evaluate response to treatment of inflammatory processes. Although the patient with DIC may have a fluid volume deficit related to hemorrhage, changes in serum sodium level are not diagnostic for DIC.

Reference: Alspach, J. G. (ed.): AACN Core Curriculum for Critical Care Nursing, 5th ed. Philadelphia, W. B. Saunders, 1998.

2–2. (**A**) The precordial leads, particularly V_1 and V_6, are most helpful in distinguishing RBBB from LBBB. Bundle branch block causes delays in impulse conduction through the affected ventricle, resulting in widening of the QRS and characteristic QRS patterns. In RBBB, the right ventricle depolarizes late and causes an R′ in lead V_1 and a wide S wave in lead V_6. In LBBB, the left bundle depolarizes late, causing a wide negative QRS in V_1 and a wide R wave in V_6.

Reference: Wright, J. E., Shelton, B. K.: Desk Reference for Critical Care Nursing. Boston, Jones & Bartlett, 1993.

2–3. (**A**) Right bundle branch block may occur in patients while floating the pulmonary artery catheter through the right ventricle. In patients with LBBB this may cause complete heart block. The nurse should have a pacing defibrillator or transcutaneous pacemaker immediately available to treat this complication. Symptoms of cardiac tamponade related to passage of the pulmonary artery catheter generally do not become apparent until after insertion. Pneumothorax is also generally diagnosed after insertion and may be diagnosed from the chest radiograph taken after insertion is complete. The complete heart block occurring in patients with LBBB is usually transient, occurring when the catheter tip is being advanced through the right atrium.

Reference: Daily, E. K., Schroeder, J. S.: Techniques in Bedside Hemodynamic Monitoring, 5th ed. St. Louis, Mosby–Year Book, 1994.

2–4. (**B**) Pain from abdominal surgery inhibits maximal inspiration, so it should be assessed for and relieved before attempting incentive spirometry or coughing and deep breathing.

Reference: Alspach, J. G. (ed.): AACN Core Curriculum for Critical Care Nursing, 5th ed. Philadelphia, W. B. Saunders, 1998.

2–5. **(C)** The patient has symptoms of atelectasis; early ambulation will help him take deep breaths by allowing his diaphragm to expand with gravitational pull. IPPB is not necessary and has not been proven to be useful for reversing atelectasis. Antipyretics are not necessary for the low-grade fever because it will resolve when the atelectasis resolves. Adequate pain control is necessary, although care needs to be taken to avoid carbon dioxide retention secondary to his preoperative pulmonary status. It is preferable to use oral pain medications.

Reference: Alspach, J. G. (ed.): AACN Core Curriculum for Critical Care Nursing, 5th ed. Philadelphia, W. B. Saunders, 1998.

2–6. **(B)** History of cigarette smoking is the most important risk factor for developing atelectasis. The other risk factors may increase the patient's risk of atelectasis but not to the extent that his smoking history does.

Reference: Alspach, J. G. (ed.): AACN Core Curriculum for Critical Care Nursing, 5th ed. Philadelphia, W. B. Saunders, 1998.

2–7. **(D)** Age, immunosuppression, and organ transplant are risk factors for pneumonia. Aspiration of gastric contents is a causative agent for pneumonia.

Reference: Kersten, L. D.: Comprehensive Respiratory Nursing: A Decision Making Approach. Philadelphia, W. B. Saunders, 1989.

2–8. **(C)** *Pseudomonas* bacteria are normal flora that are opportunistic. They take advantage of patients whose immune responses are compromised, such as patients who are intubated or have a tracheostomy. *Pseudomonas* is not considered a community-acquired infection, nor does it occur with inappropriate antibiotic use. It is not considered idiopathic because its origin is known.

Reference: Alspach, J. G. (ed.): AACN Core Curriculum for Critical Care Nursing, 5th ed. Philadelphia, W. B. Saunders, 1998.

2–9. **(C)** This temporary pacemaker is failing to capture, as demonstrated by atrial pacemaker spikes without P waves and ventricular pacemaker spikes without a corresponding QRS complex. Initial treatment would therefore include placing the patient in the last position of complete capture, checking the integrity of all connections, and increasing the mA, or output, to provide a stronger pacing impulse. The myocardium around the pacing electrode may become edematous and require higher pacing thresholds. There is no evidence of sensing problems because the pacing spikes appear where ventricular activity is absent and do not compete with intrinsic ventricular beats.

Reference: Dossey, B. M., Guzzetta, C. E., Kenner, C. V.: Critical Care Nursing, Body-Mind-Spirit. Philadelphia, J.B. Lippincott, 1992.

2–10. **(C)** After ingestion of lye, there may be minimal damage to the lips, mouth, and pharynx, as the substance bypasses these structures, but severe damage to the esophagus, where it remains longer. In contrast, swallowed acid causes its most severe injury to dependent portions of the stomach, again related to duration of exposure.

Reference: Wilson, R. F.: Thoracic injuries. *In* Shoemaker, W. C., Ayres, S. M., Grenvik, A., Holbrook, P. R. (eds.): Textbook of Critical Care, 3rd ed. Philadelphia, W. B. Saunders, 1995.

2–11. **(D)** The increase in PR interval indicates a need for care plan revision related to increasing block during activity. Appropriate responses to therapy are noted in the increase in heart rate after withholding digoxin and in maintaining blood pressure when placed supine. Slowing of heart rate during bowel movements is a normal vasovagal response.

Reference: Thelan, L. A., Davie, J. K., Urden, L. D., Lough, M. E.: Critical Care Nursing, Diagnosis and Management, 2nd ed. St. Louis, Mosby–Year Book, 1994.

2–12. (**B**) Rebleeding is most common within the first 1 or 2 days after the initial rupture of an arteriovenous malformation with the incidence decreasing over time. Vasospasm generally occurs 3 to 10 days after the subarachnoid hemorrhage. Hydrocephalus, another complication of aneurysmal rupture, typically occurs days to weeks after subarachnoid hemorrhage. Intracranial pressure generally does not rise until compensatory mechanisms fail.

Reference: Alspach, J. G. (ed.): AACN Core Curriculum for Critical Care Nursing, 5th ed. Philadelphia, W. B. Saunders, 1998.

2–13. (**A**) This patient is showing rapid progression from stage I signs of hepatic encephalopathy to stage III-IV hepatic encephalopathy. Cerebral edema is a major cause of death in patients with fulminant hepatic failure and stage IV encephalopathy. Signs of increased intracranial pressure would include impaired or absent pupillary reflexes, hypertension, hyperventilation, and bradycardia (a late sign). Profound hypoglycemia occurs in approximately half of patients with fulminant hepatic failure owing to loss of glycogen stores and impaired hepatic glucose release. This can accentuate hepatic coma.

Reference: Kucharski, S. A.: Fulminant hepatic failure. Crit. Care. Nurs. Clin. North Am. 5:141–151, 1993.

2–14. (**B**) Elevated "v" waves are seen in mitral regurgitation, papillary muscle ischemia, and elevated pulmonary venous pressure. They represent continued atrial filling during ventricular systole. In pulmonary edema the increased pulmonary venous pressure and left ventricular failure cause elevations in wedge pressure. Right ventricular failure and hypovolemia would cause findings of low pulmonary pressures. Tricuspid regurgitation would cause large "v" waves in right atrial tracings but would not be reflected in the PCWP tracing.

Reference: Daily, E. K., Schroeder, J. S.: Techniques in Bedside Hemodynamic Monitoring, 5th ed. St. Louis, Mosby–Year Book, 1994.

2–15. (**D**) Cloudy lung fields and interstitial edema are signs of heart failure. Elevated hemidiaphragms are associated with abdominal distention and shallow respirations. Total whiteout of lung fields is a sign of adult respiratory distress syndrome or pulmonary edema. In left ventricular failure, the cardiac silhouette is typically larger, not smaller, owing to cardiomegaly.

Reference: Kinney, M. R., Packa, D. R.: Andreoli's Comprehensive Cardiac Care, 8th ed. St. Louis, Mosby–Year Book, 1996.

2–16. (**C**) Hypertension is the leading cause of diastolic dysfunction. In diastolic dysfunction the cardiac silhouette and ejection fraction may be normal or borderline. Both diastolic and systolic dysfunction result in symptoms of heart failure; however, in systolic dysfunction left ventricular hypertrophy results in cardiomegaly and an enlarged cardiac silhouette. Right ventricular failure would not cause dyspnea and symptoms of lung congestion and interstitial edema. Myocardial contusion would cause elevated ST segments on ECG.

Reference: Bnow, R. D., Udelson, J. E.: Left ventricular diastolic dysfunction as a cause of CHF: Mechanism and management. Ann. Intern. Med. 117:502–510, 1992.

2–17. (**D**) Positive inotropes such as digoxin are not used in diastolic dysfunction. In diastolic dysfunction the primary problem is delayed diastolic relaxation. Treatment with positive inotropes that increase systolic ejection may worsen failure. Negative inotropic medications such as beta blockers and calcium channel blockers are used in diastolic dysfunction to slow the heart rate, treat ischemia, and decrease cardiac work. Education regarding exercise and rest will improve functional status.

Reference: Beattie, S., Pike, C.: Left ventricular diastolic dysfunction: A case report. Crit. Care Nurs. 16:37–52, 1996.

2–18. (**A**) Iatrogenic complications from invasive lines and catheters are the most frequent source of iatrogenic infection; therefore, they are removed as soon as the patient's condition permits. Meticulous cannula drive line care also assists in preventing iatrogenic infection from organisms on the skin surface. Antibiotic use is governed by the organism and the white blood cell count. Standard or barrier precautions are used during patient contact and dressing changes. Masks are not necessary for noninvasive contacts.

Reference: Braunwald, E. (ed.): Heart Disease: A Textbook of Cardiovascular Medicine. Philadelphia, W. B. Saunders, 1997.

2–19. (**C**) Intubation bypasses the protective defenses of the upper and lower airway and places the patient at risk for pneumonia. Mechanical ventilation itself is not a risk for pneumonia, although the presence of an endotracheal tube is. Intravenous fluid therapy should help the defenses by keeping the mucus layer of the airways hydrated. A PEG tube would prevent aspiration of feedings from the stomach.

Reference: Alspach, J. G. (ed.): AACN Core Curriculum for Critical Care Nursing, 5th ed. Philadelphia, W. B. Saunders, 1998.

2–20. (**A**) Calcium chloride or calcium gluconate may be given intravenously when hyperkalemia is severe and dysrhythmias are present. In a hyperkalemic state, calcium will immediately stabilize the cell membranes from depolarization, thereby decreasing the potential for dysrhythmias. Additional measures must be taken to permanently eliminate the excess potassium from the body, because calcium's protective effect lasts approximately 30 minutes. The administration of sodium bicarbonate and dextrose 50% and insulin will temporarily move potassium back into the cells; this effect will last 2 to 3 and 4 to 6 hours, respectively. The hypokalemic effect of the administration of dextrose 50% and insulin takes 20 to 30 minutes to achieve. Sodium polystyrene will eliminate potassium utilizing the gastrointestinal system, but this process takes several hours to achieve the desired outcome.

Reference: Baer, C. L.: Acute renal failure. In Kinney, M. R., Packa, D. R., Dunbar, S. B. (eds.): AACN's Clinical Reference for Critical Care Nursing, 3rd ed. St. Louis, Mosby–Year Book, 1993.

2–21. (**A**) The first dose of activated charcoal is 50 to 100 g given with a cathartic to empty the stomach of its contents. This is followed by 20 to 50 g given at 2- to 4-hour intervals without a cathartic in order to act on any drug retained in gastrointestinal tissues.

Reference: Clancy, C., Litovitz, T. L.: Poisoning. In Shoemaker, W. C., Ayres, S. M., Grenvik, A., Holbrook, P. R. (eds.): Textbook of Critical Care, 3rd ed. Philadelphia, W. B. Saunders, 1995.

2–22. (**B**) Angiotensin converting enzyme (ACE) inhibitors such as captopril directly block the conversion of angiotensin I to angiotensin II. Digoxin and digitalis glycosides have an inhibitory effect on the renin-angiotensin system. Loop diuretics such as furosemide and bumetanide increase renin-angiotensin activity by decreasing preload.

Reference: Young, J. B.: Contemporary management of patients with heart failure. Med. Clin. North Am. 79:1171–1187, 1995.

2–23. (**C**) The effectiveness of interventions to prevent potentially fatal cerebral edema in patients with fulminant hepatic failure is evaluated by monitoring for signs of increasing intracranial pressure (ICP). An initial sign of elevated ICP is hypertension. Other signs include increased muscle tone in the extremities, hyperventilation, and dilated pupils.

Reference: Kucharski, S. A.: Fulminant hepatic failure. Crit. Care. Nurs. Clin. North Am. 5:141–151, 1993.

2–24. (**C**) Complete injury of the spinal cord causes irreversible loss of sensory and motor function below the level of the lesion. An incomplete (partial) lesion will cause varying degrees of motor and sensory loss below the level of the lesion. Incomplete lesions result in mixed losses of motor and sensory function because some spinal cord tracts remain intact. The posterior columns of the sensory system convey position and vibration as well as a degree of deep touch sensation. Brown-Séquard syndrome is a hemisection of the spinal cord that results in ipsilateral loss of motor, position (proprioception), and vibratory sensation, with a contralateral loss of pain and temperature perception. Central cord syndrome is manifested by a greater motor weakness in the upper extremities with varying sensory loss. Anterior cord syndrome is manifested by a complete loss of motor, pain, and temperature sensation below the level of the lesion with a sparing of proprioception, vibration, and touch.

Reference: Alspach, J. G. (ed.): AACN Core Curriculum for Critical Care Nursing, 5th ed. Philadelphia, W. B. Saunders, 1998.

2–25. (**D**) During treatment of diabetic ketoacidosis with hydration and insulin there is typically a rapid decline in plasma potassium concentration, particularly during the first few hours of treatment. Increased entry of potassium into the intracellular compartment, thus decreasing serum potassium levels, causes hyperpolarization across the cell membrane and reduces excitability of the cells. The resting membrane potential falls below normal; thus the cell requires a larger stimulus to reach threshold and cause depolarization. The cell then requires a longer time to repolarize to baseline value. Cardiac dysrhythmias induced by hypokalemia are varied and include both atrial and ventricular premature contractions, tachyarrhythmias, and sinus bradycardia. Serious dysrhythmias are usually not evident until plasma potassium is less than 3 mEq/L. Hypokalemia is potentially the most life-threatening electrolyte derangement occurring during the treatment of diabetic ketoacidosis.

References: Clochesy, J. M., Breu, C., Cardin, S., et al. (eds.): Critical Care Nursing, 2nd ed. Philadelphia, W. B. Saunders, 1996.
Kitabchi, A. E., Wall, B. M.: Diabetic ketoacidosis. Med. Clin. North Am. 79:9–37, 1995.

2–26. (**D**) Bleeding in a critically ill patient with no prior history of prolonged bleeding should alert the critical care nurse to the need for further investigation. This is especially true if the patient has any of the four predisposing signs of disseminated intravascular coagulation (DIC): hypoxemia, acidemia, hypotension, or stasis of capillary blood flow. The two pathophysiologic components of DIC include thrombosis and hemorrhage. Thrombosis of major vessels and organs results in acidosis, and hemorrhage results in volume loss and hypotension.

Reference: Bell, T.: Disseminated intravascular coagulation: Clinical complexities of aberrant coagulation. Crit. Care Nurs. Clin. North Am. 5:389–410, 1993.

2–27. (**A**) The cough reflex is a protective mechanism for the lower, not upper, airway. Protective mechanisms of the upper airway include nasopharyngeal filtration, mucosal adherence, saliva, bacterial interference, and secretory IgA.

Reference: Alspach, J. G. (ed.): AACN Core Curriculum for Critical Care Nursing, 5th ed. Philadelphia, W. B. Saunders, 1998.

2–28. (**A**) Both asthma and COPD are considered obstructive airway diseases and show decreased FEV_1, FVC, and PEF. Asthma, however, is characterized by reactive airways that will respond to bronchodilators.

Reference: Kersten, L. D.: Comprehensive Respiratory Nursing: A Decision Making Approach. Philadelphia, W. B. Saunders, 1989.

2–29. (**B**) Although all patients on a ventilator are at risk for contracting pneumonia, this patient's greatest risk at this point is for inspissated secretions (mucus plugging). Patients in status asthmaticus have an increased respiratory rate and tidal volume that dehydrates the tracheobronchial tree. This results in mucus so thick that airways may become occluded. Because he is on a ventilator, he cannot experience a respiratory arrest, although he can stop breathing spontaneously. Barotrauma is always a possibility but does not represent the greatest risk for this patient.

Reference: Kersten, L. D.: Comprehensive Respiratory Nursing: A Decision Making Approach. Philadelphia, W. B. Saunders, 1989.

2–30. (**C**) Lorazepam reduces the seizure potential and agitation associated with cocaine overdose. Haloperidol may be cautiously administered to patients who are paranoid or violent, but this drug should not be the initial treatment because it reduces the seizure threshold. Naloxone is used for opioid intoxication and has no effect on cocaine receptors. Flumazenil is for benzodiazepine reversal and likewise has no effect on cocaine receptors.

Reference: Schnoll, S. H.: Drug abuse, overdose and withdrawal syndromes. *In* Shoemaker, W. C., Ayres, S. M., Grenvik, A., Holbrook, P. R. (eds.): Textbook of Critical Care, 3rd ed. Philadelphia, W. B. Saunders, 1995.

2–31. (**A**) Vasodilators and diuretics are the primary methods used to reduce preload in heart failure. Furosemide and bumetamide are loop diuretics. Amiloride is a potassium-sparing diuretic. Nitroprusside, minoxidil, and nitroglycerin are vasodilators. Captopril and enalapril are angiotensin converting enzyme inhibitors, which also have vasodilating activities. Sodium restriction is a nonpharmacologic method to decrease preload. Positive inotropic medications such as digoxin and dobutamine improve contractility but do not vasodilate or diurese to decrease preload. Beta blockers, in general, do not decrease preload by diuresis or vasodilation. A relatively new beta blocker, however, called carvedilol has alpha-blocking properties and is associated with mild vasodilation.

Reference: Armstrong, P. W., Moe, G. W.: Medical advances in the treatment of congestive heart failure. Circulation 88:2941–2949, 1993.

2–32. (**B**) Angiotensin II is a potent vasoconstrictor. ACE inhibitors interrupt the pathophysiologic cascade in heart failure and inhibit the vasoconstrictive effects of angiotensin II and aldosterone. Aldosterone causes retention of water and sodium. ACE inhibitors block these neurohormonal activities. When combined with diuretics and salt restriction, ACE inhibitors act to limit the effects of the RAAS. Digoxin has an inhibitory effect on the RAAS. Potassium replacement, beta blockers, and calcium channel blockers do not influence the RAAS.

Reference: Futterman, L. G., Lemberg, L.: Management of congestive heart failure: Is the role of positive inotropic therapy fading? Am. J. Crit. Care 5:455–460, 1996.

2–33. (**D**) Blood in the balloon catheter signifies balloon rupture, and the catheter should no longer be used. The pulmonary artery diastolic pressure must be used for further estimates of left-sided heart pressures. Changing the syringe instead of removing it may enable another nurse to attempt wedging the catheter. Injection of air into the catheter may result in pulmonary air embolism. Aspiration of blood is unnecessary to diagnose balloon rupture.

Reference: Darovic, G. O.: Hemodynamic Monitoring: Invasive and Noninvasive Clinical Application, 2nd ed. Philadelphia, W. B. Saunders, 1995.

2–34. (**B**) A ventilation/perfusion scan is usually ordered in clinically stable patients suspected of having a pulmonary embolism, although it is not definitive. It shows the matching of ventilation and perfusion and will identify areas of decreased perfusion when intravenous dye is used. ECG and chest radiography are usually normal in a pulmonary embolus, except in the case of a massive pulmonary embolus. Spirometry would not be useful because it measures ventilation, not perfusion.

Reference: Alspach, J. G. (ed.): AACN Core Curriculum for Critical Care Nursing, 5th ed. Philadelphia, W. B. Saunders, 1998.

2–35. (**A**) All might be appropriate, but because the patient is clinically stable, heparin is the most appropriate. Streptokinase or tissue plasminogen activator is usually used for recent, massive pulmonary embolus with hemodynamic compromise. If a venous Doppler study shows continuing thrombosis, a vena caval umbrella would be appropriate.

Reference: Kinney, M. R., Packa, D. R., Dunbar, S. B. (eds.): AACN's Clinical Reference for Critical Care Nursing, 3rd ed. St. Louis, Mosby–Year Book, 1993.

2–36. (**C**) Pituitary tumors are often removed through a transsphenoidal approach to avoid extensive and direct manipulation of brain tissue. Elevating the head of the bed to between 15° and 30°, if vital signs permit, is the generally accepted intervention for headache. This position allows for venous drainage of the head and decreased intracranial pressure. Because the brain itself is generally tolerant to pain, low doses of non-narcotic analgesics may be sufficient for pain relief. Narcotic analgesics should be avoided if possible because they may dilate cerebral blood vessels, thus increasing intracranial pressure. Fluid intake should be maintained to prevent dehydration, which may exacerbate postoperative headache levels. Overstimulation may cause agitation in the patient; however, some stimulation provides the necessary catalyst for the reticular activating system to maintain regulation of visceral functions.

Reference: Clochesy, J. M., Breu, C., Cardin, S., et al. (eds.): Critical Care Nursing, 2nd ed. Philadelphia, W. B. Saunders, 1996.

2–37. (**C**) Severe, unrelenting left upper quadrant abdominal pain is the clinical hallmark of acute pancreatitis. Angina presents as crushing, tight, retrosternal pain that persists from 1 to 15 minutes. Pulmonary emboli are characterized by sharp, stabbing pain over the affected lung that persists for minutes to hours. Fulminant hepatitis presents with vague, prodromal symptoms, aches, and malaise rather than pain.

References: Krumberger, J. M.: Acute pancreatitis. Crit. Care Nurs. Clin. North Am. 5:185–202, 1993. Scher, H. E.: Chest pain: Developing rapid assessment skills. Orthop. Nurs. 14(3):30–34, 1995.

2–38. (**D**) The patient would benefit from furosemide and morphine to decrease afterload and preload in the presence of extremely high pulmonary pressures. Nitroprusside should not be titrated to the wedge pressure because the patient has mitral regurgitation, as evidenced by the murmur. Digoxin is not indicated from the presentation.

Reference: Roach, J. M., Stajduhar, K. C., Torrington, K. G.: Right upper lobe pulmonary edema caused by acute mitral regurgitation. Chest 103:1286–1288, 1993.

2–39. (**A**) Fluoroscopy or an overpenetrated chest radiograph confirms knotting of the pulmonary artery catheter. Other symptoms include excessive catheter length and resistence during removal of the catheter. The normal length of the catheter from the right or left internal jugular artery is 40 to 50 cm. Catheter knotting often occurs when the catheter is advanced and withdrawn frequently during insertion. Inability to obtain a pulmonary capillary wedge waveform may be caused by retrograde slippage of the catheter into the pulmonary trunk or right ventricle. Low pressures or a clot at the tip of the catheter may cause damping that does not improve with flushing the catheter.

Reference: Darovic, G. O.: Hemodynamic Monitoring: Invasive and Noninvasive Clinical Application, 2nd ed. Philadelphia, W. B. Saunders, 1995.

2–40. (**C**) Hypomagnesemia can cause the following ECG changes: tachycardia, cardiac dysrhythmias, prolonged QT interval, broadened T waves with diminished amplitude, and shortened ST segment. Muscle weakness, tremors, positive Chvostek's and Trousseau's signs, tetany, seizures, cardiac dysfunction, anorexia, and dysphagia are also symptoms of hypomagnesemia. Hyponatremia causes headaches, lethargy, irritability, seizures, and muscle weakness. Hyperchloremia causes muscle weakness, lethargy, decreased level of consciousness, and rapid, deep respiration. Hypercalcemia produces a shortened QT interval, muscle weakness, depression, stupor, anorexia, and cardiac dysrhythmia.

Reference: Baer, C. L.: Fluid and electrolyte balance. *In* Kinney, M. R., Packa, D. R., Dunbar, S. B. (ed.): AACN's Clinical Reference for Critical Care Nursing, 3rd ed. St. Louis, Mosby–Year Book, 1993.

2–41. (**A**) Premature ventricular contractions and ventricular tachycardia are associated with cocaine overdose. Beta blockers are used to treat these ventricular arrhythmias associated with cocaine intoxication/overdose to block stimulation of beta$_1$ (myocardial) sites and slow heart rate. Calcium channel blockers are indicated when there is evidence of ischemic injury. Nitroglycerin does not act on the conduction system and therefore has no antiarrhythmic properties. Digoxin, which slows conduction through the atrioventricular node, is typically used to treat atrial rather than ventricular tachyarrhythmias.

Reference: Schnoll, S. H.: Drug abuse, overdose and withdrawal syndromes. *In* Shoemaker, W. C., Ayres, S. M., Grenvik, A., Holbrook, P. R. (eds.): Textbook of Critical Care, 3rd ed. Philadelphia, W. B. Saunders, 1995.

2–42. **(C)** The normal value for mean arterial pressure (MAP) is 70 to 105 mm Hg. The normal value for the pulmonary capillary wedge pressure (PCWP) is 4 to 12 mm Hg. PCWPs of greater than 12 mm Hg are elevated. The normal value for cardiac index is 2.5 to 4.2 L/min/m². A cardiac index of 2.0 or 1.9 is low.

Reference: Thelan, L. A., Davie, J. K., Urden, L. D., Lough, M. E.: Critical Care Nursing, Diagnosis and Management, 2nd ed. St. Louis, Mosby–Year Book, 1994.

2–43. **(B)** Cardiopulmonary, cerebral, renal, and peripheral tissue perfusion must be frequently assessed in hypertensive crisis. Administration of vasodilating medications and diuretics may alter results of urine tests, skin turgor, and capillary refill. Early symptoms of decreased perfusion include changes in level of consciousness, breath sounds, crackles, prolonged capillary refill, and decreased urinary output. Urine specific gravity is not helpful if the patient is receiving diuretics. Urinary protein demonstrates existing renal failure and is not specific for hypertensive crisis.

Reference: Wright, J. E., Shelton, B. K.: Desk Reference for Critical Care Nursing, Boston, Jones & Bartlett, 1993.

2–44. **(D)** Continuous pressure monitoring via an arterial line and use of infusion pumps is necessary for patient comfort and control of antihypertensive infusions. A quiet environment is preferred to decrease sensory stimuli and to prevent abrupt increases in pressure from stimulation and anxiety.

Reference: Wright, J. E., Shelton, B. K.: Desk Reference for Critical Care Nursing, Boston, Jones & Bartlett, 1993.

2–45. **(D)** Blood flow is greatest to the lower lobes; therefore, they are more frequently involved.

Reference: Alspach, J. G. (ed.): AACN Core Curriculum for Critical Care Nursing, 5th ed. Philadelphia, W. B. Saunders, 1998.

2–46. **(C)** Because of its rapid onset of action and short half-life, nitroprusside (a vasodilator) is administered to decrease the pulmonary artery pressures (afterload) and increase the cardiac output. Prostacyclin (PGE₂, also a vasodilator) might also be useful, but its effects on the pulmonary vasculature are not as well known. Nitroglycerin (also a vasodilator) administered by patch would take too long to act, and the dosage is not controllable. Diuresis would decrease the pressures by decreasing the intravascular volume, but the low cardiac output would preclude using this therapy.

Reference: Kersten, L. D.: Comprehensive Respiratory Nursing: A Decision Making Approach. Philadelphia, W. B. Saunders, 1989.

2–47. **(A)** A saddle embolus sits at the bifurcation of the pulmonary artery. The high right-sided pressure keeps the lumens of the right and left pulmonary artery open. Decreasing the PAP and right ventricular pressures allows the saddle to close off the pulmonary artery, and total hemodynamic collapse ensues. Right and left ventricular wall infarcts are unlikely because the decreasing pressures should have improved myocardial contractility. Air embolism is unlikely because the patient was responding to the medication.

Reference: Kinney, M. R., Packa, D. R., Dunbar, S. B. (eds.): AACN's Clinical Reference for Critical Care Nursing, 3rd ed. St. Louis, Mosby–Year Book, 1993.

2–48. **(D)** Hypertension is a particularly significant risk factor for a cerebral embolic event in the elderly, as was shown in the Framingham study. Although previous stroke, cardiac disease, diabetes, transient ischemic attacks, hyperlipidemia, blood viscosity, and oral contraceptives are known risk factors for cerebrovascular events, hypertension is the greatest risk factor for embolic stroke and is directly related to the magnitude of blood pressure. Any patient with hypertension, especially those with labile hypertension, should be monitored aggressively for this complication.

Reference: Clochesy, J. M., Breu, C., Cardin, S., et al. (eds.): Critical Care Nursing, 2nd ed. Philadelphia, W. B. Saunders, 1996.

2–49. **(C)** Medications containing opiates such as morphine may falsely elevate the amylase level because they may cause spasm of the sphincter of Oddi. This stimulates secretion of pancreatic enzymes, which enter the systemic circulation via portal vein blood. Non–opiate-containing analgesics such as meperidine, levorphanol tartrate, and fentanyl have been recommended for analgesia in pancreatitis because they do not cause spasm of the sphincter of Oddi.

Reference: Krumberger, J. M.: Acute pancreatitis. Crit. Care Nurs. Clin. North Am. 5:185–202, 1993.

2–50. **(B)** Laboratory values of the patient with diabetic ketoacidosis classically include a glucose level greater than 250 mg/dl, low pH, low bicarbonate, ketones in the blood and urine, variable osmolality, and slightly low sodium. The values in (A) are the typical laboratory values of a patient with hyperglycemic hyperosmolar nonketotic syndrome, and those in (C) and (D) are not associated with any specific condition.

Reference: Kitabchi, A. E., Wall, B. M. Diabetic ketoacidosis. Med. Clin. North Am. 79:9–37, 1995.

2–51. **(D)** Heparin interrupts the DIC cycle in two ways. The first is due to its antithrombin effect. Excessive amounts of thrombin can potentially stimulate coagulation and fibrinolysis. Heparin enhances antithrombin III activity, and antithrombin III effectively neutralizes the free circulating thrombin. When thrombin is neutralized by the effects of heparin, less fibrin is formed. The anticoagulant effect of heparin is the second reason for heparin administration in DIC. Heparin does not alter clots that have already formed, but it prevents microvascular obstruction by thrombi and minimizes platelet aggregation. Administration of heparin in DIC slows the coagulation cycle, allowing the body to replenish platelets and clotting factors.

References: Alspach, J. G. (ed.): AACN Core Curriculum for Critical Care Nursing, 5th ed. Philadelphia, W. B. Saunders, 1998.
Bell, T.: Disseminated intravascular coagulation: Clinical complexities of aberrant coagulation. Crit. Care Nurs. Clin. North Am. 5:389–410, 1993.

2–52. **(A)** After ingestion of ethylene glycol, patients are often asymptomatic early and the history of ingestion may be in doubt. Meanwhile, toxic metabolites are being formed, and these eventually result in anion gap acidosis and osmolar gap. Toxicology screens do not routinely test for ethylene glycol. Thus, initiation of therapy to block ethylene glycol metabolism is indicated by history alone until a definitive diagnosis is made.

Reference: Clancy, C., Litovitz, T. L.: Poisoning. In Shoemaker, W. C., Ayres, S. M., Grenvik, A., Holbrook, P. R. (eds.): Textbook of Critical Care, 3rd ed. Philadelphia, W. B. Saunders, 1995.

2–53. **(B)** Although the systemic hypoxia and ischemia associated with drowning or near-drowning affects all organs, morbidity and mortality are primarily due to the irreversible cerebral ischemia effects.

Reference: Goodwin, S. R., Boysen, P. G., Modell, J. H.: Near drowning: Adults and children. In Shoemaker, W. C., Ayres, S. M., Grenvik, A., Holbrook, P. R. (eds.): Textbook of Critical Care, 3rd ed. Philadelphia, W. B. Saunders, 1995.

2–54. **(B)** Nitroprusside gives the best control in lowering the blood pressure because its actions are immediate and controlled by titration. Nifedipine is contraindicated in CVA because the rapid fall in blood pressure it produces may precipitate or worsen cerebral ischemia. Diazoxide is contraindicated in cerebral ischemia because of the rapid and unpredictable decrease in blood pressure it causes. Methyldopa is not used in hypertension complicated by CVA because of its sedative effects.

Reference: Khan, M. G.: Heart Disease Diagnosis and Therapy. Baltimore, Williams & Wilkins, 1996.

2–55. **(B)** Effective treatment for hypertensive crisis includes restoring blood pressure to normal levels and preventing end organ failure and other complications. The most frequent complications associated with hypertensive crisis are renal failure, myocardial infarction, cerebrovascular accidents, and encephalopathy. The normal Glasgow Coma Scale score is 15, indicating prevention of neurologic complications. The normal values for serum creatinine kinase (CK) are 96 to 140 U/L in females and 38 to 174 U/L in males. Normal CK totals implies that CK-MB fractions are also normal, implying that myocardial infarction as a complication of hypertensive crisis has not occurred. The normal serum (venous) pH is 7.31 to 7.41. During hypertensive crisis, the activation of the renin-angiotensin-aldosterone system causes the exchange of sodium for potassium and results in hypokalemia and metabolic alkalosis. Treatment of hypertension with diuretics may further lower the serum potassium level and raise pH. The normal values for creatinine are 0.7 to 1.3 mg/dl in males and 0.6 to 1.2 mg/dl in females. The creatinine value of 1.8 mg/dl is elevated, indicating that there is a possibility of renal impairment related to hypertensive crisis.

Reference: Thelan, L. A., Davie, J. K., Urden, L. D., Lough, M. E.: Critical Care Nursing, Diagnosis and Management, 2nd ed. St. Louis, Mosby–Year Book, 1994.

2–56. **(B)** The most apparent sign of a flail chest is paradoxical movement of the chest wall: depression of portions of the chest wall on inspiration while the rest of the chest wall moves outward. A chest radiograph is useful in diagnosing rib fractures but not presence or absence of flailing. The patient's history may be helpful to establish the type of injury. Arterial blood gases are nonspecific for a flail chest.

Reference: Kinney, M. R., Packa, D. R., Dunbar, S. B. (eds.): AACN's Clinical Reference for Critical Care Nursing, 3rd ed. St. Louis, Mosby–Year Book, 1993.

2–57. **(B)** The treatment of choice for diaphragmatic rupture is surgical repair. Positive- and negative-pressure ventilators are temporizing measures, and positive-pressure ventilation is preferable because there is less movement of the diaphragm. The phrenic nerve pacer is not indicated because the diaphragm muscle is functional but not intact.

Reference: Kersten, L. D.: Comprehensive Respiratory Nursing: A Decision Making Approach. Philadelphia, W. B. Saunders, 1989.

2–58. **(B)** Cardiogenic shock is associated with elevated pulmonary capillary wedge pressures and the development of abnormal heart tones. Extra heart sounds (S_3–S_4) are generally not heard with hypovolemia. A PCWP of 20 mm Hg indicates left ventricular failure or fluid overload. Septic warm shock and anaphylactic shock are associated with hypovolemia.

Reference: Ruppert, S. D., Kernicki, J. G., Dolan, J. T.: Dolan's Critical Care Nursing, 2nd ed. Philadelphia, F. A. Davis, 1996.

2–59. (**B**) Signs of hyponatremia include hypotension, tachycardia, thready peripheral pulse, hyperpnea, headache, vertigo, confusion, hyperreflexia, seizures, coma, anorexia, vomiting, diarrhea, decreased urine output, anuria, fever, and loss of skin turgor. Dehydration, flushed skin, and hypertension are signs of hypernatremia. Ileus, dysrhythmias, and prolonged QT interval are signs of hypocalcemia. Hypercalcemia can cause hypertension, bradycardia, and slurred speech.

Reference: Tucker, S. M., Canobbio, M. M., Paquette, E. V., Wells, M. F.: Patient Care Standards: Collaborative Practice Planning Guides, 6th ed. St. Louis, Mosby–Year Book, 1996.

2–60. (**A**) The priority intervention for patients with hyponatremia is to institute seizure precautions. When the serum sodium concentration falls below 120 mEq/L, the patient is at high risk for the development of central nervous system effects related to hyponatremia. These effects may range from confusion to convulsions and coma. In the event of convulsive activity, having instituted seizure precautions will maintain patient safety and allow for the establishment of a patent airway. Limiting activity, measuring intake and output, and controlling pain are also appropriate but are not priority interventions.

Reference: Baer, C. L.: Fluid and electrolytes. *In* Kinney, M. R., Packa, D. R., Dunbar, S. B. (eds.): AACN's Clinical Reference for Critical Care Nursing, 3rd ed. St. Louis, Mosby–Year Book, 1993.

2–61. (**C**) The risk of toxic megacolon in patients with ulcerative colitis is dramatically increased with opiate administration, hypokalemia, anticholinergic drugs, and barium enema. The clinical presentation is severe abdominal pain, distention, and tympany. Bowel sounds will be hypoactive and stools will be reduced in number, followed by bloody diarrhea. The significance of a history of ulcerative colitis in patients with nongastrointestinal critical illness is often underestimated. Peptic ulcer, hepatic failure, and costochondritis do not present with sudden abdominal pain, distention, or tympany.

Reference: Doughty, D. B., Jackson, D. B.: Gastrointestinal Disorders. St. Louis, Mosby–Year Book, 1993.

2–62. (**D**) The most likely explanation for the pulmonary infiltrates, crackles, secretions, hypoxemia, and CO_2 retention is pulmonary contusion. This is a direct result of the anterior portion of the lung striking the steering wheel with direct force. There was no sign of pneumothorax or hemothorax on the chest radiograph, and it is unlikely that adult respiratory distress syndrome has developed this rapidly.

Reference: Kinney, M. R., Packa, D. R., Dunbar, S. B. (eds.): AACN's Clinical Reference for Critical Care Nursing, 3rd ed. St. Louis, Mosby–Year Book, 1993.

2–63. (**A**) Correction of the hypoxemia and hypercarbia is the first step in treatment and is accomplished by intubation and mechanical ventilation. A chest tube is not indicated, and prophylactic antibiotic therapy has not proven useful for pulmonary contusion. A bronchoscopy may be indicated at some point if vigorous chest therapy and nasotracheal suctioning are not effective in clearing secretions.

Reference: Kinney, M. R., Packa, D. R., Dunbar, S. B. (eds.): AACN's Clinical Reference for Critical Care Nursing, 3rd ed. St. Louis, Mosby–Year Book, 1993.

2–64. (**A**) The paradoxical chest wall movement is characteristic of a flail. Removal from positive-pressure ventilation allows spontaneous breathing. During inspiration, the chest wall on the affected side moves inward. During expiration, it moves outward. He may be in pain, but that is not the cause of his deterioration. Adult respiratory distress syndrome and diaphragmatic herniation are unlikely because his condition is improving. Diaphragmatic herniation would have been apparent on a chest radiograph.

Reference: Kinney, M. R., Packa, D. R., Dunbar, S. B. (eds.): AACN's Clinical Reference for Critical Care Nursing, 3rd ed. St. Louis, Mosby–Year Book, 1993.

2–65. (**D**) The PCWP in a patient with cardiogenic shock should be maintained at 18 mm Hg to optimize preload. Fluid administration will increase the PCWP to 18 mm Hg without increasing the systemic vascular resistance. Dobutamine does not increase preload. Nitroglycerin decreases preload. Dopamine, in doses greater than 7 μg/kg/min, increases systemic vascular resistance, which would increase cardiac work. At doses less than 7 μg/kg/min it may decrease preload through renal and mesenteric vasodilation.

Reference: Khan, M. G.: Heart Disease Diagnosis and Therapy. Baltimore, Williams & Wilkins, 1996.

2–66. (**A**) Dobutamine increases contractility without affecting systemic vascular resistance. Norepinephrine and dopamine at doses greater than 6 μg/kg/min cause peripheral vasoconstriction. Digoxin is too weak as an inotropic agent to be effective in cardiogenic shock.

Reference: Khan, M. G.: Heart Disease Diagnosis and Therapy. Baltimore, Williams & Wilkins, 1996.

2–67. (**B**) Inflation of the balloon pump should occur at the beginning of diastole, after the left ventricle has ejected its stroke volume and is passively filling with more blood. When inflated, the IABP then displaces the blood in the aorta, causing an increase in diastolic pressure that improves coronary artery perfusion. Deflation at the end of diastole just before ventricular systole ensures that the ventricle ejects against a greatly decreased preload.

Reference: Kinney, M. R., Packa, D. R.: Andreoli's Comprehensive Cardiac Care, 8th ed. St. Louis, Mosby–Year Book, 1996.

2–68. (**B**) Pressure gradients between 40 and 120 mm Hg by Doppler echocardiography signify severe aortic stenosis. Evidence of left ventricular hypertrophy on the ECG with or without hypertension indicates severe aortic stenosis. Dilation of the left ventricle is more frequently seen in aortic regurgitation. Right-axis deviation ($+180°$ to $90°$) is found in severe mitral stenosis.

Reference: Khan, M. G.: Heart Disease Diagnosis and Therapy. Baltimore, Williams & Wilkins, 1996.

2–69. (**B**) The first step with near-drowning, as with all patients, is to establish a patent airway. Although drugs and alcohol frequently play a part in near-drowning, testing for them is not the first priority. Rewarming should be considered if the near-drowning occurred in cold weather or if the patient was immersed for a prolonged period of time. Water does not enter the lungs in all near-drowning events; therefore, this option would not be a priority.

Reference: Alspach, J. G. (ed.): AACN Core Curriculum for Critical Care Nursing, 5th ed. Philadelphia, W. B. Saunders, 1998.

2–70. (**C**) A body burn injury of major extent, even without a facial burn or smoke inhalation, markedly increases upper airway edema because of massive fluid shifts into interstitial spaces, especially because large amounts of fluids are infused during burn shock.

Reference: Demling, R. H.: Management of the burn patient. *In* Shoemaker, W. C., Ayres, S. M., Grenvik, A., Holbrook, P. R. (eds.): Textbook of Critical Care, 3rd ed. Philadelphia, W. B. Saunders, 1995.

2–71. (**C**) Atrioventricular sequential pacing is the preferred mode of dysrhythmia control in the postoperative cardiac surgical patient because it increases cardiac output and index by supplying atrial kick. Increasing the rate to 80 beats/min would also serve to increase the cardiac output. Lidocaine suppresses ventricular ectopic beats but may further depress the myocardium and decrease cardiac output. Lidocaine is generally administered if premature ventricular contractions are six or more per minute. Potassium supplementation is routinely given to cardiac surgical patients to maintain the serum potassium level at 4.2 to 4.8 mEq/L to prevent myocardial irritability, but it does not improve cardiac index.

Reference: Kinney, M. R., Packa, D. R.: Andreoli's Comprehensive Cardiac Care, 8th ed. St. Louis, Mosby–Year Book, 1996.

2–72. (**A**) Unilateral neglect is often related to cerebral impairment in the right hemisphere. Patients experience consistent inattention to stimuli on the affected side, have inadequate self-care, position themselves inappropriately on the affected side, attempt to move or get up without assistance, and do not recognize affected body parts as part of their body. Because these patients do not look toward the affected side and have homonymous hemianopsia (visual loss in the same half of each visual field), it is not appropriate to position objects in the affected visual field.

References: Alspach, J. G. (ed.): AACN Core Curriculum for Critical Care Nursing, 5th ed. Philadelphia, W. B. Saunders, 1998.
Hickey, J. V.: The Clinical Practice of Neurological and Neurosurgical Nursing, 3rd ed. Philadelphia, J. B. Lippincott, 1992.

2–73. (**C**) The goal of surgical resection of necrotic bowel is the removal of nonviable tissue and maximum retention of viable tissue. Verification of tissue viability is a priority, but progression of tissue damage can occur after surgical resection has taken place. Progression of tissue damage can result in nonviable tissue at the anastomosis. Infected pseudocyst and coagulopathy are complications of acute pancreatitis. Surgical stress may cause mild metabolic acidosis due to lactic acid production.

References: Krumberger, J. M.: Acute pancreatitis. Crit. Care Nurs. Clin. North Am. 5:185–202, 1993.
Quinn, A. D.: Acute mesenteric ischemia. Crit. Care Nurs. Clin. North Am. 5:171–175, 1993.

2–74. (**C**) A classic sign of aortic rupture is differences in pulses and blood pressure between upper and lower extremities. Differences in blood pressure between the right and left arm may also occur. A ruptured ventricular aneurysm may cause pain similar to myocardial infarction but is associated with symptoms of tamponade. Tamponade would not cause a pressure difference between arms or between upper and lower extremities. A ruptured abdominal aneurysm would cause a decrease in pressure of the lower extremities but not a difference between the right and left arms.

Reference: Ruppert, S. D., Kernicki, J. G., Dolan, J. T.: Dolan's Critical Care Nursing: Clinical Management Through the Nursing Process. Philadelphia, F. A. Davis, 1996.

2–75. (**C**) The first priority is to improve circulating volume and tissue perfusion. Then the other choices need to be addressed.

Reference: Kitabchi, A. E., Wall, B. M. Diabetic ketoacidosis. Med. Clin. North Am. 79:9–37, 1995.

2–76. (**B**) Frequent pulmonary toilet helps to prevent pulmonary congestion. Patients who have had aortic surgery are generally ventilated for 36 to 72 hours postoperatively. Blood gas analysis and oxygen saturation monitoring do not prevent or treat pulmonary congestion.

Reference: Moore, W. S.: Vascular Surgery: A Comprehensive Review. Philadelphia, W. B. Saunders, 1993.

2–77. (**A**) A 750- to 1500-ml fluid loss is considered a moderate fluid loss. During this stage, compensatory mechanisms are elicited as protective mechanisms and hypovolemic shock is reversible. Symptoms include decreased cardiac output, increased heart rate, narrowed pulse pressure, elevated diastolic pressure, respiratory alkalosis, hypoxemia, and decreased urinary output. Jugular veins are flat in hypovolemia. With greater or prolonged fluid loss, metabolic acidosis occurs.

Reference: Thelan, L. A., Davie, J. K., Urden, L. D., Lough, M. E.: Critical Care Nursing, Diagnosis and Management, 2nd ed. St. Louis, Mosby–Year Book, 1994.

2–78. (**C**) Even though the patient has a high alcohol level (in most states 0.08 to 0.1 is considered legally intoxicated), the proximate cause of his hypoxemia is most likely aspiration secondary to impaired reflexes. The ventilator would correct for hypoventilation. Pulmonary embolism is possible but is not the most likely explanation because aspiration is common when the airway is not protected.

Reference: Alspach, J. G. (ed.): AACN Core Curriculum for Critical Care Nursing, 5th ed. Philadelphia, W. B. Saunders, 1998.

2–79. (**D**) The most appropriate initial intervention for aspiration of stomach contents would be corticosteroid administration to decrease the inflammatory response to the aspirated material. Antibiotic therapy may be indicated later if an infectious process develops. Vigorous pulmonary hygiene is also indicated but is not the priority at this time. Supine position should be avoided because it predisposes to aspiration.

References: Alspach, J. G. (ed.): AACN Core Curriculum for Critical Care Nursing, 5th ed. Philadelphia, W. B. Saunders, 1998.
Britto, J., Demling, R. H.: Aspiration lung injury. New Horizons 1:435–439, 1993.

2–80. (**C**) Burn patients respond to major burn injury by resetting their core body temperature at about 38°C and will shiver when unable to maintain that temperature. Shivering increases the metabolic rate, which is already increased in response to the burn, by another 20% or more. Thus measures such as external heating are provided to stop the patient's shivering.

Reference: Roberts, S. L.: Multisystem deviations. *In* Critical Care Nursing: Assessment and Intervention. Stamford, Conn., Appleton & Lange, 1996.

2–81. (**B**) The most common complication of renal trauma is the destruction of renal tissue with associated renal failure. Once destruction of renal tissue occurs, renal failure is permanent and patients often require long-term dialysis management. Hemodialysis is the method of choice in the initial injury period. These patients may become candidates for renal transplant, but only after confirmation of end-stage renal disease.

Reference: Cook, L.: Genitourinary injuries and renal management. *In* Cardona, V. D., Hurn, P. D., Mason, P. J., et al. (eds.): Trauma Nursing: From Resuscitation Through Rehabilitation, 2nd ed. Philadelphia, W. B. Saunders, 1994.

2–82. (**A**) Defining characteristics of hypovolemic shock related to blood loss are heart rate greater than 100 beats/min, cardiac output less than 5.0 L/min, and PCWP less than 6 mm Hg.

Reference: Thelan, L. A., Davie, J. K., Urden, L. D., Lough, M. E.: Critical Care Nursing, Diagnosis and Management, 2nd ed. St. Louis, Mosby–Year Book, 1994.

2–83. (**C**) Patients who receive multiple transfusions or refrigerated blood and large amounts of intravenous fluids at room temperature may become hypothermic. To prevent this occurrence, blood warmers should be used on transfusions and high-rate intravenous fluids. Pressure cuffs increase the rate of transfusion, but with rapid transfusion rates reactions may not be apparent until after the volume has been infused. Citrate in bank blood may cause hypocalcemia in patients who receive multiple transfusions; however, calcium chloride is generally administered after each third or fourth unit of blood has transfused. Blood samples for a complete blood cell count should not be drawn earlier than 30 minutes after transfusion.

Reference: Darovic, G. O.: Hemodynamic Monitoring: Invasive and Noninvasive Clinical Application, 2nd ed. Philadelphia, W. B. Saunders, 1995.

2–84. (**D**) The principal clot-specific therapeutic agent used in thrombolytic therapy for stroke is tissue-type plasminogen activator (tPA). Its principal lytic action is to convert plasminogen to plasmin (fibrinolysin), whose enzymatic action breaks down fibrin threads and fibrinogen, thus lysing the clot. tPA has an extremely short half-life of about 5 minutes. Hemorrhage is a possible side effect, but the risk is decreased if used within the first 90 to 180 minutes (1.5 to 3 hours) of an evolving stroke. Risk of hemorrhage is increased 6 hours after its administration.

Reference: Barker, E. (ed.): Neuroscience Nursing. Mosby–Year Book, St. Louis, 1994.

2–85. (**A**) Although many critical care nurses prefer their patients to be supine, the most comfortable position for a patient with severe abdominal pain is semi-Fowler's, in which the patient is sitting upright with the knees drawn up to the abdomen. This position enhances drainage of fluid to the pelvic region where treatment of fluid or abscess is easiest to manage. It also minimizes abdominal muscle irritation. Prone, supine, and Sims' position are associated with abdominal muscle irritation and general dispersion of the contaminated fluid.

Reference: Luckmann, J., Sorensen, K. C. (eds.): Medical Surgical Nursing, 4th ed. Philadelphia, W. B. Saunders, 1993.

2–86. (**A**) Patients with wet drowning are more likely to be obtunded and have aspirated. A CPAP mask should not be used in patients who are obtunded and therefore may not be appropriate for patients with wet drowning. Mechanical ventilation, PEEP, and rewarming may be interventions for resuscitation of both types of drowning.

Reference: Kinney, M. R., Packa, D. R., Dunbar, S. B. (eds.): AACN's Clinical Reference for Critical Care Nursing, 3rd ed. St. Louis, Mosby–Year Book, 1993.

2–87. (**C**) Transient episodes of this type are characteristic of loculated pneumothoraces that occur in scarred areas of the lungs such as in severe/chronic adult respiratory distress syndrome, repeated spontaneous episodes of pneumothorax, and in patients who require increased peak pressures to maintain adequate ventilation. The scarred lung tissue prevents the classic signs of tracheal deviation. A chest tube should be placed directly into the area of lung collapse. Arterial blood gas analysis may be useful but would probably have returned to normal. An ECG and ventilation/perfusion scan would not assist in the diagnosis.

Reference: Kersten, L. D.: Comprehensive Respiratory Nursing: A Decision Making Approach. Philadelphia, W. B. Saunders, 1989.

2–88. (**B**) All of the above are appropriate measures to decrease the risk of bronchopleural fistula. In this patient situation, however, decreasing the inspiratory time would decrease the time available for oxygen diffusion to occur and his oxygenation would therefore diminish.

Reference: Alspach, J. G. (ed.): AACN Core Curriculum for Critical Care Nursing, 5th ed. Philadelphia, W. B. Saunders, 1998.

2–89. (**A**) Normal saline is the most appropriate choice of the fluids listed. Lactated Ringer's solution, which contains potassium, should not be administered when the serum potassium value is elevated. Fresh frozen plasma is given to replace clotting factors. Packed cells are not indicated for the hematocrit of 47%, which is normal.

Reference: Ruppert, S. D., Kernicki, J. G., Dolan, J. T.: Dolan's Critical Care Nursing: Clinical Management Through the Nursing Process. Philadelphia, F. A. Davis, 1996.

2–90. (**D**) Sepsis affects the integrity of cell membranes, allowing extracellular sodium to enter the cells and intracellular potassium to escape. A shift such as the one above (decreasing serum sodium level and increasing serum potassium level) suggests the possibility of early sepsis. Electrolytes do not reflect blood loss. Starting intravenous fluids may be necessary, but crystalloids would be indicated.

Reference: Roberts, S. L.: Multisystem deviations. *In* Critical Care Nursing: Assessment and Intervention. Stamford, Conn., Appleton & Lange, 1996.

2–91. (**D**) Patients with COPD develop spontaneous pneumothoraces secondary to tissue destruction and bullae formation. The bullae rupture easily and positive-pressure ventilation increases the risk of a pneumothorax. Pneumonia would cause tracheal deviation toward the affected side. COPD alone and pulmonary embolus would not produce tracheal deviation or minimal to absent breath sounds.

Reference: Alspach, J. G. (ed.): AACN Core Curriculum for Critical Care Nursing, 5th ed. Philadelphia, W. B. Saunders, 1998.

2–92. (**C**) Patients with COPD who have spontaneous pneumothoraces and are placed on mechanical ventilation are at risk of developing a bronchopleural fistula. The positive pressures of the ventilator provide a diffusion gradient for the air and keep the fistula patent. Troubleshooting the system is necessary, however, to rule out the chest tube being pulled out of the chest wall. A displaced or plugged chest tube or kinked tubing would result in no bubbling in the water-seal chamber.

Reference: Boggs, R. L., Wooldridge-King, M. (eds.): AACN Procedure Manual for Critical Care, 3rd ed. Philadelphia, W. B. Saunders, 1993.

2–93. (**C**) Echocardiography is the most specific diagnostic test for pericarditis. Chest radiographic findings with normal heart size are nondiagnostic. ST segment changes may be found across the precordial leads in pericarditis but are nonspecific. Pleuritic chest pain that increases on inspiration is a nonspecific finding in pericarditis.

Reference: Heger, J. W., Roth, R. F., Niemann, J. T., Criley, J. M. Cardiology, 3rd ed. Baltimore, Williams & Wilkins, 1994.

2–94. (**A**) Indomethacin or aspirin may be given to patients with pericarditis for their anti-inflammatory effects. Nonsteroidal anti-inflammatory drugs (NSAIDs), such as ibuprofen, may interfere with the healing of infarcted tissue. Anticoagulants are contraindicated because of the potential for tamponade. Corticosteroids are given late in therapy and more specifically for tuberculin pericarditis or recurrent pericarditis due to immune causes.

Reference: Khan, M. G.: Heart Disease: Diagnosis and Therapy. Baltimore, Williams & Wilkins, 1996.

2–95. (**D**) Diabetes insipidus is caused by a decreased secretion of antidiuretic hormone (ADH). Patients with this syndrome excrete copious amounts of dilute urine, as much as 10 L daily. Urine specific gravity for these patients is low (1.001 to 1.005); they complain of polyuria, and the serum osmolarity is elevated. Patients with syndrome of inappropriate secretion of antidiuretic hormone (SIADH) have a low serum osmolarity, dilutional hyponatremia, and decreased urinary output with a concomitant increased specific gravity. The laboratory values presented indicate a water diuresis consistent with diabetes insipidus because the plasma sodium is in the high normal range (normal = 140 to 145 mEq/L), the plasma osmolarity is elevated (normal = 280 to 285 mOsm/L), the urine specific gravity is low (normal = 1.010 to 1.020), and urine output is excessive relative to fluid intake.

Reference: Hickey, J. V.: The Clinical Practice of Neurological and Neurosurgical Nursing, 3rd ed. Philadelphia, J. B. Lippincott, 1992.

2–96. (**A**) Treatment of diabetes insipidus focuses on replacing lost fluids, administration of antidiuretic hormone, monitoring urinary output and specific gravity, and monitoring electrolyte values. Hypertensive hypervolemic therapy, sometimes referred to as triple H therapy (hypervolemia, hemodilution, and hypertension) may be used. This volume expansion and induced hypertension can be beneficial when attempting to prevent or reverse neurologic degeneration as a result of lost autoregulation from vasospasm. It is desirable to reduce the hematocrit in this patient because viscous blood carries an increased risk for further damage. Nimodipine, a calcium channel antagonist, improves patient outcomes because it may reduce the incidence of cerebral infarct. The patient's laboratory data indicated osmolarity and serum sodium levels that are normal; thus an infusion of 0.9% normal saline is not appropriate because that solution is generally administered for rapid fluid resuscitation in patients who are hyponatremic.

References: Barker, E. (ed.): Neuroscience Nursing, St. Louis, Mosby–Year Book, 1994.
Clochesy, J. M., Breu, C., Cardin, S., et al. (eds.): Critical Care Nursing, 2nd ed. Philadelphia, W. B. Saunders, 1996.

2–97. (**D**) This patient presents with classic signs of mesenteric ischemia and/or bowel infarction. Angiography provides optimal visualization of the mesenteric circulation to diagnose this condition. The presence of emboli, thrombi, or vasospasm provides the differential diagnosis. Radiography, endoscopy, and laparoscopy are of limited value because these tests may appear normal in the presence of necrosis of bowel mucosa.

Reference: Quinn, A. D.: Acute mesenteric ischemia. Crit. Care Nurs. Clin. North Am. 5:171–175, 1993.

2–98. (**B**) Values for the QT interval depend on heart rate. In general, as the heart rate increases, both the RR interval and the QT interval shorten.

Reference: Ruppert, S. D., Kernicki, J. G., Dolan, J. T.: Dolan's Critical Care Nursing: Clinical Management Through the Nursing Process. Philadelphia, F. A. Davis, 1996.

2–99. (**C**) Elevating extremities, promoting physical activity as clinically indicated, and promoting hemodynamic stability by monitoring and correcting fluid, electrolyte, and osmolality imbalances will result in mobilization of edema fluid and improved peripheral tissue perfusion. During this phase of burn injury, oxygen consumption is increased to meet the hypermetabolism associated with burn injury and the hemoglobin is decreased owing to destruction of red blood cells at the time of burn injury and to hemodilution as edema fluid is mobilized. Gastric motility is restored but is not related to peripheral tissue perfusion.

Reference: Roberts, S. L.: Multisystem deviations. *In* Critical Care Nursing: Assessment and Intervention. Stamford, Conn., Appleton & Lange, 1996.

2–100. (**B**) Intravenous insulin can be discontinued once ketoacidosis is resolved, as evidenced by a rising bicarbonate level and negative ketones in the urine and blood. Subcutaneous insulin must be started, however, to prevent relapse of the ketoacidosis.

Reference: Alspach, J. G. (ed.): AACN Core Curriculum for Critical Care Nursing, 5th ed. Philadelphia, W. B. Saunders, 1998.

2–101. (**A**) Some activation of the coagulation cascade occurs in TTP. Fibrin split product levels will increase but usually not enough to prolong the partial thromboplastin time or prothrombin time. Hemoglobin and hematocrit are usually decreased in TTP. Lactic dehydrogenase is elevated in TTP due to increased hemolysis.

Reference: Kajs-Wyllie, M.: Thrombotic thrombocytopenic purpura: Pathology, treatment, and related nursing care. Crit. Care Nurs. 15(6):44–51, 1995.

2–102. (**B**) The critical care nurse should anticipate that a lumbar puncture will be performed cautiously, and cerebrospinal fluid samples will be obtained for the presence, type, and antibiotic sensitivity of organisms. A lumbar puncture is necessary to make the diagnosis of meningitis. Computed tomography is also necessary to ensure that a mass lesion is not present. Neither magnetic resonance imaging nor electroencephalography is standard practice. Patients may require mechanical ventilation as a result of respiratory distress, but endotracheal intubation rather than tracheostomy may suffice. An electroencephalogram is the primary diagnostic tool for encephalitis.

Reference: Clochesy, J. M., Breu, C., Cardin, S., et al. (eds.): Critical Care Nursing, 2nd ed. Philadelphia, W. B. Saunders, 1996.

2–103. (**C**) The "a" wave is produced by the retrograde conduction of the pressure wave caused by atrial contraction to the jugular veins. Atrial contraction must be present for "a" waves to occur. Constant cannon "a" waves are seen in AV nodal re-entry WPW reciprocating tachycardia because of simultaneous atrial and ventricular contraction. Flutter waves replace "a" waves in atrial flutter, and there are more P waves than QRS complexes. The "a" waves may be intermittent in AV junctional rhythms and occur only after P waves with atrial contraction.

Reference: Kinney, M. R., Packa, D. R.: Andreoli's Comprehensive Cardiac Care, 8th ed. St. Louis, Mosby–Year Book, 1996.

2–104. (**D**) The strip represents supraventricular tachycardia. Carotid massage is a vagal maneuver that slows conduction from the atria to the AV node and increases AV nodal delay of the impulse to the ventricles. This generally slows tachycardias, which are caused by impulses originating above the AV junction. Ventricular rhythms are not slowed by carotid massage because the impulse originates in the ventricles and carotid massage is effective only in rhythms originating above the AV junction. The rate in nonparoxysmal AV junctional tachycardia is generally 60 to 100 beats/min with a ventricular rate of 60 to 130/min. AV junctional tachycardias are not affected by carotid massage because they originate in the AV node and there is no conduction delay as occurs in impulses that arrive at the AV node from the atria.

Reference: Kinney, M. R., Packa, D. R.: Andreoli's Comprehensive Cardiac Care, 8th ed. St. Louis, Mosby–Year Book, 1996.

2–105. (**A**) The four major pathophysiologic mechanisms responsible for acute respiratory failure include hypoventilation, ventilation/perfusion mismatch, shunt, and diffusion impairment.

Reference: Alspach, J. G. (ed.): AACN Core Curriculum for Critical Care Nursing, 5th ed. Philadelphia, W. B. Saunders, 1998.

2–106. (**C**) Family history of emphysema with and without a smoking history is an indicator of possible genetic involvement. Despite the smoking history and growing up with passive smoke, the early age at onset is strongly suggestive of alpha$_1$-antitrypsin deficiency as the cause for emphysema. Carboxyhemoglobin and methemoglobin levels test for abnormal hemoglobins, not specifically for emphysema. Carboxyhemoglobin level will be elevated with smoking, and methemoglobin value will be elevated with high levels of nitrates. A theophylline level would not be useful unless a patient was taking the drug.

Reference: Alspach, J. G. (ed.): AACN Core Curriculum for Critical Care Nursing, 5th ed. Philadelphia, W. B. Saunders, 1998.

2–107. (**A**) Pulmonary function tests measure the ability to move air in and out of the lungs. Bronchodilators would alter the results so are withheld before these tests: 6 hours for inhaled bronchodilators, 12 hours for short-acting theophylline, and 24 hours for long-acting theophylline drugs. Anxiolytics would depress the respiratory drive and are contraindicated. Oxygen may be continued throughout the test, and it is not necessary to be NPO, although a large meal should not be eaten within 2 hours of the test.

Reference: Kersten, L. D.: Comprehensive Respiratory Nursing: A Decision Making Approach. Philadelphia, W. B. Saunders, 1989.

2–108. (**C**) Mobitz type I heart block occurs with progressive delayed conduction from the sinoatrial node to the atrioventricular node causing an increasing PR interval until a dropped beat occurs and the process begins again. The major potential problem in Mobitz I heart block is progression of heart block. Mobitz type I heart block is usually self-limiting and causes no symptoms. Atropine and transcutaneous pacing are initiated only if the patient exhibits symptoms such as mental status changes or hypotension. Activity generally does not increase the degree of block or cause syncope.

Reference: Wright, J. E., Shelton, B. K.: Desk Reference for Critical Care Nursing, Boston, Jones & Bartlett, 1993.

2–109. (**A**) Rapid deceleraton and two-point lap belts create compressive forces that cause rupture of the solid viscera. An understanding of the mechanism of injury helps to determine the location, type, and degree of injury in trauma. Low-velocity penetration injuries (knife) or high-velocity penetration injuries (rifles or shotguns) are more likely to cause hollow viscus injury, laceration to major vessels, and/or bone fragmentation that causes enough tissue damage for cavitation wounds. Cavitation wounds occur from bone fragmentation within a missile path.

Reference: Lawrence, D. M.: Gastrointestinal trauma. Crit. Care Nurs. Clin. North Am. 5:127–140, 1993.

2–110. (**D**) Vasoactive mediators create a flushed appearance owing to peripheral vasodilation. A later stage of hypodynamic or cold septic shock is associated with cold and clammy skin. Even though the patient may have an elevated core temperature, the lack of perfusion to peripheral areas will prevent hot and sweaty skin. Cyanosis is the result of tissue hypoxia, not hypoperfusion.

Reference: Clochesy, J. M.: Patients with systemic inflammatory response syndrome. *In* Clochesy, J. M., Breu, C., Cardin, S., et al. (eds.): Critical Care Nursing. Philadelphia, W. B. Saunders, 1996.

2–111. (**A**) A VVIR or VVI pacemaker is the most appropriate treatment for this patient with atrial fibrillation and a slow ventricular rate. The VVI pacemaker will maintain the ventricular rate to prevent bradycardia. DDD pacemakers track and pace according to the upper atrial rate. In atrial fibrillation the DDD pacemaker paces at the rapid atrial rate, which may increase myocardial demands and cause symptoms of failure or infarction. Although beta blockers are used to control atrial fibrillation, slow ventricular rates preclude their use in this case.

Reference: Braunwald, E. (ed.): Heart Disease: A Textbook of Cardiovascular Medicine. Philadelphia, W. B. Saunders, 1997.

2–112. (**B**) Intravenous amiodarone is given as a slow initial bolus of 5 to 10 mg/kg over 20 to 30 minutes, followed by a continuous infusion of 1 g/day. Another method of administration is to deliver 2 to 2.5 mg/min for 12 hours and then decrease to 0.7 mg/min as a constant infusion. Bolus doses of 1 to 3 mg may be given for breakthrough dysrhythmias during continuous infusion.

Reference: Kupersmith, J., Deedwania, P. C.: The Pharmacologic Management of Heart Disease. Baltimore, Williams & Wilkins, 1997.

2–113. (**D**) Mechanical ventilation is provided to support gas exchange, increase lung volumes, and reduce the work of breathing. Hyperinflation of the lungs is not normally provided through mechanical ventilation. Intubation and mechanical ventilation may predispose to pneumonia rather than prevent it.

Reference: Alspach, J. G. (ed.): AACN Core Curriculum for Critical Care Nursing, 5th ed. Philadelphia, W. B. Saunders, 1998.

2–114. (**C**) SIMV provides a minimum ventilatory rate while allowing patient-triggered breaths. Pressure support and CPAP require an adequate respiratory rate and are usually used in weaning. IRV is an advanced method of ventilation whereby inspiration (I) is longer than expiration (E) (normally the I:E ratio is 1:1.5 to 2). It is not necessary in this situation and may cause harmful effects by altering hemodynamics.

Reference: Alspach, J. G. (ed.): AACN Core Curriculum for Critical Care Nursing, 5th ed. Philadelphia, W. B. Saunders, 1998.

2–115. (**B**) Lidocaine is considered a first-line drug for wide-complex tachycardia. Synchronized cardioversion is a treatment for both ventricular tachycardia (VT) and supraventricular tachycardia (SVT). Adenosine is very short acting and is considered safe to administer in both SVT and VT. Verapamil is not given in wide-complex tachycardias of indeterminate origin because it can cause hypotension and asystole in patients with ventricular rhythms.

Reference: Huszar, R. J.: Basic Dysrhythmias: Interpretation and Management. St. Louis, Mosby–Year Book, 1994.

2–116. (**A**) Fever due to right lower lobe pneumonia is the likely cause of the sinus tachycardia in this patient. The heart rate generally increases by 4 beats/min for every 1°F rise in temperature.

Reference: Kinney, M. R., Packa, D. R.: Andreoli's Comprehensive Cardiac Care, 8th ed. St. Louis, Mosby–Year Book, 1996.

2–117. (**C**) Predischarge, the patient is generally brought back to the electrophysiology laboratory to have function of the AICD checked in a controlled environment where he can also experience the sensation of the "shock." Testing function requires that the dysrhythmia is induced. The supraventricular or ventricular tachycardia that is induced may lead to hypotension and cardiac arrest; therefore, it is not performed at the bedside or in the physician's office during postdischarge follow-up. There is no guarantee that treadmill stress testing will induce the dysrhythmia to be terminated by the AICD, and the electrophysiology laboratory is a safer environment in which to test the device.

Reference: Kinney, M. R., Packa, D. R.: Andreoli's Comprehensive Cardiac Care, 8th ed. St. Louis, Mosby–Year Book, 1996.

2–118. (**A**) Phenytoin (Dilantin) and phenobarbital are frequently given in combination to patients to prevent seizures. The therapeutic range for phenytoin is 9 to 20 µg/ml.

Reference: Alspach, J. G. (ed.): AACN Core Curriculum for Critical Care Nursing, 5th ed. Philadelphia, W. B. Saunders, 1998.

2–119. (**C**) Signs and symptoms of anaphylaxis can begin within 20 minutes after exposure to the allergen. The sooner the signs, the more severe the reaction. An early sign is a feeling of being warm. Later, urticaria, pruritus, and angioedema may occur. The individual may complain of a "sense of impending doom." Airway compromise and cardiovascular collapse occur in later stages. Antibiotic administration does not influence conditions associated with delirium tremens, seizures, or anxiety.

Reference: Jones, K.: Shock. *In* Clochesy, J. M., Breu, C., Cardin, S., et al. (eds.): Critical Care Nursing. Philadelphia, W. B. Saunders, 1996.

2–120. (**A**) Intrarenal failure is characterized by a normal BUN:creatinine ratio of 10:1. During intrarenal failure there is direct injury to the renal tissue that affects the glomeruli, tubules, or interstitium. Prerenal failure is characterized by a BUN:creatinine ratio of 20:1. This type of renal failure is caused by decreased renal blood flow, which leads to decreased glomerular filtration and solute retention; however, there is no structural damage. If blood flow is re-established, kidney function will recover. Postrenal failure has a variable BUN:creatinine ratio and is caused by an obstruction of the flow of urine.

Reference: Carlson, K. K.: Acute renal failure. *In* Urban, N. A., Krumberger, J. M., Winkelman, C. (eds.): Guidelines for Critical Care Nursing. St. Louis, Mosby–Year Book, 1995.

2–121. (**D**) One of the most lethal abdominal injuries is trauma to the large bowel complicated by sepsis due to fecal contamination of the abdomen. Malabsorption syndrome occurs if more than 200 cm of small bowel has been damaged. Hemorrhage is precipitated by liver, spleen, and stomach injuries and is not associated with large bowel trauma. Biliary fistula is associated with liver and small bowel trauma.

References: Lawrence, D. M.: Gastrointestinal trauma. Crit. Care Nurs. Clin. North Am. 5:127–140, 1993.
Toto, K. H., Yucha, C. B.: Magnesium: homeostasis, imbalances, and therapeutic uses. Crit. Care Nurs. Clin. North Am. 6:767–781, 1994.

2–122. (**C**) The most likely cause of the patient's inability to wean is chronic respiratory distress syndrome, which is characterized by decreased tissue compliance, increased pulmonary vascular resistance, fibrotic appearance in the lung tissue, and hypoxemia. Although pneumonia, pneumothorax, and diaphragm fatigue may affect weaning, they would not present as these clinical findings. There was no pneumothorax or pneumonia findings on the chest radiograph report. Diaphragmatic fatigue would result in increased carbon dioxide, and lung compliance would not be decreased.

Reference: Alspach, J. G. (ed.): AACN Core Curriculum for Critical Care Nursing, 5th ed. Philadelphia, W. B. Saunders, 1998.

2–123. (**D**) In this patient situation, decreasing her dead space would decrease the $Paco_2$ and facilitate weaning. Tracheostomy may be implemented to remove secretions, decrease dead space, bypass upper airway obstruction, prevent or limit aspiration, and deliver ventilation over an extended period of time.

Reference: Alspach, J. G. (ed.): AACN Core Curriculum for Critical Care Nursing, 5th ed. Philadelphia, W. B. Saunders, 1998.

2–124. (**B**) There is no need to sedate this patient and that may impair the weaning process. Her physical impairments would make it difficult for her to use the alphabet board. The artificial larynx would have to be held to her neck, which would make it more difficult to use. The easiest method would be changing to a speaking tracheostomy or using the speaking valve (Passey-Muir) on the existing tracheostomy.

Reference: Kersten, L. D.: Comprehensive Respiratory Nursing: A Decision Making Approach. Philadelphia, W. B. Saunders, 1989.

2–125. (**B**) Vigorous treatment of HHNK with insulin in the presence of inadequate fluid replacement increases the risk of vascular thrombosis by shifting water out of the blood stream into the cells. As insulin reduces blood glucose and hypertonicity, the protective effect of hypertonicity on blood volume is lost and water flows out of the vasculature into the cells. The resulting volume contraction increases blood viscosity and increases the risk of thromboembolism. The cornerstone of therapy in HHNK is aggressive early volume replacement.

Reference: Lorber, D.: Nonketotic hypertonicity in diabetes mellitus. Med. Clin. North Am. 79:39–52, 1995.

2–126. (**B**) Skin tests serve as a barometer of immune function. The immune response mediates the normal response to skin test antigens. Immunosuppressed patients may have delayed reactions to skin testing. Leukocytosis reflects a normal functioning of the immune system in response to bacterial or viral invasion. Pneumonia is a condition that occurs as a complication rather than as a sign of immunosuppression.

Reference: Alspach, J. G. (ed.): AACN Core Curriculum for Critical Care Nursing, 5th ed. Philadelphia, W. B. Saunders, 1998.

2–127. (**D**) Application of the pacemaker magnet causes the pacemaker to pace at a preset rate, which allows the evaluation of capture. Carotid massage and Valsalva maneuvers decrease the intrinsic rate by slowing sinoatrial node discharge and increasing atrioventricular block. If the rate obtained is slower than the lower limit rate, capture can be observed. Exercise and chest wall stimulation are maneuvers used to evaluate sensing capability by raising the rate above the lower limit rate.

Reference: Kinney, M. R., Packa, D. R.: Andreoli's Comprehensive Cardiac Care, 8th ed. St. Louis, Mosby–Year Book, 1996.

2–128. (**A**) Ventricular dysrhythmias and atrial fibrillation are the two most common dysrhythmias found in hypertrophic cardiomyopathy. Ventricular dysrhythmias in hypertrophic cardiomyopathy are often refractory to conventional agents such as lidocaine and procainamide. Amiodarone appears to be useful in controlling both atrial and ventricular tachydysrhythmias in hypertrophic cardiomyopathy. Positive inotropic medications such as digoxin are contraindicated in hypertrophic cardiomyopathy. Adenosine is used for supraventricular tachsdysrhythmias such as in Wolff-Parkinson-White syndrome.

Reference: Stewart, J. T., McKenna, W. J.: Management of dysrhythmias in hypertrophic cardiomyopathy. Cardiovasc. Drugs Ther. 8:95–99, 1994.

2–129. (**C**) Vasodilators do not improve contractility, but they improve cardiac output and cardiac performance by decreasing preload and vascular resistance. Calcium channel blockers also slow heart rate and improve diastolic filling time and ejection fraction. The improvement in cardiac performance and reduction of symptoms of heart failure increase survival rates.

Reference: Kinney, M. R., Packa, D. R.: Andreoli's Comprehensive Cardiac Care, 8th ed. St. Louis, Mosby–Year Book, 1996.

2–130. (**B**) Microbial translocation refers to gastrointestinal flora moving from the gut into the systemic circulation, thus causing sepsis. Nutritional factors contributing to microbial translocation include malnutrition and the infusion of total parenteral nutrition. Although a decreased level of consciousness can increase the incidence of aspiration and pulmonary sepsis, microbial translocation refers to an intestinal source of the organism.

Reference: Clochesy, J. M.: Patients with systemic inflammatory response syndrome. *In* Clochesy, J. M., Breu, C., Cardin, S., et al. (eds.): Critical Care Nursing. Philadelphia, W. B. Saunders, 1996.

2–131. (**C**) Pulsus paradoxus is a sign of cardiac tamponade. Although distended neck veins are also a classic sign of tamponade, they may be flat if blood loss is significant. In pneumothorax and hemothorax, breath sounds would not be clear bilaterally. Aortic transection would not cause a paradoxical pulse.

Reference: Rosenthal, M. A., Ellis, J. I.: Cardiac and mediastinal trauma. Emerg. Med. Clin. North Am. 13:887–899, 1995.

2–132. (**A**) Phenytoin (Dilantin), when given as a loading dose for status epilepticus, should be administered intravenously over 40 to 60 minutes. The usual loading dose is 15 to 20 mg/kg, or an average of about 1 g. Phenytoin should never be administered faster than 50 mg/min in adults and no faster than 3 mg/min/kg in children. The maximum dose in a 24-hour period is 1 g. The acceptable routes for administration of phenytoin are oral and intravenous. Although the drug literature states that phenytoin may be given intramuscularly, this route of administration is not recommended because absorption rates are inconsistent and the drug is irritating to the tissues. When given orally, phenytoin is absorbed slowly from the gastrointestinal tract, taking 8 to 12 hours to reach peak blood concentration.

Reference: Hickey, J. V.: The Clinical Practice of Neurological and Neurosurgical Nursing, 3rd ed. Philadelphia, J. B. Lippincott, 1992.

2–133. **(D)** Profound hypotension, minimal urine output, and pulse over 140 beats/min are the clinical signs of hemorrhagic blood loss that exceeds 40% of total blood volume. With blood loss less than 15%, the patient will have a normal pulse, normal urine output, and normal blood pressure with orthostatic hypotension. A blood loss of 15% to 30% results in pulse over 100 beats/min, urine output of 25 to 30 ml/hr, and normal blood pressure with decreased pulse pressure. A blood loss of 30% to 40% is associated with a resting pulse over 120 beats/min, low urine output, and hypotension.

References: Kerber, K.: The adult with bleeding esophageal varices. Crit. Care Nurs. Clin. North Am. 5:153–162, 1993.
Klein, D.: Physiologic response to traumatic shock. AACN Clin. Issues Crit. Care Nurs. 1:508–521, 1990.

2–134. **(C)** Acute respiratory failure is defined by the failure of the pulmonary system to maintain elimination of CO_2 and delivery of adequate oxygen, leading to an increased $PaCO_2$ and decreased PaO_2.

Reference: Alspach, J. G. (ed.): AACN Core Curriculum for Critical Care Nursing, 5th ed. Philadelphia, W. B. Saunders, 1998.

2–135. **(B)** The hallmarks of respiratory distress syndrome include increased right-to-left shunting of blood through the lungs (normal is 5%) without being oxygenated, increased physiologic dead space, decreased lung compliance, and increased resistance to blood flow through the lungs.

Reference: Alspach, J. G. (ed.): AACN Core Curriculum for Critical Care Nursing, 5th ed. Philadelphia, W. B. Saunders, 1998.

2–136. **(B)** The cardiac index is decreased, systemic vascular resistance is increased, and hematocrit is acceptable. The patient is hypovolemic. The choice of fluid would be normal saline. Dopamine is contraindicated in hypovolemia. Fifty milliliters of salt-poor albumin would not restore volume rapidly and is indicated when extravascular volume is increased. Transfusion is not indicated for a hematocrit of 32% because hemodilution lowers blood viscosity and improves blood flow.

Reference: Wright, J. E., Shelton, B. K.: Desk Reference for Critical Care Nursing. Boston, Jones & Bartlett, 1993.

2–137. **(C)** The ankle index is obtained by dividing the ankle pressure by the brachial pressure. The normal ankle index should be 1.0 or greater. Patients with aortoiliac occlusive disease often have a normal ankle pressure and ankle index at rest. The ankle pressure and ankle index, however, fall during exercise owing to claudication.

Reference: Moore, W.: Vascular Surgery: A Comprehensive Review. Philadelphia, W. B. Saunders, 1993.

2–138. **(B)** The aorta is cross-clamped during aortic surgery. This may result in impairment of renal function, which is best assessed by monitoring urinary output, specific gravity, blood urea nitrogen, and creatinine.

Reference: Wright, J. E., Shelton, B. K.: Desk Reference for Critical Care Nursing. Boston, Jones & Bartlett, 1993.

2–139. **(B)** Dopamine, administered in conjunction with crystalloids for volume replacement, acts as a vasoconstrictor to increase systemic pressures, thereby increasing tissue perfusion. The capillary leak continues for at least 24 hours even with optimal therapy, and to date no reversal mechanisms are known. Serum osmolality is within normal range in shock. Oxygen consumption will actually increase as oxygen is taken up by the perfused cells.

Reference: Jones, K.: Shock. *In* Clochesy, J. M., Breu, C., Cardin, S., et al. (eds.): Critical Care Nursing. Philadelphia, W. B. Saunders, 1996.

2–140. (**C**) Hyperkalemia is the most common reason for the initiation of dialysis in patients with acute renal failure. Of all of the potential electrolyte disorders, hyperkalemia is considered to be the most life threatening, secondary to the effects of potassium on the heart, which may lead to the development of potentially lethal dysrhythmias. Fluid overload may be managed with diuretics and fluid restriction. Hyponatremia will be corrected with the management of the patient's fluid volume. Metabolic acidosis can be corrected with the administration of sodium bicarbonate, if it becomes profound.

Reference: Carlson, K. K.: Acute renal failure. *In* Urban, N. A., Krumberger, J. M., Winkelman, C. (eds.): Guidelines for Critical Care Nursing. St. Louis, Mosby–Year Book, 1995.

2–141. (**D**) High-frequency ventilation can be implemented on any ventilator by increasing the respiratory rate and decreasing the tidal volume. The delivered breath then travels by diffusion to the alveoli. IVOX and $ECCO_2R$ are experimental, and ECMO has been shown to have no advantage in adults over conventional mechanical ventilation. The last three options are only performed in select centers, and the patient is not stable enough to be transferred.

References: Dellinger, R. P.: Clinical trials in adult respiratory distress syndrome. *In* Dellinger, R. P. (ed.): New Horizons 1:584–592, 1993.
Gattinoni, L., Pesenti, A., Bombino, M., et al.: Role of extracorporeal circulation in adult respiratory distress syndrome management. *In* Dellinger, R. P. (ed.): New Horizons 1:603–612, 1993.

2–142. (**D**) The improvement in the patient's oxygenation is due to increased diffusion of oxygen to the functional lung units provided by high-frequency ventilation. Her lung compliance would not be affected, but pressures needed to deliver the volume would be decreased, thus reducing the risk of barotrauma. Because she is already sedated and chemically paralyzed, her oxygen needs would not be affected. Patients who are alert and assist with breathing have reported a reduced need to breathe, but it does not apply in this clinical situation.

Reference: Alspach, J. G. (ed.): AACN Core Curriculum for Critical Care Nursing, 5th ed. Philadelphia, W. B. Saunders, 1998.

2–143. (**C**) All of these are possible causes. Because the mean PAP is stable, however, the most likely explanation is that a lower tidal volume and mean airway pressure have produced a lower intrathoracic pressure and that has translated into a lower wedge pressure. The mean PAP would remain stable because it reflects pressures within the pulmonary artery.

Reference: Alspach, J. G. (ed.): AACN Core Curriculum for Critical Care Nursing, 5th ed. Philadelphia, W. B. Saunders, 1998.

2–144. (**C**) Encephalopathy is the end result of other diseases or pathologic conditions on the brain and not a disease in itself. There are numerous diagnostic and laboratory tests that can be used as an adjunct in the assessment of intracranial pressure as a result of encephalopathy. Cerebrospinal fluid levels of glucose may aid in the diagnosis. Blood urea nitrogen levels are not always consistent with uremic encephalopathy. Serum ammonia levels may aid in the diagnosis of hepatic encephalopathy; however, in patients with metabolic encephalopathy it is more important to rule out water intoxication. Total body water is composed of intracellular fluid (ICF) and extracellular fluid (ECF). The most important determinant of ECF is its sodium content. As serum osmolarity rises, intracellular water moves to the ECF and may result in edema. Thus, serum osmolarity along with serum sodium levels are most important to determine if there is a risk for increased intracranial pressure. Normal serum osmolarity levels should be between 280 and 295 mOsm/L.

References: Hickey, J. V.: The Clinical Practice of Neurological and Neurosurgical Nursing, 3rd ed. Philadelphia, J. B. Lippincott, 1992.
Clochesy, J. M., Breu, C., Cardin, S., Whittaker, A. A.: Critical Care Nursing, 2nd ed. Philadelphia, W. B. Saunders, 1996.

2–145. (**D**) The most important goal in treating an acute gastric hemorrhage is to control the bleeding. Prostaglandins may be useful in supporting gastric defense mechanisms but are not useful in acute hemorrhage. Reduction of portal hypertension may reduce the venous pressure, which contributes to bleeding esophageal varices. Reducing enzyme stimulation is indicated for pancreatitis rather than for gastrointestinal bleeding.

References: Prevost, S. S., Oberlie, A.: Stress ulceration in the critically ill patient. Crit. Care Nurs. Clin. North Am. 5:163–169, 1993.
Urban, N., et al.: Guidelines for Critical Care Nursing. St. Louis, Mosby–Year Book, 1995.

2–146. (**A**) Low-molecular-weight dextran is often used after vascular surgery as an antithrombotic agent that improves blood flow and volume. Aspirin inhibits platelet aggregation but has no effect on blood flow. Atenolol is a beta blocker that is cardioselective and has minimal effect on peripheral beta$_2$ receptors that decrease vasoconstriction. Nitroglycerin vasodilates but has no antithrombotic effect.

Reference: Thelan, L. A., Davie, J. K., Urden, L. D., Lough, M. E.: Critical Care Nursing, Diagnosis and Management, 2nd ed. St. Louis, Mosby–Year Book, 1994.

2–147. (**B**) A major side effect of dextran infusion is anaphylaxis, which is indicated by the wheezing, hypotension, and reddened skin. It should be discontinued. Until the blood pressure recovers, the nitroglycerin should also be decreased to maintain blood pressure. Increasing the bicarbonate infusion may cause alkalosis, which would diminish the oxygen available to tissues.

Reference: Moore, W. S.: Vascular Surgery: A Comprehensive Review. Philadelphia, W. B. Saunders, 1993.

2–148. (**A**) T waves invert in ischemia because of altered repolarization. ST segment elevation indicates a pattern of injury. Q waves indicate infarction and changes in the pattern of depolarization.

Reference: Dossey, B. M., Guzzetta, C. E., Kenner, C. V.: Critical Care Nursing, Body-Mind-Spirit. Philadelphia, J. B. Lippincott, 1992.

2–149. (**C**) Patients with sepsis are at risk for developing disseminated intravascular coagulation (DIC), a syndrome caused by the presence of large quantities of plasmin and thrombin in the systemic circulation. Plasmin breaks down fibrin, producing fibrin degradation products. The D-dimer test confirms the presence of fibrin split products. Confirmatory tests for DIC include D-dimer greater than 2.0 mg/ml, low platelet count, and elevated prothrombin time/partial thromboplastin time. DIC patients are at risk for significant bruising and hematoma formation from standard nursing care, and plans to protect the skin with padding, avoiding shaving, and limiting venipuncture are indicated. The other responses are not specific to the implications of an elevated D-dimer level.

Reference: Roberts, S. L.: Multisystem deviations. *In* Critical Care Nursing: Assessment and Intervention. Stamford, Conn., Appleton & Lange, 1996.

2–150. (**C**) The patient with mild hypoglycemia has symptoms that reflect effects on the autonomic nervous system. These include tremors, sweating, anxiety, and warmness. Beta-adrenergic blocking agents, such as metoprolol and propranolol, can blunt the display of the autonomic nervous system symptoms of hypoglycemia. The other medications listed have no effect on these symptoms, but lidocaine toxicity can produce central nervous system symptoms that mimic severe hypoglycemia, such as lethargy and seizures.

Reference: Service, F. J.: Hypoglycemia. Med. Clin. North Am. 79:1–8, 1995.

2–151. (**C**) A patient with blood type A can receive type A or type O blood. Blood type remains the same after liver transplantation. Although institutional practices for blood transfusions after transplantation may vary related to the use of filters and cell washing, the patient's ABO compatibility does not change from its preoperative status. Adequate immunosuppression therapy is not a requirement for blood transfusion.

References: Alspach, J. G. (ed.): AACN Core Curriculum for Critical Care Nursing, 5th ed. Philadelphia, W. B. Saunders, 1998.
Coffland, F. I., Shelton, D. M.: Blood component replacement therapy. Crit. Care Nurs. Clin. North Am. 5:543–556, 1993.

2–152. (**D**) The five-lead system is used with ST segment monitoring. The chest lead for optimal anterior wall observations should be V_2 or V_3. The optimal lead for circumflex artery monitoring is lead III; for occlusion of the right coronary artery, the optimal leads are III or aVF.

Reference: Thelan, L. A., Davie, J. K., Urden, L. D., Lough, M. E.: Critical Care Nursing, Diagnosis and Management, 2nd ed. St. Louis, Mosby–Year Book, 1994.

2–153. (**A**) Early reperfusion is demonstrated by ST segment elevation, which resolves rapidly, and the accelerated development and resolution of Q waves. ST segment elevation and Q waves as well as T wave inversion are the typical evolutionary changes associated with acute myocardial infarction.

Reference: Kinney, M. R., Packa, D. R.: Andreoli's Comprehensive Cardiac Care, 8th ed. St. Louis, Mosby–Year Book, 1996.

2–154. (**C**) ST segment elevation and tall T waves in II, III, and aVF indicate acute inferior wall myocardial infarction (MI). ST segment elevation and tall T waves in I, aVL, and V_{5-6} would indicate acute lateral wall MI. ST segment elevation and tall T waves in V_{3-4} would indicate acute anterior wall MI. Posterior MI is recognized by reciprocal changes (ST segment depression and tall R waves) in V_{1-3}.

Reference: Thelan, L. A., Davie, J. K., Urden, L. D., Lough, M. E.: Critical Care Nursing, Diagnosis and Management, 2nd ed. St. Louis, Mosby–Year Book, 1994.

2–155. (**A**) Papillary muscle rupture may complicate inferior wall MI because the right coronary artery supplies both the inferior wall and the posterior papillary muscle. Ventricular septal rupture occurs with the same frequency in both anterior and inferior wall MIs. Both are associated with development of a holosystolic murmur. In tamponade, heart tones are muffled but breath sounds are clear. Anterior wall MI demonstrated by ST segment elevation in the anterior leads is associated with left ventricular failure, but the development of pulmonary edema is not abrupt. Right ventricular MI, demonstrated by ST segment elevation in leads V_3R and V_4R, causes hypovolemic symptoms of shock.

Reference: Darovic, G. O.: Hemodynamic Monitoring: Invasive and Noninvasive Clinical Application. Philadelphia, W. B. Saunders, 1995.

2–156. (**D**) Hyperventilation has been used in the past to control ICP but has recently been associated with a reduction in cerebral oxygen saturation as a result of vasoconstriction that leads to reduced cerebral blood flow and worsened clinical outcomes. Sedation with narcotics, benzodiazepines, or propofol should be used only in patients who have an ICP monitor in place. Although loop diuretics such as furosemide may be used to control ICP, they are usually used in conjunction with osmotic diuretics such as mannitol as an effective means of reducing ICP through osmotic diuresis and improving cerebral microcirculation. Barbiturate therapy, a last step in the control of increased ICP, is used only after all conventional methods have proved ineffective. It is generally initiated when the ICP is greater than 30 mm Hg for more than 30 minutes with a cerebral perfusion pressure of less than 70 mm Hg or an ICP of greater than 40 mm Hg in the absence of other hemodynamic parameters.

Reference: Alspach, J. G. (ed.): AACN Core Curriculum for Critical Care Nursing, 5th ed. Philadelphia, W. B. Saunders, 1998.

2–157. (**A**) Because natural prostaglandin synthesis is inhibited by NSAIDs and aspirin, synthetic prostaglandins are recommended for stress ulcers that occur with long-term use of these drugs. Unprescribed use of over-the-counter NSAIDs for pain management and aspirin for cardiovascular prophylaxis has surged in recent years. Consequently, the importance of matching ulcer therapy with ulcer etiology is extremely important. Lidocaine, calcium channel blockers, and warfarin may all potentially interact with H2-receptor antagonists used for ulcer treatment. The function of each of the drugs is unpredictably prolonged.

Reference: Prevost, S. S., Oberlie, A.: Stress ulceration in the critically ill patient. Crit. Care Nurs. Clin. North Am. 5:163–169, 1993.

2–158. (**B**) In right ventricular MI the right ventricle is unable to contribute to the forward flow of blood to the lungs, causing clear breath sounds and hypotension. Anterior wall MIs are more commonly associated with hypotension and pulmonary edema. Right ventricular MI is most frequently associated with occlusion of the right coronary artery, which supplies both the sinoatrial and atrioventricular nodes in most persons, making them prone to bradydysrhythmias and heart block.

Reference: Thelan, L. A., Davie, J. K., Urden, L. D., Lough, M. E.: Critical Care Nursing, Diagnosis and Management, 2nd ed. St. Louis, Mosby–Year Book, 1994.

2–159. (**B**) Fresh frozen plasma (FFP) is administered to patients in septic shock to restore host defenses such as complement. FFP administration does expand circulating volume; but if that is the treatment goal, crystalloid administration is the method of choice. Likewise, if albumin is low, the preferred therapy is administration of albumin. Although septic patients often have coagulation disorders, treatment of its specific etiology may or may not indicate administration of FFP.

Reference: Roberts, S. L.: Multisystem deviations. In Critical Care Nursing: Assessment and Intervention. Stamford, Conn., Appleton & Lange, 1996.

2–160. **(A)** Mannitol, an osmotic diuretic, causes vasodilatation of the renal vessels and expands vascular volume by enhancing movement of fluid from the interstitial space. Mannitol is often used prophylactically in an effort to protect the kidney in suspected acute renal failure (ARF). Once ARF has been established, mannitol can contribute to fluid overload in the patient who has lost excretory renal function. It is important to avoid the use of potassium-sparing diuretics, like spironolactone, because the patient with renal failure will have diminished ability to eliminate potassium. Loop diuretics, such as furosemide and bumetanide, are used more commonly after ARF has been established. They work by blocking sodium reabsorption in the renal tubules, thereby enhancing excretion of sodium and water; this may reduce fluid overload and frequency of dialysis in the patient with ARF.

Reference: Carlson, K. K.: Acute renal failure. *In* Urban, N. A., Krumberger, J. M., Winkelman, C. (eds.): Guidelines for Critical Care Nursing. St. Louis, Mosby–Year Book, 1995.

2–161. **(B)** Corticosteroids have not been proven efficacious in the treatment of the acute phase of respiratory distress syndrome but may have a role in the chronic phase. In the chronic phase of respiratory distress syndrome, corticosteroids may decrease inflammation of airways and reduce the extent of fibrotic damage.

Reference: Alspach, J. G. (ed.): AACN Core Curriculum for Critical Care Nursing, 5th ed. Philadelphia, W. B. Saunders, 1998.

2–162. **(B)** Patients with right ventricular (RV) infarction are very sensitive to decreases in blood volume. Decreases in RV volume further decrease left ventricular preload and cause decreased systemic and coronary perfusion. Dopamine is contraindicated because it may cause increased pump failure. Nitroglycerin and ACE inhibitors further decrease RV preload so they are contraindicated in RV failure.

Reference: Khan, M. G.: Heart Disease Diagnosis and Therapy. Baltimore, Williams & Wilkins, 1996.

2–163. **(B)** Large inferior wall MIs are most often associated with extension to right ventricular MIs. If lead V_4R is used to monitor a patient with evolving MI of the inferior wall, ST segment changes indicative of right ventricular MI can best be seen. At the fifth intercostal space in the left anterior axillary and left midaxillary line, the lateral wall is viewed. The right sternal border at the fourth intercostal space (lead V_3R) is not considered to be as accurate as lead V_4R in detecting right ventricular MI.

Reference: Kinney, M. R., Packa, D. R.: Andreoli's Comprehensive Cardiac Care, 8th ed. St. Louis, Mosby–Year Book, 1996.

2–164. **(C)** Recombinant tissue plasminogen activator (rt-PA) may be given more than once and may follow administration of SSK. Because of its allergic predisposition, SSK is only given once. Urokinase is given via the intracoronary route but is not given systemically.

Reference: Kinney, M. R., Packa, D. R.: Andreoli's Comprehensive Cardiac Care, 8th ed. St. Louis, Mosby–Year Book, 1996.

2–165. **(D)** The average return to work date for PTCA patients is 7 days. The patient's fears are realistic, and giving the patient factual information without discounting the risks is an appropriate nursing intervention. Although the nurse should aid the development of trust, general comments predicting the outcome of a procedure are not appropriate. Although the patient should be encouraged to speak with the physician about return to work plans, specifying that he do so after the procedure supports the fear of a possible negative outcome.

Reference: Kern, M. J., Deligonul, U.: The Interventional Cardiac Catheterization Handbook. St. Louis, Mosby–Year Book, 1996.

2–166. (**D**) Contraindications to administration of beta blockers include bronchospasm, heart failure, and heart block. PCWP greater than 20 mm Hg, rales, and wheezes suggest bronchospasm or left ventricular failure. A PR interval of 0.24 indicates the development of first-degree heart block. Propranolol should be withheld until consultation with the physician determines that a lower dosage should be administered or the dose withheld. A lower dose may be indicated to prevent beta blocker withdrawal ischemia.

Reference: Kinney, M. R., Packa, D. R., Dunbar, S. B.: AACN's Clinical Reference for Critical Care Nursing, 3rd ed. St. Louis, Mosby–Year Book, 1993.

2–167. (**B**) A nitroglycerin drip should be initiated to increase coronary artery diameter and improve blood flow. The APTT and heparin rate are appropriate so no change in the heparin rate is necessary. If the patient will be able to return to the cardiac catheterization laboratory for repeat PTCA in 2 hours, surgery is not a consideration. The family should be notified after the patient-centered activities are completed to decrease their anxiety.

Reference: Kern, M. J., Deligonul, U.: The Interventional Cardiac Catheterization Handbook. St. Louis, Mosby–Year Book, 1996.

2–168. (**D**) Basilar skull fractures account for nearly 20% of all skull fractures. It is important for the critical care nurse to recognize subjective symptoms and objective signs that indicate this type of fracture. A basilar skull fracture may involve the anterior, middle, or posterior fossa. Patients with basilar fractures may complain of a sensation of a salty or sweet taste due to altered receptors mediated through the facial, glossopharyngeal and/or vagus nerve from the brain stem. Anterior fossa basilar fractures may present with a cerebrospinal fluid (CSF) rhinorrhea whereas middle fossa fractures present with CSF otorrhea. Paresthesias are more commonly associated with parietal lobe injuries, whereas diplopia, or double vision, generally arises as a result of occipital lobe injuries.

Reference: Clochesy, J. M., Breu, C., Cardin, S., et al. (eds.): Critical Care Nursing, 2nd ed. Philadelphia, W. B. Saunders, 1996.

2–169. (**C**) The esophageal balloon will normally be inflated to between 20 and 45 mm Hg. The lowest balloon pressure necessary to control bleeding is selected based on the principle of capillary closing pressure. This will vary over time based on the patient's current pressures and position. Normal capillary pressure on the arterial side ranges from 30 to 40 mm Hg. Esophageal balloon pressure greater than 45 mm Hg puts the patient at risk for esophageal necrosis and perforation. Balloon pressure less than 20 mm Hg is not likely to stop venous bleeding.

Reference: Kerber, K.: The adult with bleeding esophageal varices. Crit. Care Nurs. Clin. North Am. 5:153–162, 1993.

2–170. (**A**) Side effects of dopamine include headache, vomiting, dyspnea, mydriasis, arrhythmias, widening QRS complex, tachycardia, aberrant conduction, bradycardia, hypotension, angina, and piloerection.

Reference: Roberts, S. L.: Cardiac deviations. In Critical Care Nursing: Assessment and Intervention. Stamford, Conn., Appleton & Lange, 1996.

2–171. (**C**) Volutrauma occurs in patients on mechanical ventilation when the inspiratory volume flows into areas of the lung that are more compliant and functional because the pressure is lower in those areas. Gas flows down a pressure gradient. This distends these structures and sometimes causes rupture. Pneumonia results from an infectious process, and a decreased cardiac output is associated with compliant lungs. Oxygen toxicity is associated with an increase in FIO_2 of more than 50% for greater than 24 hours.

Reference: Tobin, M. J. (ed.): Principles and Practice of Mechanical Ventilation. New York, McGraw-Hill, 1994.

2–172. (**D**) Calcium channel blockers are given during PTCA for patients with vasospastic angina. They are generally given for approximately 2 weeks to 3 months after PTCA to prevent vasoconstriction and vasospasm, which would induce ischemia in incompletely revascularized regions. Nitroglycerin and beta blockers do not reduce spasm. ACE inhibitors reduce vasoconstriction but not spasm.

Reference: Kern, M. J., Deligonul, U.: The Interventional Cardiac Catheterization Handbook. St. Louis, Mosby–Year Book, 1996.

2–173. (**C**) Flank or low back pain in a PTCA patient may indicate a retroperitoneal hemorrhage. The additional peritoneal signs of urgency and radiation of pain to the abdomen on turning increase the likelihood of this complication. The heparin drip should be stopped to prevent further bleeding. The abdominal and flank pain are most likely not related to referred myocardial pain or to urinary problems related to Foley catheter use, so the furosemide and nitroglycerin will not decrease the discomfort. Morphine should be used cautiously in the bleeding patient because of its hypotensive effects.

Reference: Kern, M. J., Deligonul, U.: The Interventional Cardiac Catheterization Handbook. St. Louis, Mosby–Year Book, 1996.

2–174. (**C**) Heparin bolus with infusion is usually attempted first when stent thrombosis as evidenced by ST segment elevation occurs. If emergent PTCA cannot be performed, systemic thrombolytic agents may be given. Atherectomy is not performed in stent thrombosis because of the potential to disturb the stent and because the procedure is contraindicated in patients receiving ongoing thrombolytic therapy.

Reference: Kern, M. J., Deligonul, U.: The Interventional Cardiac Catheterization Handbook. St. Louis, Mosby–Year Book, 1996.

2–175. (**A**) Priority nursing interventions for a patient with diabetes insipidus include meticulous recording of intake and output, body weight, urine specific gravity, plasma, and urine osmolality. These parameters are the best indicators of the patient's state of fluid balance, which is critical to evaluate in diabetes insipidus in which antidiuretic hormone is lacking; the body cannot conserve water, and urine output is markedly increased. Central venous pressure measurement is another tool used to evaluate volume status, but compensatory vasoconstriction may produce pressure readings that are misleadingly high relative to the amount of volume lost, and not all of these patients may have a central line. The monitoring of electrolytes is not the top priority because these may not initially be affected in diabetes insipidus.

Reference: Alspach, J. G. (ed.): AACN Core Curriculum for Critical Care Nursing, 5th ed. Philadelphia, W. B. Saunders, 1998.

2–176. (**C**) Veno-occlusive disease (VOD) is a complication of BMT, as are infections and renal failure. Immunosuppressive therapy is necessary after BMT. VOD is caused by obstruction resulting in reduced hepatic function and manifested by increased bilirubin, increased ammonia, and decreased clotting factors. Infection may be asymptomatic, but fever is the first indicator. Renal failure during the postoperative phase would be manifested by alterations in blood urea nitrogen, creatinine, and fluid status. Cyclosporine therapy is usually administered during this period, and its most common side effect is nephrotoxicity.

References: Wahrenberger, A.: Pharmacologic immunosuppression: Cure or curse? Crit. Care Nurs. Q. 17(4):27–36, 1995.
Wujcik, D., Ballard, B., Camp-Sorrell, D.: Selected complications of allogenic bone marrow transplantation. Semin. Oncol. Nurs. 10:28–41, 1994.

2–177. (**A**) In VOD, therapy should optimize hepatic blood flow and minimize fluid distribution into the interstitial and peritoneal spaces; central vascular volume can be optimized with albumin. Normal saline is generally avoided because of its sodium content. Colony-stimulating factor is useful to treat neutropenia after transplantation. Total body irradiation is a common pretransplant conditioning therapy.

References: Franco, T., Gould, D. A.: Allogenic bone marrow transplantation. Semin. Oncol. Nurs. 10:3–11, 1994.
Wujcik, D., Ballard, B., Camp-Sorrell, D.: Selected complications of allogenic bone marrow transplantation. Semin. Oncol. Nurs. 10:28–41, 1994.

2–178. (**D**) A decreased level of consciousness indicates neurologic deterioration; thus it has the highest priority in nursing care. It is generally the earliest clinical finding and occurs as a result of sensitivity to a decreased oxygen supply by the cerebral cortex. An additional rationale for determining a patient's level of consciousness is that terminal arteries may be compromised as a result of brain injury, resulting in decreased oxygen supply to the cerebral cortex.

Reference: Hickey, J. V.: The Clinical Practice of Neurological and Neurosurgical Nursing, 3rd ed. Philadelphia, J. B. Lippincott, 1992.

2–179. (**C**) Epinephrine increases systolic blood pressure but may decrease diastolic blood pressure. The proximal port of the pulmonary artery catheter is not used for infusion of epinephrine if hemodynamic parameters are being measured. The solution should be clear, not brown, which would indicate oxidation. A mixture of 1 ampule 1:1000 in 250 ml produces a concentration of 4 μg/ml, the standard preparation of epinephrine infusion.

Reference: Roberts, S. L.: Cardiac deviations. *In* Critical Care Nursing: Assessment and Intervention. Stamford, Conn., Appleton & Lange, 1996.

2–180. (**D**) CAVH is contraindicated in patients with a systolic blood pressure less than 60 mm Hg, hematocrit greater than 45%, or an inability to tolerate high volume fluid exchanges. A hematocrit greater than 45% can potentially cause the hemofilter to clot due to the increased viscosity of the blood.

Reference: Baer, C. L.: Acute renal failure. *In* Kinney, M. R., Packa, D. R., Dunbar, S. B. (eds.): AACN's Clinical Reference for Critical-Care Nursing, 3rd ed. St. Louis, Mosby–Year Book, 1993.

2–181. **(B)** The four major complications of balloon tamponade of esophageal varices are ruptured esophagus, asphyxia secondary to pharyngeal obstruction, aspiration, and erosion of the gastric wall. Complaints of substernal pain that is aggravated by ventilation are indicative of esophageal perforation. The chest movement associated with ventilation is believed to extend the exposure of esophagogastric juices through the rupture and/or further strain smooth muscle at the site of the tear. The balloon does not enter the bowel, so bowel obstruction is not a complication of this therapy.

Reference: Kerber, K.: The adult with bleeding esophageal varices. Crit. Care Nurs. Clin. North Am. 5:153–162, 1993.

2–182. **(D)** Corticosteroids have been proposed as useful in chronic respiratory distress to decrease the chronic inflammation that leads to fibrosis. Corticosteroids have been shown to be ineffective in sepsis and have not been shown to be effective in pneumonia or thrombotic pulmonary embolus.

Reference: Meduri, G. U.: Late adult respiratory distress syndrome. New Horizons 1:563–577, 1993.

2–183. **(C)** Coronary angiography gives the best indication of coronary artery flow. Medications can be administered during catheterization to simulate sympathetic stimulation, and various views of coronary perfusion may be examined. Exercise stress testing gives information on coronary flow because it pertains to ECG changes. M-mode echocardiography views cardiac wall, chambers, valves, and great vessels. MUGA scans are used to assess ventricular performance.

Reference: Kinney, M. R., Packa, D. R.: Andreoli's Comprehensive Cardiac Care, 8th ed. St. Louis, Mosby–Year Book, 1996.

2–184. **(A)** ECG signs of unstable angina include transient ST segment elevation or depression and T wave inversion that resolve with pain relief or within 12 hours. Transient inverted U waves may also be seen in unstable angina. Persistence of ST segment elevation or depression for over 12 hours suggests that the patient has had a non–Q wave myocardial infarction. Q waves indicate that an infarction has occurred.

Reference: Braunwald, E. (ed.): Heart Disease: A Textbook of Cardiovascular Medicine. Philadelphia, W. B. Saunders, 1997.

2–185. **(B)** The compression device precludes palpation of the site for hematoma. Palpation of the pedal pulse on the affected extremity ensures that compression tamponades bleeding but does not impede distal flow. Assessment of potential tamponade or dissection is ongoing but is not intensified at the time of sheath removal.

Reference: Thelan, L. A., Davie, J. K., Urden, L. D., Lough, M. E.: Critical Care Nursing, Diagnosis and Management, 2nd ed. St. Louis, Mosby–Year Book, 1994.

2–186. **(A)** On angiography, lesions with less than 75% occlusion are associated with unstable angina. Lesions of 75% occlusion or greater are associated with infarction from total occlusion or with the development of collateral circulation. Twenty percent occlusion or near normal coronary arteries generally reflect coronary artery spasm as the cause of angina.

Reference: Crawford, M.: Current Diagnosis and Treatment in Cardiology. Norwalk, Conn., Appleton & Lange, 1995.

2–187. (**B**) The immediate goals of treatment for a patient with unstable angina are to relieve pain and prevent ischemia or infarction. Evaluation of the cause of symptoms and the reduction of risk factors may be attempted after the patient has been stabilized and is free of pain.

Reference: Braunwald, E., Mark, D. B., Jones, R. H., et al.: Unstable Angina: Diagnosis and Management. Clinical Practice Guideline Number 10. ACHPR Publication No. 94–0602. Rockville, Md.: Agency For Health Care Policy and Research and the National Heart, Lung and Blood Institute, Public Health Service, U.S. Department of Health and Human Services, March 1994.

2–188. (**B**) Evaluation of chest pain and prevention of myocardial ischemia always take priority. Evaluation of risk factors and patient education may be provided after the patient is stable.

Reference: Matrisciano, L.: Unstable angina: An overview. Crit. Care Nurs. 12(12):30–40, 1992.

2–189. (**B**) Calcium channel blockers may be used to control ischemic symptoms in unstable angina. Nifedipine has been shown to increase the risk of myocardial infarction because it is primarily a peripheral vasodilator with little effect on coronary blood flow. Verapamil decreases heart rate and conduction and vasodilates coronary and smooth muscle. Diltiazem is a potent coronary artery vasodilator and moderately decreases atrioventricular nodal conduction. Felodipine has less negative inotropic effects than verapamil, nifedipine, and diltiazem and is more vasoselective for coronary and vascular smooth muscle.

Reference: Braunwald, E., Mark, D. B., Jones, R. H., et al.: Unstable Angina: Diagnosis and Management. Clinical Practice Guideline Number 10. ACHPR Publication No. 94–0602. Rockville, Md.: Agency for Health Care Policy and Research and the National Heart, Lung and Blood Institute, Public Health Service, U.S. Department of Health and Human Services. March 1994.

2–190. (**B**) Cardiogenic shock produces hypotension, increased afterload (SVR), and elevated preload (PCWP). Effective therapy will increase the MAP, decrease the afterload, and decrease preload. As a result, CO will increase.

Reference: Roberts, S. L.: Multisystem deviations. *In* Critical Care Nursing: Assessment and Intervention. Stamford, Conn., Appleton & Lange, 1996.

2–191. (**A**) To prevent contamination by oxygenated blood from the capillaries, the mixed venous blood gas sample must be drawn slowly at a rate of 1 ml/min. Blood taken from a wedged pulmonary artery catheter would be a capillary blood gas and highly oxygenated. The blood gas sample must be obtained from the distal port of the pulmonary artery catheter to be a true "mixed" venous sample.

References: Boggs, R. L., Wooldridge-King, M. (eds.): AACN Procedure Manual for Critical Care, 3rd ed. Philadelphia, W. B. Saunders, 1993.
Morris, A., Chapman, R.: Wedge pressure confirmation by aspiration of pulmonary capillary blood. Crit. Care Med. 13:736–741, 1985.

2–192. (**A**) Cerebral injury results in a disrupted cerebral blood supply and cerebral edema. Monitoring the edema with an intracranial pressure monitoring device and subsequent calculation of cerebral perfusion pressure are important. Elevating the head of the bed to between 30° and 45° has become a standard practice, but some research suggests that patients with severe intracranial hypertension should be maintained in a flat position to increase cerebral perfusion pressure. Research findings in this area continue to be inconclusive. Neither the side-lying nor prone position has been demonstrated to either reduce or maintain intracranial pressure. Elevating the head of the bed to 30° remains the standard of practice to reduce intracranial pressure in the majority of patients.

Reference: Feldman, Z., Kanter, M. J., Robertson, C. S., et al.: Effect of head elevation on intracranial pressure and cerebral blood flow in head-injured patients. J Neurosurg 77:651–652, 1992.

2–193. (**B**) Vasopressin therapy reduces portal venous pressure by stimulating smooth muscle contraction in the splanchnic arterial bed. Vasopressin also causes vasoconstriction of the coronary, mesenteric, and peripheral arteries. Coronary artery vasoconstriction can result in angina, dysrhythmias, and myocardial infarction. Potent vasoconstriction elevates blood pressure. Vasopressin also increases water reabsorption by the kidney. This can result in water intoxication (not dehydration). Uterine cramping is stimulated by oxytocin therapy. The similarity of the trade names Pitocin and Pitressin should be noted.

Reference: Kerber, K.: The adult with bleeding esophageal varices. Crit. Care Nurs. Clin. North Am. 5:153–162, 1993.

2–194. (**B**) Direct pressure on the insertion site will slow blood flow around the catheter site and tamponade bleeding so that clot formation may occur and the bleeding will stop. Ice may cause vasoconstriction to a moderate degree to slow bleeding but will not stop bleeding as effectively as tamponade. Heparin infusion should not be stopped because it prevents thrombus formation in the coronary vessels. Applying pressure above the site with sheaths in place has minimal effect because the sheath may become compressed and act as an obstacle to direct tamponade.

Reference: Ruppert, S. D., Kernicki, J. G., Dolan, J. T.: Dolan's Critical Care Nursing: Critical Management Through the Nursing Process. Philadelphia, F. A. Davis, 1996.

2–195. (**B**) Calcium channel blockers, such as amlodipine, have the least effect on mortality in cardiac ischemia. The most important medications at this point are the nitrates and the beta blockers, such as atenolol. Headache is a side effect of nitroglycerin, a potent vasodilator, and decreasing the dosage should improve the blood pressure and relieve the headache.

Reference: Braunwald, E., Mark, D. B., Jones, R. H., et al.: Unstable Angina: Diagnosis and Management. Clinical Practice Guideline Number 10. ACHPR Publication No. 94–0602. Rockville, Md.: Agency For Health Care Policy and Research and the National Heart, Lung and Blood Institute, Public Health Service, U.S. Department of Health and Human Services. March 1994.

2–196. (**A**) The plan for preventing activity intolerance includes patient education regarding self-monitoring. The patient who is observed taking his own pulse during activity demonstrates a skill necessary to prevent increases in heart rate, which may cause activity intolerance and chest pain. Physical activity should be avoided after meals, when blood flow is directed to the stomach and digestion. The heart rate should be maintained below 120 beats/min with activity. One-half hour of sedentary activity does not adequately demonstrate activity tolerance.

Reference: Kinney, M. R., Packa, D. R.: Andreoli's Comprehensive Cardiac Care, 8th ed. St. Louis, Mosby–Year Book, 1996.

2–197. (**D**) An increase in the CK2 indicates myocardial ischemia/infarction. The current therapy should be re-evaluated to determine if the patient's condition warrants more aggressive treatment such as percutaneous transluminal coronary angioplasty or thrombolytic therapy to prevent further increases in the ischemic zone. Heparin dosage changes should be made when indicated by APTT results. Before increasing nitroglycerin therapy, the nurse should evaluate the ECG to rule out the possibility of right ventricular infarction.

Reference: Crawford, M. H.: Current Diagnosis and Treatment in Cardiology. Norwalk, Conn., Appleton & Lange, 1995.

2–198. (**B**) According to research on families of critical care patients, the most important need that the critical care nurse can meet is the need for information. Other critical care family needs include support, comfort, proximity, and assurance.

Reference: Bartz, C.: Families in critical care: Environment, needs, and barriers to care. *In* Shoemaker, W. C., Ayres, S. M., Grenvik, A., Holbrook, P. R. (eds.): Textbook of Critical Care, 3rd ed. Philadelphia, W. B. Saunders, 1995.

2–199. (**C**) Intrarenal failure is characterized by urine sodium greater than 30 mEq/L (due to loss of sodium reabsorption by the kidney), urine osmolality less than 350 mOsm/L, and a specific gravity of less than 1.010 (due to loss of the concentrating ability of the kidney). A creatinine clearance less than 85 ml/min is consistent with renal failure. Prerenal failure is characterized by a urine sodium less than 10 mEq/L, urine osmolality greater than 500 mOsm/L, and a specific gravity greater than 1.015. In post or obstructive renal failure, the urine sodium is greater than 20 mEq/L, urine osmolality is less than 350 mOsm/L, and the specific gravity is approximately 1.010.

Reference: Carlson, K. K.: Acute renal failure. *In* Urban, N. A., Krumberger, J. M., Winkelman, C. (eds.): Guidelines for Critical Care Nursing. St. Louis, Mosby–Year Book, 1995.

2–200. (**A**) Laboratory findings for a patient with SIADH include a serum sodium level of less than 130 mEq/L and a serum osmolality of less than 275 mOsm/L. Other laboratory values, such as blood urea nitrogen, creatinine, hematocrit, and albumin, may also be decreased. The diagnosis of SIADH is suspected in any patient with these laboratory results.

Reference: Clochesy, J. M., Breu, C., Cardin, S., et al. (eds.): Critical Care Nursing, 2nd ed. Philadelphia, W. B. Saunders, 1996.

CORE REVIEW TEST 3

3–1. A patient diagnosed with leukemia has received her first dose of chemotherapy. After chemotherapy, her serum uric acid level is 7.4 mg/dl. In addition to this laboratory finding, which of the following serum laboratory values indicate a life-threatening complication of chemotherapy?

A. Potassium = 6.0 mEq/L, phosphorus = 6.0 mg/dl, and calcium = 12.0 mg/dl.
B. Potassium = 2.5 mEq/L, phosphorus = 5.5 mg/dl, and calcium = 12.0 mg/dl.
C. Potassium = 3.0 mEq/L, phosphorus = 2.5 mg/dl, and calcium = 7.0 mg/dl.
D. Potassium = 6.0 mEq/L, phosphorus = 7.0 mg/dl, and calcium = 6.0 mg/dl.

3–2. Microembolism in the patient who has had an aortic aneurysm repair is demonstrated by

A. Myoglobinuria and decreased urine output.
B. Abdominal distention and absent bowel sounds.
C. Development of flank and groin pain.
D. Small patchy white areas on the plantar aspect of the foot.

3–3. Blood pressure control in the patient with acute aortic dissection would include which of the following?

A. Nitroprusside.
B. Dopamine.
C. Dobutamine.
D. Amrinone.

3–4. The leading cause of lung contusion is

A. Bomb blast.
B. Shotgun blast.
C. Falls from high elevations.
D. High-speed vehicular crashes.

3–5. Which of the following would be consistent with a diagnosis of hemothorax?

A. Subcutaneous emphysema, increased breath sounds.
B. Tracheal deviation away from injured side, tympany on percussion.
C. Dullness to percussion, decreased breath sounds.
D. Decreased vocal fremitus, ipsilateral hyperresonance.

3–6. When assessing a patient with blunt chest trauma, the critical care nurse should anticipate

A. The need for mechanical ventilation.
B. That severity of injury may not be obvious.
C. Development of adult respiratory distress syndrome.
D. Development of pulmonary embolus.

3–7. The preferred treatment for a self-limiting hemothorax is

A. Chest tube insertion.
B. Fluid administration.
C. Mechanical ventilation.
D. Transfusion.

3–8. An 85-year-old woman is resuscitated by CPR from a cardiopulmonary arrest. On a chest radiograph, costochondral separation is noted on the sternum bilaterally. This produces a flail chest when she breathes spontaneously; the patient is agitated and restless. What ventilatory support should be implemented for this patient?

A. Synchronized intermittent mandatory ventilation (SIMV) and positive end-expiratory pressure (PEEP).
B. Continuous mandatory ventilation (CMV).
C. Continuous positive airway pressure (CPAP).
D. Intermittent positive-pressure breathing (IPPB).

3–9. Which pulmonary capillary wedge pressure (PCWP) indicates hypovolemia?

A. 10 mm Hg.
B. 15 mm Hg.
C. 4 mm Hg.
D. 2 mm Hg.

3–10. A comatose near-drowning victim is admitted to the ICU after salt water aspiration. Initial assessment would be expected to demonstrate

A. Volume overload and hypernatremia.
B. Hypovolemia and hyponatremia.
C. Hypovolemia and hypernatremia.
D. No significant fluid and electrolyte changes.

3–11. Which of the following hematocrits indicates that blood loss is the cause of hypovolemia in a postoperative patient?

A. 54%.
B. 47%.
C. 37%.
D. 30%.

3–12. A 43-year-old patient with hemorrhage into the subarachnoid space as a result of a cerebral aneurysm is scheduled for surgery. Subarachnoid precautions for this patient include which of the following?

A. Bed rest, head of bed flat, quiet environment.
B. Head of bed elevated, anticonvulsants, vasodilators.
C. Bed rest, stool softeners, limitation of stimulation.
D. Head of bed elevated, bedside commode, fluid restriction.

3–13. Which of the following patient conditions is associated with hypomagnesemia?

A. Gastritis.
B. Colitis.
C. Pancreatitis.
D. Active ulcer disease.

3–14. The initial treatment for hypovolemic shock includes

I. Administering vasopressors to maintain blood pressure.
II. Administering crystalloid to keep pulmonary capillary wedge pressure greater than 6 and less than 15 mm Hg.
III. Elevating the legs to increase preload.
IV. Sedation to decrease tissue oxygen demands and anxiety if the systolic blood pressure is greater than 95 mm Hg.

A. I, II, and III.
B. II, III, and IV.
C. I, III, and IV.
D. I, II, and IV.

3–15. A 500-ml fluid bolus has been administered to a 28-year-old patient in hypovolemic shock who now has a blood pressure of 74/60 mm Hg. Arterial blood gas results drawn during the infusion demonstrate a pH of 7.30, PaO_2 of 88 mm Hg, $PaCO_2$ of 30 mm Hg, and HCO_3 of 20 mEq/L. The hematocrit is 35%. Which of the following would the nurse anticipate performing?

A. Administer 100 mEq of sodium bicarbonate with the fluid bolus.
B. Initiate a dopamine infusion to maintain the systolic blood pressure greater than 100 mm Hg.
C. Administer 1 unit of type-specific blood.
D. Administer a second bolus of 500 ml lactated Ringer's solution.

3–16. The most common findings in myocarditis include which of the following?

I. Preceding viral illness.
II. Palpitations.
III. Tachycardia out of proportion to fever.
IV. ECG changes similar to evolving myocardial infarction.

A. I, II, and III.
B. II, III, and IV.
C. I, III, and IV.
D. I, II, and IV.

3–17. Treatment for heart failure in a patient with myocarditis includes

I. Modified bed rest.
II. Lidocaine to suppress ventricular dysrhythmias.
III. Angiotensin converting enzyme (ACE) inhibitors to decrease afterload.
IV. Corticosteroids in the early phase of treatment.

A. I only.
B. I, II, and III.
C. I, III, and IV.
D. I and III.

3–18. Prolongation of the PR interval above 0.2 second indicates

A. Delayed sinus node firing.
B. First-degree atrioventricular block.
C. His bundle conduction delay.
D. Mobitz type II heart block.

3–19. The extent of pulmonary injury in aspiration is determined by all of the following *except*

A. pH of the aspirate.
B. Volume of the aspirate.
C. Decreased level of consciousness.
D. Size of the particles.

3–20. The most important aspect in assessing renal trauma is

A. Performing a primary survey.
B. Obtaining a complete history.
C. Performing a secondary survey.
D. Completing diagnostic testing.

3–21. A patient with a measured carboxyhemoglobin level of 40% to 60% is most likely experiencing

A. No symptoms.
B. Headache and confusion.
C. Disorientation and nausca.
D. Hallucinations and combativeness.

3–22. Carotid massage is ineffective in slowing the rate of which of the following dysrhythmias?

A. Atrial flutter.
B. Wolff-Parkinson-White reciprocating tachycardia.
C. Atrioventricular (AV) junctional rhythm.
D. Atrial tachycardia.

3–23. Surgery for acute volvulus is the treatment for

A. A telescoping of one bowel segment into the next.
B. An outpocketing of the colon lumen.
C. A colonic carcinoma.
D. A 180° twist in a bowel segment.

3–24. A patient with a subarachnoid hemorrhage has the following laboratory data. The critical care nurse would be most concerned about

A. $Paco_2$ of 36 mm Hg.
B. $Paco_2$ of 55 mm Hg.
C. Urine specific gravity of 1.018.
D. Serum sodium of 140 mEq/L.

3–25. Which of the following reactions exhibited by the family of a patient in a hyperglycemic hypertonic nonketotic (HHNK) coma are most important for the critical care nurse to remember when teaching the family about the condition?

A. Decreased sense of personal effectiveness.
B. Decreased ability to make decisions and solve problems.
C. Decreased ability to concentrate and utilize incoming information.
D. Decreased sensitivity or awareness of the environment.

3–26. A patient is admitted to the ICU after bone marrow transplant with a neutrophil count of 425/μl, and 1 hour later a fever is detected. Which of the following would be the most appropriate first action?

A. Administer broad-spectrum antibiotics.
B. Administer colony-stimulating factor.
C. Obtain blood cultures.
D. Obtain sputum cultures.

3–27. A 26-year-old man is admitted for observation after a near-drowning accident when he fell into a fast-moving river and was unable to pull himself out. In planning care for this patient, the nurse needs to be aware that freshwater drowning tends to result in

A. Hypocapnia.
B. Alkalosis.
C. Hemodilution.
D. Hemoconcentration.

3–28. The most important objective in preventing chronic aspiration in intubated patients is to prevent pneumonia. Mechanisms of prevention include use of

A. A percutaneous endogastric (PEG) tube.
B. Nasogastric suction.
C. Corticosteroid therapy.
D. Prophylactic antibiotic therapy.

3–29. A patient with a tracheostomy has been started on tube feedings through a nasogastric tube. Suctioned tracheal secretions have changed from thin white in small amounts to moderate amounts of cream-colored secretions. Which of the following assessments is the most appropriate to evaluate for regurgitation and aspiration?

A. Check for glucose in the tracheal secretions.
B. Place blue food coloring in tube feedings.
C. Obtain a chest radiograph.
D. Perform a swallowing study.

3–30. The primary reason why burn patients receive acetaminophen rather than aspirin to control fever is because aspirin may

A. Promote stress ulcer formation.
B. Produce vasodilatation.
C. Decrease renal blood flow.
D. Increase capillary permeability.

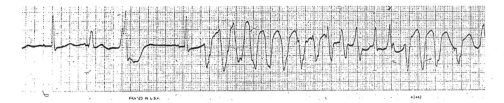

Questions 3–31 and 3–32 relate to the rhythm strip above.

3–31. The dysrhythmia indicated in the center of the lead II ECG tracing above is best described as

A. Supraventricular tachycardia.
B. Ventricular tachycardia.
C. Accelerated idioventricular rhythm.
D. Torsades des pointes.

3–32. Immediate treatment for this dysrhythmia should include administration of which medication?

A. Lidocaine.
B. Amiodarone.
C. Sotolol.
D. Magnesium.

3–33. To prevent ventricular ectopy in a post–cardiac surgical patient, the plan of care should include which of the following?

I. Maintain serum potassium level greater than 4.2 mEq/L and less than 5.0 mEq/L.
II. Maintain oxygen saturation greater than 95%.
III. Lidocaine, 1 mg/kg bolus for premature ventricular contractions greater than 6/min.
IV. Asynchronous ventricular pacing at a rate of 80 beats/min.

A. I and II.
B. I, II, and III.
C. II and III.
D. I, II, and IV.

3–34. Differences in physical findings between an open pneumothorax and a tension pneumothorax include

A. Direction of tracheal deviation.
B. Tympany.
C. Subcutaneous emphysema.
D. Decreased vocal fremitus.

3–35. The critical care nurse should anticipate that initial treatment of a tension pneumothorax would consist of

A. Insertion of a chest tube.
B. Insertion of a large-gauge needle.
C. Bronchoscopy.
D. Thoracoscopy.

3–36. When caring for a patient with acute intracranial hemorrhage, the critical care nurse will

A. Administer long-acting sedatives to prevent restlessness and agitation.
B. Administer platelet-aggregating agents to prevent bleeding.
C. Maintain head of the bed elevation at less than 15°.
D. Provide a quiet, dimly lit environment.

3–37. For patients with bowel infarction, early institution of enteral nutrition is preferred whenever possible to

A. Eliminate pathogenic organisms.
B. Enhance the immune protection of the gut.
C. Promote macrophage phagocytosis.
D. Dilute bacterial endotoxin.

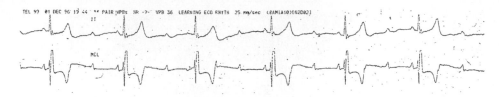

3–38. The definitive treatment for an alert 80-year-old patient with the dysrhythmia noted above is

A. Transcutaneous pacemaker immediately available.
B. Administer atropine boluses of 0.5 mg IV push whenever the patient becomes symptomatic.
C. Equipment for transvenous pacemaker insertion available at the bedside.
D. Permanent pacemaker implantation.

3–39. Treatment of supraventricular tachycardia includes which of the following medications?

A. Lidocaine.
B. Procainamide.
C. Bretyllium.
D. Verapamil.

3–40. In the patient with acute renal failure, signs of hypervolemia include

A. Increased pulmonary artery pressure (PAP), increased cardiac output/cardiac index (CO/CI), paradoxical pulse.
B. Increased PAP, increased CO/CI, widened pulse pressure.
C. Decreased PAP, decreased CO/CI, paradoxical pulse.
D. Increased PAP, decreased CO/CI, widened pulse pressure.

3–41. A burn patient in the postresuscitation phase is receiving enteral feedings in addition to an oral diet. The nurse notes increasing polyuria, and the patient complains of thirst. The nurse needs to

A. Keep meticulous records of intake and output.
B. Obtain a fingerstick blood sample to determine the patient's serum glucose level.
C. Assess the patient's diet for excess salt intake.
D. Send urine specimen for culture and sensitivity.

3–42. When a patient has developed an atrial tachycardia, the physician orders carotid massage. The nurse should first

A. Apply firm pressure to the carotid artery in a circular motion.
B. Auscultate the carotid artery before applying any pressure.
C. Massage both right and left carotid arteries.
D. Apply firm direct pressure first on one side and then on the other.

3–43. In reviewing the medications administered to a patient with an automatic implantable cardioverter-defibrillator (AICD), the nurse knows which of the following medications will increase the efficiency of the AICD by decreasing the energy requirements for internal defibrillation?

A. Sotolol.
B. Amiodarone.
C. Verapamil.
D. Procainamide.

3–44. In a patient with an implantable cardioverter-defibrillator (ICD) that fires appropriately during a tachycardia episode, but fails to convert the dysrhythmia, the nurse performs direct-current countershock. Which of the following evaluates the potential cause of the ICD failure?

    I. Chest radiograph.
    II. 12 lead ECG.
    III. Review of current medications.
    IV. Application of the magnet over the ICD generator.

    A. I and II.
    B. I, II, and III.
    C. I, II, and IV.
    D. II, III, and IV.

3–45. A patient with a chest tube for pneumothorax is weaned off the ventilator over a few days, is extubated, and then increases his activity level. He continues to have an air leak, however. What intervention could be implemented for this problem before his discharge?

    A. Use a Heimlich valve and drainage bag.
    B. Return weekly for evacuation of air and fluid.
    C. Pleurodesis.
    D. Thoracotomy to repair the leak.

3–46. Which of the following would be consistent with a diagnosis of pneumothorax?

    A. Subcutaneous emphysema, dullness to percussion.
    B. Decreased vocal fremitus, equal chest expansion.
    C. Ipsilateral hyperresonance, decreased breath sounds.
    D. Tracheal deviation, increased breath sounds.

3–47. What are the two most common processes involved in patients in acute respiratory failure?

    A. Pulmonary edema, adult respiratory distress syndrome.
    B. Neuromuscular disease, chronic obstructive pulmonary disease.
    C. Increased lung vascular water, impaired ventilation.
    D. Pneumothorax, cerebrovascular accident.

3–48. A 25-year-old patient is admitted after an automobile crash. Neurodiagnostic studies show a basal skull fracture of the middle fossa. Assessment of the patient reveals both halo and Battle's signs. The critical care nurse is most concerned about the possibility of

    A. Spinal cord injury.
    B. Jugular venous compression.
    C. Seizures.
    D. Meningitis.

3–49. A 72-year-old patient was admitted 5 days ago to the ICU with an acute myocardial infarction. His ECG shows new onset of atrial fibrillation. The patient is now complaining of acute abdominal pain that is different from the initial chest pain. The abdomen is firm. Bowel sounds are absent. Which of the following operative therapies can be expected?

    A. Pyloroplasty and vagotomy.
    B. Temporary ileostomy.
    C. Mesenteric embolectomy.
    D. Transverse colostomy.

3–50. An ICU patient with severe hypoglycemia should receive

    A. Two 8-ounce glasses of orange juice.
    B. A 50-ml bolus of 50% dextrose IV.
    C. Glucagon, 1 mg, IM or SQ.
    D. A 50-ml bolus of 5% dextrose IV.

3–51. A patient who has had a bone marrow transplant has produced 900 ml of green, watery, guaiac-positive diarrhea during the past 12 hours. The most appropriate intervention is

A. Initiating fluid replacement.
B. Avoiding analgesics.
C. Instituting broad-spectrum antibiotic therapy.
D. Stopping immunosuppression therapy.

3–52. In evaluating a burn patient with progressive chemical tracheobronchitis after resuscitation the nurse observes for

A. Increasing dynamic compliance.
B. Decreasing ventilation/perfusion shunt.
C. Increasing minute ventilation.
D. Decreasing pulmonary edema.

3–53. A septic patient is not responding to crystalloid resuscitation and remains hypotensive. An infusion of dopamine and antibiotic coverage is initiated. The patient's ECG shows a widening QRS complex. The most likely cause for this ECG finding is

A. Reduced venous return.
B. Myocardial ischemia.
C. Dopamine side effect.
D. Anaphylaxis.

3–54. The care plan for nursing management of a patient with hypertrophic cardiomyopathy after percutaneous laser myoplasty should include monitoring which of the following potential problems?

  I. Potential for cardiac dysrhythmias.
 II. Potential for septal rupture.
III. Potential for decreased cardiac output.
 IV. Potential for cerebrovascular accident.

A. I and II.
B. I, II, and III.
C. II, III, and IV.
D. I, II, III, and IV.

3–55. Education of the patient undergoing dynamic cardiomyoplasty regarding the timing of electrical stimulation of the latissimus dorsi muscle includes which of the following information?

A. Electrical stimulation begins 2 weeks after surgery.
B. Electrical stimulation begins on the first postoperative day.
C. Electrical stimulation begins on the third postoperative day.
D. Electrical stimulation begins when the incision is healed and the patient is hemodynamically stable.

Questions 3–56 and 3–57 relate to the following situation.

3–56. A 76-year-old woman with emphysema has been intubated for 3 weeks secondary to pneumonia. Orders have been written to wean her from the ventilator. She has had two previous failed weaning attempts, one of which progressed to extubation. Which of the following are predictors that this attempt will be successful?

A. She is psychologically prepared and cooperative.
B. She is able to triple her minute ventilation.
C. Her spontaneous tidal volume is less than 5 ml/kg.
D. Her respiratory rate is greater than 35 breaths/min.

3–57. Which of the following weaning methods might be most successful for this patient?

A. T-tube trial.
B. Pressure support ventilation.
C. Intermittent mandatory ventilation.
D. Extubation.

3–58. A patient whose chest struck the steering wheel in a high-speed motor vehicle crash has a respiratory rate of 40 breaths/min with coarse rales throughout all lung fields. ECG findings include right-axis deviation and right bundle branch block. Blood pressure is 80 mm Hg by palpation and a holosystolic murmur is auscultated. These findings suggest

    A. Septal rupture.
    B. Mitral valve rupture.
    C. Aortic valve rupture.
    D. Tricuspid valve rupture.

3–59. The diet for a patient with acute renal failure usually consists of

    A. Increased protein, decreased sodium, increased calories.
    B. Decreased protein, increased sodium, decreased calories.
    C. Increased protein, increased sodium, decreased calories.
    D. Decreased protein, decreased sodium, increased calories.

3–60. In acute renal failure, treatment to correct metabolic acidosis is begun when the patient's serum bicarbonate level drops below

    A. 30 mEq/L.
    B. 25 mEq/L.
    C. 20 mEq/L.
    D. 15 mEq/L.

3–61. In the emergency department, a 27-year-old patient presents with gunshot wounds in the right upper quadrant/flank area of the abdomen. The patient's abdomen is rigid with rebound tenderness. Bowel sounds are absent. Which of the following are most likely to be injured?

    A. Lungs and spleen.
    B. Pancreas and duodenum.
    C. Liver and gallbladder.
    D. Stomach and descending colon.

3–62. A clinically stable patient with chronic obstructive pulmonary disease (COPD) is being weaned off the ventilator. Current settings are FIO_2 of 30%, synchronized intermittent mandatory ventilation of 2 with a spontaneous rate of 20 breaths/min, positive end-expiratory pressure of 8, and spontaneous tidal volume of 350 ml. Arterial blood gas results show pH, 7.38; $PaCO_2$, 52 mm Hg; PaO_2, 38 mm Hg; SaO_2, 70%; and HCO_3, 32 mEq/L. What is the most likely explanation for these arterial blood gas analysis results?

    A. Respiratory alkalosis.
    B. Venous blood gas.
    C. Hypoventilation.
    D. Cardiac failure.

3–63. A 73-year-old man with a diagnosis of chronic obstructive pulmonary disease (COPD) was admitted yesterday in acute respiratory failure. He is intubated, on a ventilator, and sedated to decrease work of breathing and oxygen needs. He has been severely disabled for 5 years, is on home oxygen, and requires total assistance with activities of daily living. His wife has been largely responsible for his care, with infrequent assistance by a daughter-in-law. His wife has not visited since she brought him to the hospital and has not called. In planning care for this patient, the most appropriate intervention would be to

    A. Hold a family conference.
    B. Call the daughter-in-law and ask her to visit.
    C. Ask the chaplain to visit the wife.
    D. Call the wife and ask how she wants to be involved in his care.

3–64. Pursed-lip breathing assists patients in all of the following except that it does *not*

    A. Slow the respiratory rate.
    B. Increase airway pressure.
    C. Mobilize secretions.
    D. Relieve dyspnea.

3–65. The patient drains 200 ml in 1 hour from a mediastinal chest tube inserted after repair of a ventricular stab wound. The physician orders the following laboratory tests: prothrombin time, partial thromboplastin time, fibrinogen, and platelets. Which of the following volume replacement orders is most appropriate while awaiting the results of these laboratory tests?

A. Autotransfuse mediastinal shed blood greater than 200 ml within 4 hours.
B. Transfuse 1 unit of packed red blood cells.
C. Transfuse 1 unit of fresh frozen plasma.
D. Infuse plasmanate, 500 ml.

3–66. Which of the following indicates an abnormal resting ankle-brachial index suggestive of advanced occlusive disease?

A. 1.2
B. 0.90.
C. 0.70.
D. 0.40.

3–67. During the first 8 hours after aortic surgery, assessments of graft patency should include assessment of

   I. Renal function.
  II. Distal perfusion.
 III. Signs of infection.
  IV. Motor and sensory function.

A. II and III.
B. I, II, and III.
C. II, III, and IV.
D. I, II, and IV.

3–68. The usual rate of urokinase infusion for thrombolysis of an occluded peripheral vessel is

A. 1000 to 4000 IU/min.
B. 10,000 to 40,000 IU/min.
C. 100,000 to 400,000 IU/min.
D. Urokinase is given by bolus, not as an infusion.

3–69. A shift to the right in the oxyhemoglobin dissociation curve indicates

A. Hemoglobin releases oxygen more readily.
B. Hemoglobin becomes fully saturated.
C. Hemoglobin binds with oxygen more tightly.
D. A respiratory alkalosis.

3–70. After steering wheel trauma to the chest, the patient may experience obstructive shock related to

A. Flail chest.
B. Tension pneumothorax.
C. Bronchial edema.
D. Myocardial infarction.

3–71. After aortic surgery the patient is on a nitroglycerin drip to maintain his systolic blood pressure between 100 and 160 mm Hg and mean arterial pressure of 75 to 95 mm Hg. The purpose of the nitroglycerin infusion is to reduce the potential for

A. Graft rupture.
B. Arterial spasm.
C. Alteration in tissue perfusion.
D. Embolization.

3–72. Which of the following characterizes status epilepticus?

A. Generalized seizure activity without regaining consciousness.
B. Brief loss of contact with the environment.
C. Akinetic movements.
D. Myoclonic movements.

3–73. An important objective of early enteral nutrition in the patient who has sustained abdominal trauma is to

A. Inhibit bile secretion.
B. Prevent bacterial translocation.
C. Avoid glutamate exposure.
D. Stimulate the hypermetabolic response.

3–74. Occlusion of the right coronary artery causes infarction of the

A. Anterior wall.
B. Anteroseptal wall.
C. Lateral wall.
D. Inferior wall.

3–75. In diabetes insipidus, select the hormone affected and the resulting changes seen in urine output and urine specific gravity.

Hormone	Urine Output	Urine Specific Gravity
A. Antidiuretic hormone	Increased	Decreased
B. Glucagon	Decreased	Increased
C. Insulin	Increased	Increased
D. Aldosterone	Decreased	Decreased

3–76. The value of continuous ST segment monitoring in a patient who has had open-heart surgery is that

A. It assists in the differentiation of supraventricular from ventricular ectopy.
B. It can help differentiate surgical pain from ischemic pain.
C. It provides cost savings from the elimination of the need for 12-lead ECGs.
D. It is invaluable in demonstrating graft patency for research purposes.

3–77. Which of the following are diagnostic of acute myocardial infarction?

A. CPK-MB, 1.0 μ/L.
B. CK total, 100 μ/L.
C. CK-MB isoforms ratio of 1:1.
D. CK-MB2/MB1 ratio of 2.0.

3–78. A 28-year-old woman 2 hours post partum is transferred from the obstetrics unit. She is dyspneic, using accessory muscles, hypotensive, confused, and coughing up small amounts of pink-tinged sputum. She has bilateral inspiratory and expiratory crackles. Her vital signs are blood pressure of 110/70 mm Hg, heart rate of 110 beats/min, and respiratory rate of 35 breaths/min. She has the following blood gas levels on 50% oxygen: pH, 7.52; $PaCO_2$, 30 mm Hg; PaO_2, 60 mm Hg; and SaO_2, 90%. Her most likely diagnosis is

A. Pulmonary thromboembolus.
B. Cardiomyopathy.
C. Respiratory distress syndrome.
D. Status asthmaticus.

3–79. A 6-year-old boy is transferred to the ICU after an industrial accident in which he inhaled unknown substances. Initial arterial blood gases drawn from an arterial line while the patient was on mechanical ventilation with an FIO_2 of 1.0 were pH, 7.25; $PaCO_2$, 40 mm Hg; PaO_2, 40 mm Hg; and SaO_2, 72%. A chest radiograph shows bilateral infiltrates. The most appropriate initial treatment for this patient would be to

A. Initiate positive end-expiratory pressure (PEEP).
B. Institute hyperbaric oxygen.
C. Institute negative-pressure ventilation.
D. Perform bronchoscopy.

3–80. A patient remains in the ICU after experiencing several bouts of respiratory failure associated with septic shock. The patient now complains of severe right upper quadrant pain. A possible cause may be

A. Cholecystitis.
B. Stress ulcer.
C. Diverticulitis.
D. Pleuritis.

3–81. Acute hemodialysis is initiated to treat acute renal failure when the following laboratory values are reached:

Blood Urea Nitrogen	Creatinine	Creatinine Clearance
A. 60 mg/dl	5 mg/dl	25 ml/min
B. 90 mg/dl	8 mg/dl	15 ml/min
C. 120 mg/dl	11 mg/dl	5 ml/min
D. 150 mg/dl	14 mg/dl	0 ml/min

3–82. Echocardiography is useful in patients with nonspecific ECG changes associated with myocardial infarction because

A. Non–Q wave myocardial infarctions are visualized as thin, dyskinetic areas that are highly mobile during systole.
B. Old myocardial infarctions are visualized as thickened areas of scar tissue.
C. It visualizes new infarcts as thickened, dyskinetic areas.
D. Left ventricular aneurysms are visualized as thick-walled, dyskinetic areas that are immobile during systole.

3–83. A patient in the CCU for acute myocardial infarction develops chest pain, syncope, and hypotension. A new holosystolic murmur is noted. A pulmonary artery catheter is inserted. The pulmonary capillary wedge pressure (PCWP) shows a large "v" wave at 30 mm Hg. The right ventricular blood gas sample oxygen saturation is 85%. The patient's condition and physical findings are consistent with a diagnosis of

A. Cardiogenic shock.
B. Right ventricular infarction.
C. Papillary muscle rupture.
D. Ventricular septal rupture.

3–84. Phenytoin (Dilantin) is ordered for a patient with generalized seizures. In planning care for this patient, the critical care nurse knows that the medication must not be abruptly stopped or withdrawn because

A. Gingival hyperplasia can result.
B. Peripheral neuropathy can develop.
C. Blood dyscrasias will develop.
D. Status epilepticus may occur.

3–85. A patient with a stress ulcer can safely resume use of

A. Ethanol.
B. H_2 blockers.
C. Salicylates.
D. Corticosteroids.

Questions 3–86 through 3–88 refer to the following situation.

3–86. A 76-year-old woman was admitted to the ICU 6 days ago in respiratory distress after a head injury. She was intubated for deteriorating oxygenation and has been on controlled mandatory ventilation with a respiratory rate of 18, FIo_2 of 50%, and PEEP of 8. In determining whether she is ready to be weaned, what parameters should be evaluated?

A. Hemodynamic status and arterial blood gases.
B. Chest radiograph and hemodynamic status.
C. Arterial blood gases and spirometry.
D. Pulmonary function tests and hemodynamic status.

3–87. Her weaning parameters are tidal volume of 200 ml, spontaneous respiratory rate of 33 breaths/min, minute ventilation of 6.6 L/min, vital capacity of 500 ml, mandatory voluntary ventilation (MVV) of 8.9 L/min, and maximum inspiratory pressure (MIP) of 12 cm H_2O. What should be the next step in the weaning process?

A. T-tube trial.
B. Increase activity level to get her into a chair.
C. Decrease the mechanical ventilation rate.
D. Transfer her to a weaning unit/ hospital.

3–88. A week later, she is on SIMV 6 with a spontaneous rate of 25 breaths/min, PEEP of 5, spontaneous tidal volume of 250 ml, vital capacity of 800 ml, MVV of 9.5 L/min, MIP of 18 cm H_2O, and FIO_2 of 45%. Her arterial blood gases are pH, 7.36; $PaCO_2$, 48 mm Hg; PaO_2, 68 mm Hg; and SaO_2, 92%. She gets out of bed twice daily with assistance, but her saturation drops at that time, requiring an increase in her FIO_2. What would be the appropriate next step in the weaning process?

   A. T-tube trial.
   B. Decrease the mechanical ventilatory rate.
   C. Ambulate the patient.
   D. Consider transfer to a weaning unit/facility.

3–89. Papillary muscle rupture is a complication most frequently associated with myocardial infarctions located in the

   A. Anterior and posterior wall.
   B. Inferior and posterior wall.
   C. Anterolateral wall.
   D. Inferoposterior and posterolateral wall.

3–90. In the septic patient, nutrition becomes a priority

   A. During the initial phase.
   B. Once the patient is hemodynamically stable.
   C. Once the adynamic ileus resolves.
   D. After the patient has been on antibiotics 48 hours.

3–91. Permissive hypercapnia is a mode of ventilation that would *not* be appropriate for patients with

   A. Asthma.
   B. Respiratory distress syndrome.
   C. Acute lung injury.
   D. Acute head injury.

3–92. A 48-year-old man with respiratory distress syndrome secondary to sepsis is intubated and placed on a ventilator. Arterial blood gases obtained on 100% oxygen are pH of 7.32, $PaCO_2$ of 55 mm Hg, PaO_2 of 37 mm Hg, and SaO_2 of 70%. What would be the most appropriate intervention to implement at this point?

   A. Administer blood.
   B. Institute positive end-expiratory pressure (PEEP).
   C. Administer inotropic agents.
   D. Administer fluid therapy.

3–93. Which of the following medications may be used as an alternative antiplatelet agent for patients with myocardial infarction who cannot take aspirin?

   A. Dipyridamole, warfarin.
   B. Ticlodipine, low-molecular-weight heparin.
   C. Dipyridamole, ticlodipine.
   D. Enteric-coated aspirin.

3–94. When acute anterior myocardial infarction causes third-degree atrioventricular (AV) block, the block is usually

   A. Transient and pacemaker insertion is unnecessary.
   B. Permanent and permanent pacemaker implant is necessary.
   C. Transient but often requires transcutaneous pacing.
   D. Transient but often requires insertion of a temporary transvenous pacemaker.

3–95. In a patient with meningitis, an intraventricular intracranial pressure (ICP) of 22 mm Hg and a calculated cerebral perfusion pressure (CCP) of 55 mm Hg indicate a

   A. Normal intraventricular pressure.
   B. Mildly increased intraventricular pressure.
   C. Moderately increased intraventricular pressure.
   D. Severely increased intraventricular pressure.

3–96. A 24-year-old patient is admitted to the neurosurgical ICU after surgical evacuation of an epidural hematoma that developed after a traumatic head injury. In report, the critical care nurse learns that the patient's intracranial pressure is elevated. Which of the following intracranial waveforms would the nurse likely observe on the monitor as a result of increased intracranial pressure?

A. A waves.
B. B waves.
C. C waves.
D. D waves.

3–97. When planning to check for the presence of occult blood in gastric drainage or stool, which of the following could cause a false-negative result on guaiac testing?

A. Cimetidine.
B. Aspirin.
C. Iron supplements.
D. Antacids.

3–98. Which of the following is the most effective treatment for a patient with an anterior wall myocardial infarction with fine rales at both bases?

A. Discontinue weaning of nitroglycerin drip and increase rate of administration to previous level.
B. Place the patient on fluid restriction.
C. Place patient on a sodium-restricted diet.
D. Perform a 12-lead ECG.

3–99. During volume replacement for septic shock, the guide to fluid requirements is based on maintaining

A. Mean arterial pressure of 60 mm Hg or greater.
B. Pulmonary artery wedge pressure of 18 mm Hg or greater.
C. Urine output greater than 30 ml/hr.
D. Lactate levels less than 3 mmol/dl.

3–100. Assessment of an ICU patient reveals a change in the level of consciousness, headache, fatigue, and weakness along with hyponatremia and elevated urine osmolality. Select the most likely nursing diagnosis.

A. Fluid volume excess related to inability to excrete water.
B. Fluid volume deficit related to inability to conserve water.
C. Alteration in thought processes related to confusion and ICU psychosis.
D. Impaired gas exchange–related hypervolemia and bed rest.

3–101. To prevent acute rejection after organ transplantation, it would be most appropriate for the nurse to

A. Ensure ABO blood group compatibility between donor and recipient.
B. Ensure negative lymphocyte cross-match between donor and recipient.
C. Administer an agent to halt the cellular immune response.
D. Administer an agent to halt the humoral immune response.

3–102. The Glasgow Coma Scale (GCS) assesses the patient's best

A. Sensory, motor, and verbal responses.
B. Eye opening, motor response, and verbal response.
C. Motor response, eye opening, and vital signs.
D. Sensory response, motor response, and eye opening.

3–103. A right precordial ECG should be obtained on patients with ECG changes indicating a(n)

A. Anterior wall myocardial infarction.
B. Anteroseptal myocardial infarction.
C. Inferior wall myocardial infarction.
D. Lateral wall myocardial infarction.

3–104. Which of the following agents are administered to prevent thrombosis and reinfarction in the patient with acute myocardial infarction?

    I. Aspirin.
    II. Heparin.
    III. Nitroglycerin.
    IV. Angiotensin-converting enzyme (ACE) inhibitors.

    A. I and II.
    B. II and III.
    C. III and IV.
    D. I and IV.

3–105. A pulmonary wedge pressure changes dramatically from one reading to the next 2 hours later, with minimal clinical changes. What would be the appropriate initial step for the nurse to take when troubleshooting this change?

    A. Inspect the system for leaks or blood/air.
    B. Obtain a chest radiograph.
    C. Check the skin to tip distance of the pulmonary artery catheter.
    D. Check the level of the transducer.

3–106. Pneumothoraces that occur in patients with respiratory distress syndrome on mechanical ventilation are secondary to

    A. Alpha$_1$-antitrypsin deficiency.
    B. Increased mean airway pressure.
    C. Coexistent chronic obstructive pulmonary disease (COPD).
    D. Atelectasis.

3–107. Isolation for tuberculosis should be considered until

    A. The chest radiograph shows the lung has cleared.
    B. Six weeks of drug therapy has been completed.
    C. There has been a clinical and bacterial response to drug therapy.
    D. The sputum culture is negative.

3–108. Which of the following is the appropriate treatment for headache in a patient on a nitroglycerin drip for anginal relief?

    A. Continue titrating the nitroglycerin until chest pain is relieved.
    B. Reduce the nitroglycerin, administer an analgesic, and then increase the nitroglycerin.
    C. Stop titration, administer analgesic, and then continue titration of nitroglycerin.
    D. Premedicate with 2 mg of morphine for each increase in nitroglycerin.

3–109. Enteral nutrition should be incorporated early in the care plan during acute gastrointestinal bleeding to reduce the risk of

    A. Constipation.
    B. Hypometabolism.
    C. Mucosal hyperplasia.
    D. Sepsis.

3–110. A septic patient receiving parenteral nutrition should receive what percent of the total caloric requirements from lipids?

    A. 1.
    B. 5.
    C. 10.
    D. 20.

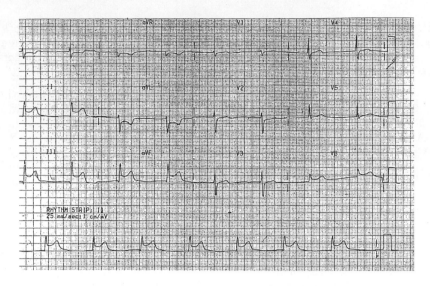

3–111. A patient is admitted to the coronary care unit after percutaneous transluminal coronary angioplasty complicated by coronary air embolism. He is on a dopamine infusion at 8 μg/kg/min, lidocaine infusion at 2 mg/min, and nitroglycerin infusion at 82 μg/min. Blood pressure is 96/60 mm Hg, and the heart rate is 119 beats/min with occasional premature ventricular contractions. Continuous ST segment monitoring is being performed. He is on 4 L of nasal oxygen, and oxygen saturation is 98%. Which of the following interventions is appropriate at this time?

A. Obtain a 12-lead ECG.
B. Maintain the patient in a left lateral position.
C. Place the patient on a 100% FIo_2 face mask.
D. Decrease dopamine infusion to 6 μg/kg/min.

3–112. The electrocardiogram above was obtained on a 72-year-old woman. The cardiologist is in attendance and states that the patient is not a candidate for thrombolytic therapy or emergent percutaneous transluminal coronary angioplasty. Current blood pressure is 84/66 mm Hg and the patient is disoriented. Which of the following interventions should the nurse anticipate at this time?

A. Emergent coronary artery bypass surgery.
B. Transthoracic pacemaker placement.
C. Administration of atropine, 0.5 mg IV.
D. Placement of a transvenous atrioventricular sequential pacemaker.

Questions 3–113 and 3–114 relate to the following situation.

3–113. A morbidly obese woman is admitted to the ICU after gastric bypass surgery. What might the nurse obtain to assist in this patient's pulmonary hygiene?

A. Suction equipment.
B. Abdominal support.
C. Nasal trumpet.
D. Arterial blood gas analysis.

3–114. Her pulse oximeter reading decreases to 89%, and her respirations increase to 26 breaths/min and are shallow. The physician orders an arterial blood gas analysis. What results would you expect?

A. Acidosis, hypocarbia, hypoxemia
B. Alkalosis, hypocarbia, hypoxemia
C. Acidosis, hypercarbia, hypoxemia
D. Alkalosis, hypercarbia, hypoxemia

3–115. The admission database contains the following information: total cholesterol, 240 mg/dl; HDL cholesterol, 25 mg/dl; one pack per day smoker; and blood pressure, 170/90 mm Hg before administration of thrombolytic therapy. The patient has been identified as unmotivated to make any risk factor modification changes and has made statements that he does not have heart disease. Which of the following interventions should be performed to motivate the patient to control the identified risk factors?

A. Focus all educational efforts on family members because the patient is clearly in denial.
B. Point out the concrete evidence of coronary artery disease such as the ECG, elevated total cholesterol level, and low HDL cholesterol level to the patient to make him recognize the danger of coronary compromise.
C. Use repetition to point out modifiable risk factors such as smoking, control of hypertension, and dietary changes during each patient contact.
D. Reinforce the dietary and non-smoking accomplishments and changes the patient is already accommodating while in the hospital.

3–116. Which of the following outcomes demonstrates appropriate patient care management during an 8-hour shift for a patient who has 2-mm ST segment elevation in lead V_1; Q waves in leads II, III, and aVF; systolic blood pressure of 90 mm Hg; and total creatine kinase of 600 μ/L?

I. Nitroglycerin infusion with systolic pressure maintained greater than 90 mm Hg.
II. Disappearance of Q waves in leads II, III, and aVF.
III. Intravenous fluid administration maintains systolic blood pressure greater than 90 mm Hg.

A. I only.
B. II only.
C. III only.
D. I and II.

3–117. Which of the following symptoms may occur in both Prinzmetal's angina and unstable angina?

I. ST segment elevation during pain episodes.
II. Angina at rest.
III. Worsening of chest pain during beta blocker use.
IV. Chest pain that occurs without identifiable stimuli.

A. I and II.
B. I, II, and III.
C. II, III, and IV.
D. I, II, and IV.

3–118. Which of the following interventions should the critical care nurse anticipate for a traumatic brain injured patient with diabetes insipidus?

A. Administration of a 10% glucose solution and a loop diuretic.
B. Administration of intravenous fluids and antidiuretic hormone.
C. Administration of a hypertonic saline solution and a loop diuretic.
D. Administration of antidiuretic hormone and fluid restriction.

3–119. Measures to improve cardiac function in the elderly patient in septic shock may include

A. Inotropic agents.
B. Vasopressors.
C. Hypertonic fluids.
D. Restricted fluids.

3–120. After the insertion of femoral access for continuous renal replacement therapy, the patient complains of sudden pain in the abdomen and back. The nurse should assess for the presence of the following:

A. Chvostek's sign.
B. Grey Turner's sign.
C. Trousseau's sign.
D. Kernig's sign.

3–121. A patient's bleeding from a duodenal ulcer has not responded to conventional therapy over the past 10 days. Recommended surgical treatment is

A. Mesenteric embolectomy.
B. Temporary ileostomy.
C. Transverse colostomy.
D. Pyloroplasty and vagotomy.

Questions 3–122 through 3–124 refer to the following situation.

3–122. An 87-year-old man is admitted from a retirement home. His symptoms are confusion, tachycardia, tachypnea, dyspnea, productive cough of yellow-colored purulent sputum, and temperature greater than 101°F. He reports having a cold last week and not feeling well ever since. His symptoms and history would be consistent with

A. Pulmonary embolus.
B. Community-acquired pneumonia.
C. Noncardiogenic pulmonary edema.
D. Congestive heart failure.

3–123. The patient is placed on an antibiotic and treated with fluids, antipyretics, and oxygen. After 48 hours, he is still having fever and chills and producing large amounts of purulent sputum. His chest radiograph shows patchy infiltrates throughout all lung fields. His oxygenation has decreased sufficiently so that he now requires intubation and mechanical ventilation. What is the most likely cause of his deterioration?

A. Septic shock.
B. Pulmonary embolus.
C. Superinfection.
D. Resistant microorganism.

3–124. In doing initial planning for his eventual discharge, what factor might affect his return to the retirement home?

A. His methacillin-resistant *Staphylococcus aureus* infection.
B. His financial status.
C. His ability to perform activities of daily living.
D. His oxygen needs after discharge.

3–125. Of the choices below, the most critical laboratory test to obtain during admission assessment that is likely to also point to the cause of an episode of diabetic ketoacidosis is a(n)

A. Anion gap.
B. Chloride.
C. Complete blood cell count.
D. Amylase.

3–126. A 67-year-old man with chronic emphysema with hypoxemia (PaO_2 = 60 mm Hg) is scheduled for surgery. Admission serum laboratory values show elevated red blood cell count (RBC), elevated hemoglobin, and normal platelet count. These laboratory values are suggestive of

A. Polycythemia vera.
B. Overproduction of erythropoietin in kidneys.
C. Underproduction of erythropoietin in kidneys.
D. Idiopathic thrombocytopenic purpura.

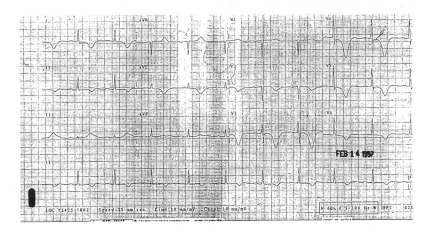

FEB 1 1997

3–127. In considering ECG changes associated with angina occurring in a patient at rest, the nurse knows that

   A. ST segment elevation occurring in fewer than three leads is not diagnostic.
   B. ST segment depression is more common in stable than in unstable angina.
   C. ST segment elevation is more common in stable than in unstable angina.
   D. ST segment elevation associated with Q waves is a symptom of chronic stable angina.

3–128. What criteria consistent with a diagnosis of unstable angina are present in the ECG above taken during an episode of chest pain in a 72-year-old man?

   A. Presence of first-degree atrioventricular block.
   B. Presence of Q waves in V_{1-2}.
   C. T-wave inversion in anterior and lateral leads.
   D. Absence of specific changes in ST segment, QRS complex, or T waves.

3–129. In formulating a care plan for a patient with unstable angina, patients with which of the following conditions need special self-assessment instructions because they frequently do not experience chest pain?

   I. Diabetes mellitus.
   II. Scleroderma.
   III. Chronic renal failure.
   IV. Cardiac transplant.

   A. I and II.
   B. II and III.
   C. III and IV.
   D. I and IV.

3–130. A patient with resolving sepsis, stable vital signs, and adequate urine output demonstrates a consistent mild elevation in blood urea nitrogen. To correct this condition, the patient receives

   A. Electrolyte supplements.
   B. Nutritional supplements.
   C. Diuretic therapy.
   D. Fluid therapy.

3–131. The nurse would plan for an emergent percutaneous transluminal coronary angioplasty in a patient with unstable angina when the

    I. Patient is stable on pharmacologic therapy.
    II. ECG demonstrates worsening ischemia.
    III. Patient exhibits symptoms of worsening failure.
    IV. Patient has recurrent or refractory ischemia.

    A. I, II, and III.
    B. II, III, and IV.
    C. I, III, and IV.
    D. I, II, III, and IV.

3–132. A patient with an acute subdural hematoma who has a depressed level of consciousness develops sustained, rapid, regular, and deep respirations. The critical care nurse knows that this patient is most likely experiencing

    A. Hydrocephalus.
    B. Transtentorial (uncal) herniation.
    C. Tonsillar herniation.
    D. Vasospasm.

3–133. A patient who has sustained multiple trauma is stabilized and on a ventilator. The patient's gastric aspirate has a pH of 1.8. Which of the following is most likely to infect this patient?

    A. Gram-negative organisms.
    B. Gram-positive organisms.
    C. Fungal organisms.
    D. Oral microflora.

Questions 3–134 and 3–135 relate to the following situation.

3–134. A 68-year-old woman is admitted to the ICU in status asthmaticus. She is on 30% oxygen by heated nebulizer. What signs and symptoms would be expected on physical examination?

    A. Rales bilaterally, pulmonary edema.
    B. Wheezing bilaterally, increased respiratory rate, accessory muscle use.
    C. Wheezing bilaterally, thick green mucus.
    D. Rhonchi, accessory muscle use.

3–135. The patient is intubated and placed on a ventilator. She requires high pressures to provide an adequate tidal volume and continues to have stiff lungs with decreased breath sounds, despite maximal bronchodilation therapy intravenously and by inhaler. What intervention might be considered at this point?

    A. Inhaled nitric oxide.
    B. Inverse ratio ventilation.
    C. Permissive hypercapnia.
    D. Pressure support ventilation.

3–136. Immediate pharmacologic therapy for unstable angina consists of administration of

    A. Sublingual nitroglycerin.
    B. Intravenous nitroglycerin.
    C. Heparin.
    D. Morphine sulfate.

3–137. Constant moderate bleeding is noted at the sheath insertion site in a patient 30 minutes after sheath removal for percutaneous transluminal coronary angioplasty (PTCA) with stent insertion. The most effective initial intervention to control bleeding is to apply

    A. Manual pressure proximal to the skin insertion site.
    B. Manual pressure directly over the skin insertion site.
    C. Manual pressure distal to the skin insertion site.
    D. A 5-lb sandbag to the site.

3–138. A patient with chest pain demonstrates symmetric T-wave inversion and 1-mm ST segment elevation in leads V_2 and V_3. The patient is given one aspirin tablet. The most appropriate medication the patient should receive next is

A. Sublingual nitroglycerin spray.
B. Heparin, 2500 units IV bolus.
C. Tissue plasminogen activator, 60 mg in 1 hour.
D. Streptokinase, 1.5 million IU over 1 hour.

3–139. Optimal response to treatment of septic shock will result in a cardiac index that is

A. 25% less than normal.
B. Within normal range.
C. 25% greater than normal.
D. 50% greater than normal.

3–140. Which of the following is related to prolonged hypophosphatemia?

A. Hypoxia.
B. Ataxia.
C. Bleeding.
D. Fatigue.

3–141. When performing oral care and suctioning an intubated patient, the nurse should wear gloves on both hands because of the risk of

A. Pneumonia.
B. Herpetic whitlow.
C. Hepatitis.
D. Aspiration.

3–142. Risk factors for venous thrombosis include all of the following *except*

A. Venous stasis.
B. Increased blood coagulability.
C. Anemia.
D. Damage to the vessel wall.

3–143. What is the advantage of a pulmonary angiogram over a ventilation/perfusion scan for pulmonary embolism?

A. It is noninvasive.
B. There is less chance of an allergic reaction to intravenous dye.
C. It can be performed in the patient's room.
D. It is more sensitive and specific for pulmonary vascular obstruction.

3–144. In planning care for a 57-year-old patient with vasospasm after clipping of an aneurysm and treatment with hypervolemic, hypertensive hemodilution and calcium channel blockers, the nurse would anticipate placement of a(n)

A. Central venous catheter.
B. Pulmonary artery catheter.
C. Left atrial catheter.
D. Intraventricular catheter.

3–145. After 10 days of ventilator dependence and hemodynamic instability, an ICU patient developed tarry stools. What complication does this indicate?

A. Stress ulcer.
B. Obstructed bile duct.
C. Erosion of the pancreas.
D. Mesenteric ischemia.

3–146. Which of the following best indicates that treatment goals for a patient with unstable angina have been achieved?

A. Relief of three pain episodes with nitroglycerin.
B. ST segment elevation and Q waves during pain episodes.
C. Absence of ST changes with pain episodes.
D. Absence of clinical and ECG changes indicative of increasing ischemia.

3–147. A patient with unstable angina has the following findings on admission: Substernal chest pain 6/10.

ECG shows sinus rhythm with deeply inverted T waves in leads II, III, aVF, and Q waves noted in V_1, V_2, and V_3.

Which of the following indicates that current therapy has prevented progression of ischemia and infarction?

A. Q waves are present in V_1, V_2, and V_3.
B. ST segment elevation is present in lead V_1 only.
C. Tall R waves are present in leads V_1 and V_2.
D. ST segment depression is present in leads V_1 and V_2.

3–148. In right bundle branch block, the QRS complex is usually

A. Negative in V_1.
B. Positive in V_6.
C. Triphasic in V_1 (rSR′).
D. Longer than 0.12 second with a slurred S wave in V_1.

3–149. When using vasopressors in treating septic shock unresponsive to crystalloid resuscitation, the dose should be titrated to the smallest dose needed to

A. Maintain mean arterial pressure (MAP) over 60 mm Hg.
B. Maintain urine output at 30 ml/hr.
C. Decrease systemic vascular resistance (SVR).
D. Increase pulmonary capillary wedge pressure (PCWP).

3–150. A patient admitted with diabetic ketoacidosis (DKA) develops increased urine output and weight loss over a 24-hour period. The critical care nurse needs to first evaluate the patient for

A. Syndrome of inappropriate antidiuretic hormone (SIADH).
B. Hyponatremia.
C. Diabetes insipidus.
D. Glucosuria.

3–151. In planning laboratory tests for a patient with suspected disseminated intravascular coagulation (DIC), the nurse knows that currently the most specific test to aid in diagnosing of DIC is

A. Fibrin degradation products (FDP).
B. Platelet count.
C. D-Dimer.
D. Thrombin time.

3–152. During carotid massage to slow supraventricular tachycardia (SVT), a patient develops ventricular standstill for 8 seconds while P waves continue to be demonstrated at a rate of 240 per minute. Patient and family education for this patient should include which of the following?

A. Instruction and demonstration of cough CPR.
B. Medication instruction regarding the use of calcium channel blockers.
C. Instruction on methods to prevent vagal stimulation.
D. Instruction in the use of self-administered vagal maneuvers to terminate future episodes of SVT.

3–153. A patient in the CCU with a permanent DDD pacemaker had been having frequent atrial premature contractions during the past 2 hours and is now in atrial fibrillation with a paced rate of 140 beats/min. Which of the following should be performed?

A. Call the physician for a digoxin loading dose order.
B. Perform synchronized cardioversion.
C. Call the cardiologist to ask if he wishes to re-program the pacemaker.
D. Continue to monitor the patient and note the reaction of the pacemaker to the rhythm change.

3–154. Which of the following indicates inappropriate DDD pacemaker function?

A. An atrial pacing spike visible at the beginning of the ventriculoatrial (VA) interval.
B. A spontaneous P wave results in a paced ventricular complex at the preset atrioventricular (AV) delay.
C. The AV interval following a sensed atrial event is shorter than the AV interval following a paced atrial event.
D. An atrial pacing spike is visible at the end of the VA interval.

3–155. Which of the following is a symptom of right ventricular failure?

A. Pulsus alternans.
B. Dyspnea.
C. Jugular venous distention.
D. Elevated pulmonary capillary wedge pressure.

3–156. In the acute phase after a T5 injury, the patient will most likely exhibit which of the following on assessment?

A. A blood pressure of 78/56 mm Hg.
B. A pulse of 138 beats/min.
C. A vital capacity of 25 ml/kg.
D. A tidal volume of 240 ml.

3–157. The following results were obtained in the emergency department on a patient who suddenly developed disoriented and combative behavior:

Elevated: blood urea nitrogen, blood alcohol
Reduced: hemoglobin/hematocrit, serum glucose, Ca^{2+}, Mg^{2+}, Na^+, K^+
Prolonged: prothrombin time

Based on these findings, which of the following would be the appropriate follow-up?

A. Serum amylase and lipase determination.
B. Serum alkaline phosphatase and aspartate aminotransferase determinations.
C. Gastric aspirate for pH and blood.
D. Peritoneal lavage.

3–158. A patient is in bed with the head of the bed elevated 45°. Using a ruler, the nurse measures the distance between the sternal angle and the point at which the nurse can see the jugular venous pulsation cease. This distance measures 6 cm and indicates

A. A normal finding.
B. Hypovolemia.
C. Right ventricular failure.
D. Left ventricular failure.

3–159. In patients with benzodiazepine overdose and possible co-ingestion of tricyclic antidepressants, flumazenil administration should be followed by observation for

A. Convulsions.
B. Ventricular arrhythmias.
C. Hypertensive crisis.
D. Jaundice.

3–160. In planning the care of a patient with a traumatic brain injury, which of the following electrolyte imbalances is likely to occur after the administration of mannitol?

A. Hyperkalemia.
B. Hypokalemia.
C. Hypernatremia.
D. Hyponatremia.

3–161. When changing the dressing on a triple-lumen central line, the tubing to the middle lumen becomes disconnected just as the patient inspires. Air immediately is pulled into the catheter. How should the patient be positioned immediately after clamping the catheter?

A. On right side with head down.
B. On left side with head up.
C. On left side with head down.
D. On right side with head up.

3–162. A patient with heart failure complicated by atrial fibrillation is receiving furosemide, captopril, amiodarone, amrinone, and renal dose dopamine. The initial chest radiograph demonstrated extensive interstitial and perivascular edema. The current radiographic report states that there are diffuse patchy infiltrates and minimal bibasilar interstitial edema. Heart rate is 80 beats/min sinus rhythm. Blood pressure is 138/76 mm Hg. Respiratory rate is 20 breaths/min unlabored. Oxygen saturation is 95% on room air despite a dusky appearance to the patient's skin. Oral temperature is 100.8°F. On admission the patient had a frequent cough productive of pink frothy sputum and currently has an occasional dry cough. The cough is most likely due to

A. Pneumonia.
B. The side effects of captopril administration.
C. Continued left ventricular failure.
D. Pulmonary fibrosis related to amiodarone administration.

3–163. In planning the care of a patient in pulmonary edema, which of the following nursing diagnoses would receive priority?

A. Alteration in fluid volume (excess).
B. Potential for alteration in gas exchange.
C. Potential for infection.
D. Decreased activity tolerance.

3–164. A patient in pulmonary edema has diuresed 3 L. Medication orders include

Nitroglycerin infusion, titrate to maintain systolic BP 90 mm Hg.
KCl 10 mEq in 1 hour for serum potassium level less than 4.2 mEq/L.
Digoxin, 0.25 mg IV each day.
Captopril, 25 mg orally qid.
Furosemide, 20 mg IV q4h.

The care plan for this patient should include which of the following?

A. Potential for hypomagnesemia, hypovolemia, digoxin toxicity.
B. Potential for digoxin toxicity, hypokalemia, hyponatremia.
C. Potential for hypovolemia, hypokalemia, hypernatremia.
D. Potential for cardiac cachexia, hypovolemia, hypernatremia.

3–165. Which of the following is an absolute contraindication to further use of an angiotensin converting enzyme (ACE) inhibitor in left ventricular failure?

A. Oropharyngeal angioedema.
B. Dizziness and angioedema.
C. Cough.
D. Blood pressure of 84/60 mm Hg.

3–166. When bolus dosing of furosemide is ineffective in diuresing a patient with heart failure, which of the following therapies may be used?

I. Administration of renal dose dopamine.
II. Continuous intravenous infusion of furosemide.
III. Administration of hydrochlorthiazide.
IV. Ultrafiltration.

A. I and II.
B. I and III.
C. II and III.
D. I, II, III, and IV.

3–167. A patient with pulmonary edema reports nausea and paresthesias after receiving a total of 120 mg of intravenous furosemide and diuresing 2 L. The cardiac monitor demonstrates sinus rhythm with occasional premature ventricular contractions (PVCs). Oxygen saturation is 97%. Treatment should include administration of

   I. Magnesium sulfate, 1 g.
   II. KCl, 10 mEq.
   III. Lidocaine, 100 mg IV.

   A. II only.
   B. III only.
   C. II and III.
   D. I and II.

3–168. A 56-year-old patient is admitted to the ICU with a diagnosis of acoustic neuroma. The patient's behavior suggests that the patient is in a situational crisis. Intervention for this problem is based on the critical care nurse's knowledge that in a situational crisis, patients

   A. Feel threatened.
   B. Have a distorted perception of the diagnosis.
   C. Perceive a lack of personal control over the event.
   D. Are unable to process thoughts.

3–169. The most sensitive indicator in assessing the severity of hepatic encephalopathy is

   A. Serum ammonia level.
   B. Papilledema.
   C. Level of consciousness.
   D. Electroencephalogram.

3–170. Toxic ingestions that produce markedly elevated methemoglobin levels should be treated by

   A. Exchange transfusion.
   B. Plasmapheresis.
   C. Hemodialysis.
   D. Peritoneal dialysis.

3–171. A 65-year-old obese woman with chronic obstructive pulmonary disease (COPD) and diabetes is in the ICU after surgery to remove two gangrenous toes on her left foot. On the second postoperative day, she becomes disoriented, restless, and anxious; her pulse oximeter reading drops slightly to 89%, which is corrected by increasing her oxygen. Her ECG and chest radiograph appear normal. The next day she coughs up blood and complains of pleuritic chest pain. The most likely explanation for these clinical findings is

   A. Tuberculosis.
   B. Pulmonary infarct.
   C. *Klebsiella* pneumonia.
   D. Heart failure.

3–172. A patient with atherosclerotic heart disease and heart failure is admitted to the ICU. Furosemide, 40 mg, was given in the emergency department, and diuresis totals 1800 ml thus far. A dobutamine drip at 10 mg/kg/min has been started. The patient's current blood pressure is 80/64 mm Hg, and heart rate is 110 beats/min. Capillary refill is 4 seconds. Admitting orders include nitroglycerin, 50 mg in 250 ml D_5W, titrate to maintain systolic blood pressure greater than 80 mm Hg; captopril, 6.25 mg orally each 8 hours. Which of the following nursing actions is most appropriate at this time?

   A. Start a nitroglycerin drip and administer captopril as ordered.
   B. Discontinue nitroglycerin drip and give captopril as ordered.
   C. Call the physician to clarify the captopril dosage, because you suspect the ordered dosage of captopril is low for this patient.
   D. Call the physician to clarify the administration of captopril for this patient who has just received 40 mg of furosemide and has had significant diuresis.

3–173. A patient with volume overload and left ventricular failure is being treated with furosemide, captopril, and digoxin but continues to have dyspnea and rales. Additional therapy for this patient should include

    I. Isosorbide dinitrate.
    II. Propranolol.
    III. Hydralazine.
    IV. Metolazone.

    A. I and II.
    B. II and III.
    C. I, III, and IV.
    D. I, II, III, and IV.

3–174. Evaluation of therapy for respiratory function in a patient with heart failure is best determined by

    A. Respiratory rate.
    B. Oxygen saturation.
    C. Arterial blood gas analysis.
    D. Chest radiography.

3–175. During the treatment of diabetic ketoacidosis, intravenous insulin can be discontinued when the

    A. Blood sugar level is normal.
    B. Serum ketones are negative.
    C. Patient is tolerating food.
    D. pH is greater than 7.3.

3–176. A common laboratory finding in disseminated intravascular coagulation (DIC) is a decrease in clotting factors. The best explanation for this finding is

    A. Activity of the intrinsic pathway.
    B. Activity of the extrinsic pathway.
    C. Decreased production of thrombin by the liver.
    D. Overstimulation of the normal coagulation cycle.

3–177. A 40-year-old woman presents with upper respiratory tract infection and complains of headache, ecchymosis, and severe epistaxis. Serum laboratory values obtained in the emergency department showed normal values for prothrombin time (PT) and partial thromboplastin time (PTT). However, hemoglobin (Hgb), hematocrit (Hct), and platelets values were decreased. Based on patient presentation and reported laboratory values, the critical care nurse would most likely suspect

    A. Disseminated intravascular coagulation (DIC).
    B. Leukemia.
    C. Thrombotic thrombocytopenic purpura (TTP).
    D. Normal values with an upper respiratory tract infection.

3–178. On assessment of a 78-year-old patient admitted to the ICU with a right frontoparietal cerebrovascular accident (CVA), the patient exhibits astereognosis. The critical care nurse knows that this finding constitutes an

    A. Inattention to objects in a visual field.
    B. Inability to dress one's self properly.
    C. Inability to determine position of body parts when moved.
    D. Inability to recognize objects placed in the hand without visual cues.

3–179. Patients with arylcyclohexylamine (PCP) intoxication need to be monitored for

    A. Acute renal failure.
    B. Cardiac arrhythmias.
    C. Hypertensive crisis.
    D. Rhabdomyolysis.

3–180. During intravenous replacement therapy for hypomagnesemia, the nurse must monitor the patient for the development of

A. Hyperventilation.
B. Seizures.
C. Myocardial ischemia.
D. Heart block.

3–181. A patient's history that suggests a cause for acute pancreatitis would be

A. Recent foreign travel.
B. Mushroom poisoning.
C. Gallstone disease.
D. Recent blood transfusion.

3–182. Streptokinase is believed to reduce obstruction by a pulmonary embolus through

A. Activation of plasminogen.
B. Activation of fibrin.
C. Blocking of fibrinogen.
D. Release of fibrin split products.

3–183. A patient with heart failure complicated by atrial fibrillation is receiving furosemide, captopril, and amiodarone. The initial chest radiograph demonstrated extensive interstitial and perivascular edema. The current radiographic report states that there are diffuse patchy infiltrates and minimal bibasilar interstitial edema present. Heart rate is 80 beats/min, sinus rhythm. Respiratory rate is 20 breaths/min, unlabored. Oxygen saturation is 95% on room air despite a dusky appearance to the patient's skin. Oral temperature is 100.8°F. On admission the patient had a frequent cough productive of pink frothy sputum and currently has an occasional dry cough. Which of the following best describes the effectiveness of the patient's pharmacologic therapy?

I. Amiodarone has been effective in controlling atrial dysrhythmias.
II. Furosemide has been effective in relieving pulmonary congestion.
III. Captopril should be discontinued because of the dry cough experienced by the patient.
IV. Amiodarone should be discontinued because of symptoms of pulmonary fibrosis.

A. I and II.
B. II and III.
C. I, II, and III.
D. I, II, and IV.

3–184. A patient in hypertensive crisis has a blood pressure of 174/110 mm Hg in both arms, both standing and supine. The patient has a heart rate of 110 beats/min; respiratory rate is 36 breaths/min with pink frothy sputum and coarse rales to mid lobe. The patient is somnolent, is oriented to person but not to place or time, and reports a severe occipital headache. An arterial catheter is inserted for continuous blood pressure monitoring. After initiating a nitroprusside infusion and administering IV furosemide, 40 mg, the nurse would anticipate assisting with which of the following diagnostic tests?

A. MRI to rule out cerebral infarction.
B. CT of the abdomen to rule out pheochromocytoma.
C. CT of the thorax to rule out aortic dissection.
D. Chest radiography to evaluate cardiac and pulmonary status.

3–185. Care planning for a patient with malignant hypertension includes monitoring for which of the following potential problems?

  I. Pheochromocytoma.
 II. Renal failure.
III. Cerebrovascular accident.
 IV. Dissection of aortic aneurysm.

A. I, II, and III.
B. II, III, and IV.
C. I, III, and IV.
D. I, II, and IV.

3–186. Sodium nitroprusside, 50 mg, in 250 ml D_5W is ordered to maintain a patient's systolic blood pressure between 100 and 150 mm Hg. The patient's current systolic blood pressure is 120/60 mm Hg. The infusion device is set to deliver 15 ml/hr. How much sodium nitroprusside is the patient receiving?

A. 9.9 μg/min.
B. 17.4 μg/min.
C. 49.5 μg/min.
D. 33.3 μg/min.

3–187. Which of the following is a realistic outcome goal that demonstrates patient readiness for transfer out of the critical care unit after aggressive treatment for hypertensive crisis?

A. Patient currently compliant with medication regimen.
B. Blood pressure controlled on oral antihypertensive.
C. Absence of renal complications of hypertension.
D. Resolution of left ventricular strain pattern on ECG.

3–188. In a patient with the following clinical findings:

MAP, 60 mm Hg
Heart rate, 129 beats/min
Cardiac index, 1.6 L/min/m²
PCWP, 18 mm Hg
CVP, 18 mm Hg
PaO_2, 95 mm Hg

cardiogenic shock is most likely due to

A. Acute anterior wall myocardial infarction.
B. Papillary muscle rupture.
C. Pulmonary embolus.
D. Cardiac tamponade.

3–189. Which of the following therapies is generally performed *first* in cardiogenic shock caused by acute myocardial infarction?

A. Cardiac surgery.
B. Coronary angioplasty.
C. Coronary angiography.
D. Intra-aortic balloon counterpulsation (IABP).

3–190. Sodium bicarbonate therapy is initiated after drug overdose associated with

A. Benzodiazepines.
B. Cocaine.
C. Acetaminophen.
D. Cyclic antidepressants.

3–191. Which of the following medications is essential to maintaining control of asthma and preventing status asthmaticus?

A. Short-acting beta$_2$ agonists.
B. Corticosteroids.
C. Short-acting theophyllines.
D. Antihistamines.

3–192. After a cerebrovascular event, the critical care nurse knows that all of the following are true *except*

A. The head of the bed may be positioned flat or elevated.
B. Hyperdilution may be ordered to reduce blood viscosity.
C. Non-narcotic analgesics are unnecessary for the acute stroke patient.
D. Gastrostomy tube feedings are the preferred route for feeding the patient with dysphagia.

3–193. The primary action of somatostatin therapy is to

A. Suppress enteric flora biotransformation of nitrogen.
B. Promote fecal nitrogen excretion.
C. Decrease pancreatic secretion in acute pancreatitis.
D. Dilate mesenteric arterioles.

3–194. Treatment of a patient in cardiogenic shock who exhibits ECG changes indicative of a massive, evolving myocardial infarction includes

A. Open-heart surgery revascularization.
B. Coronary angioplasty.
C. Intravenous administration of angiotensin converting enzyme (ACE) inhibitors.
D. Intravenous administration of calcium channel blockers.

3–195. Effectiveness of administration of vasoactive medications in a patient with cardiogenic shock is evidenced by

I. Improved cardiac output.
II. Increased systemic vascular resistance.
III. Decreased pulse pressure.
IV. Decrease in dysrhythmias.

A. I and II.
B. II and III.
C. III and IV.
D. I and IV.

3–196. The widened P wave seen in lead II of a patient with mitral stenosis is due to

A. Left ventricular dysfunction.
B. Atrioventricular (AV) junction delay.
C. Left atrial enlargement.
D. Right atrial enlargement.

3–197. Pharmacologic management of mitral stenosis with symptoms of heart failure may include

I. Prophylactic antibiotics.
II. Digitalis glycosides to treat atrial fibrillation.
III. Warfarin (Coumadin) for anticoagulation.
IV. Beta blockers to reduce tachycardia.

A. I only.
B. I and II.
C. I, II, and III.
D. I, II, III, and IV.

3–198. A patient is admitted after acute atenolol ingestion. The nurse will prepare the patient for

A. Calcium administration.
B. Glucose infusion.
C. Transvenous pacing.
D. Potassium administration.

3–199. A patient is admitted to the ICU with a diagnosis of gastrointestinal bleeding. The patient has an order to receive 6 units of packed red blood cells. After administration of these blood products, the patient should be monitored for which of these electrolyte imbalances?

A. Hypercalcemia.
B. Hypokalemia.
C. Hyperphosphatemia.
D. Hypomagnesemia.

3–200. To determine the effectiveness of treatment of diabetic ketoacidosis, the best laboratory values to evaluate are

A. Urine pH and serum glucose.
B. Serum glucose and serum pH.
C. Urine glucose and serum glucose.
D. Serum ketones and serum pH.

3–1. (**D**) The four hallmarks of acute tumor lysis syndrome (ATLS) are hyperuricemia, hyperkalemia, hyperphosphatemia, and hypocalcemia. ATLS can occur when large numbers of tumor cells are rapidly destroyed and is a special concern after the first chemotherapy dose. With chemotherapy, tumor cells are lysed, releasing cellular contents into the blood stream, which results in the serum abnormalities. Normal serum laboratory values are potassium, 3.5 to 5.5 mEq/L; phosphorus, 3.0 to 4.5 mg/dl; and calcium, 8.5 to 10.5 mg/dl.

Reference: Alspach, J. G. (ed.): AACN Core Curriculum for Critical Care Nursing, 5th ed. Philadelphia, W. B. Saunders, 1998.

3–2. (**D**) Small patchy white areas on the plantar aspect of the foot are a sign of microembolism in the patient who has had an aortic aneurysm repaired. They are caused by atheromatous debris released during surgery. Myoglobinuria is common after aneurysm repair surgery because previously obstructed flow to skeletal muscle that causes muscle necrosis releases myoglobin. The danger of myoglobinuria is the potential for acute blockage of renal tubules leading to acute renal failure. Ileus, demonstrated by abdominal distention and absent bowel sounds, is often seen for approximately 4 days after an aortic aneurysm repair due to manipulation of the abdominal organs and edema at the anastomosis site. Pain in the lower abdomen, flank, and groin is a common symptom of iliac artery aneurysm rupture, or it may reflect bleeding into the abdomen from surgical sites.

Reference: Moore, W. S.: Vascular Surgery, A Comprehensive Review. Philadelphia, W. B. Saunders, 1993.

3–3. (**A**) Blood pressure control in acute aortic dissection is aimed at lowering the blood pressure to prevent further dissection or rupture. Nitroprusside is a potent vasodilator that lowers arterial blood pressure. Dopamine selectively vasodilates at low, or renal, dosages and causes vasoconstriction and elevated blood pressure at infusion rates greater than 7 μg/kg/min. Dobutamine is an inotropic agent that does not affect the blood pressure directly. Amrinone has effects similar to dopamine, with vasodilating as well as inotropic effects; however, it does not have the immediate effect of nitroprusside in the control of blood pressure.

Reference: Khan, M. G.: Heart Disease Diagnosis and Therapy. Baltimore, Williams & Wilkins, 1996.

3–4. (**D**) Although all of these can result in lung contusion, the frequency of high-speed vehicular crashes far surpasses the others.

Reference: Kinney, M. R., Packa, D. R., Dunbar, S. B. (eds.): AACN's Clinical Reference for Critical Care Nursing, 3rd ed. New York, McGraw-Hill, 1993.

3–5. (**C**) Physical assessment findings of a hemothorax include dullness to percussion, decreased breath sounds, tracheal deviation away from the affected side, and decreased vocal fremitus.

Reference: Alspach, J. G. (ed.): AACN Core Curriculum for Critical Care Nursing, 5th ed. Philadelphia, W. B. Saunders, 1998.

3–6. (**B**) Severe internal injuries such as pulmonary contusion may not correlate with the patient's external appearance. Mechanical ventilation may be needed but can sometimes be avoided. Adult respiratory distress syndrome and pulmonary embolus may eventually develop but are not clinically important at this point.

Reference: Kinney, M. R., Packa, D. R., Dunbar, S. B. (eds.): AACN's Clinical Reference for Critical Care Nursing, 3rd ed. St. Louis, Mosby–Year Book, 1993.

3–7. (**A**) Chest tube insertion will relieve the compression of a self-limiting hemothorax. Fluid and blood administration may be necessary for a massive hemothorax. Mechanical ventilation is usually not necessary because the pressure in the chest seals off the leak and the pneumothorax does not increase in size.

Reference: Kinney, M. R., Packa, D. R., Dunbar, S. B. (eds.): AACN's Clinical Reference for Critical Care Nursing, 3rd ed. St. Louis, Mosby–Year Book, 1993.

3–8. (**A**) SIMV with PEEP has the advantage of providing support so the patient does not "fight" the ventilator and pressure changes needed to generate breaths are minimized. CMV may result in subatmospheric intrathoracic pressure when attempting to breathe and increase pain and chest wall movement. IPPB is not appropriate for prolonged ventilation. CPAP requires spontaneous breathing, which, in this patient, may increase chest wall displacement.

Reference: Kinney, M. R., Packa, D. R., Dunbar, S. B. (eds.): AACN's Clinical Reference for Critical Care Nursing, 3rd ed. New York, McGraw-Hill, 1993.

3–9. (**D**) The normal PCWP is 4 to 12 mm Hg. A value of 15 mm Hg is elevated and that of 2 mm Hg is low, as one would anticipate with hypovolemia.

Reference: Kinney, M. R., Packa, D. R., Dunbar, S. B. (eds.): AACN's Clinical Reference for Critical Care Nursing, 3rd ed. St. Louis, Mosby–Year Book, 1993.

3–10. (**D**) Animals subjected to total immersion until death in fresh water will exhibit volume overload and hyponatremia whereas those immersed in salt water with subsequent aspiration will exhibit hypovolemia and hypernatremia. However, humans who survive long enough to reach the hospital rarely exhibit these fluids and electrolyte derangements.

Reference: Goodwin, S. R., Boysen, P. G., Modell, J. H.: Near drowning: Adults and children. *In* Shoemaker, W. C., Ayres, S. M., Grenvik, A., Holbrook, P. R. (eds.): Textbook of Critical Care, 3rd ed. Philadelphia, W. B. Saunders Co., 1995.

3–11. (**D**) The normal hematocrit is 37% to 47% in women and 40% to 54% in men. Administration of fluids during surgery may dilute the hematocrit values slightly. A value as low as 30% definitely points to blood loss as the cause for hypovolemia.

Reference: Ruppert, S. D., Kernicki, J. G., Dolan, J. T.: Dolan's Critical Care Nursing: Clinical Management Through the Nursing Process. Philadelphia, F. A. Davis, 1996.

3–12. (**C**) Medical management of the patient requiring subarachnoid precautions includes bed rest with the head of the bed elevated to promote venous return and cerebrospinal fluid outflow. Bedside commode privileges may be permitted. Stool softeners, limiting visitors and other stimuli, and maintaining a quiet, dimly lit environment minimize stress and, thus, rebleeding. Anticonvulsants are generally not indicated. Lowering the blood pressure through use of vasodilators may precipitate ischemia or stroke. Fluid intake of as much as 2.5 to 3 L may be recommended to maintain normovolemia.

Reference: Barker, E. (ed.): Neuroscience Nursing. Mosby–Year Book, St. Louis, 1994.

3–13. (**C**) More than 50% of critically ill patients may have hypomagnesemia of various causes that could lead to arrhythmias, metabolic deficits, neuromuscular changes, and psychoses. In pancreatitis, the normal insulin stimulation of cellular magnesium uptake is disrupted. Colitis, gastritis, and active ulcer disease are associated with hypermagnesemia, owing to enhanced magnesium absorption. Although hypermagnesemia is less common than hypomagnesemia, most of these patients do not have their magnesium imbalance identified. Because hypermagnesemia can lead to refractory hypotension and respiratory arrest, identification of hypermagnesemia is critically important. Asthma and myocardial infarction are associated with hypomagnesemia.

Reference: Toto, K. H., Yucha, C. B.: Magnesium: Homeostasis, imbalances, and therapeutic uses. Crit. Care Nurs. Clin. North Am. 6:767–781, 1994.

3–14. (**B**) Hypovolemia must be corrected before administration of vasopressors. Crystalloid fluids are generally administered because they provide large volume with few adverse effects and are inexpensive. Raising the legs will help by elevating preload. Reducing anxiety with sedation if the blood pressure is sufficient will decrease further decompensation related to increased myocardial oxygen demand. Vasopressors increase myocardial oxygen consumption.

Reference: Thelan, L. A., Davie, J. K., Urden, L. D., Lough, M. E.: Critical Care Nursing, Diagnosis and Management, 2nd ed. St. Louis, Mosby–Year Book, 1994.

3–15. (**D**) Hematocrits of 30% to 33% are often maintained in shock states to decrease blood viscosity; therefore, lactated Ringer's solution would be the intravenous fluid of choice. It is also mildly alkalotic, which would improve the metabolic acidosis reflected by the low HCO_3 level of 20 mEq/L. Restoration of volume restores blood pH in most cases. Sodium bicarbonate is not generally given to correct alkalosis unless the pH is below 7.20. Dopamine is contraindicated in hypovolemia. Type-specific blood is given in emergencies when there is insufficient time to type and cross-match blood for a bleeding patient. It would not be given to a patient with a hematocrit above 30%.

Reference: Darovic, G. O.: Hemodynamic Monitoring: Invasive and Noninvasive Clinical Application, 2nd ed. Philadelphia, W. B. Saunders, 1995.

3–16. (**A**) Preceding viral illness occurs in 85% of cases of myocarditis. In addition, palpitations are reported by 33% of patients and tachycardia often exists out of proportion to fever. Q waves and ST and T wave changes may mimic myocardial infarction but do not evidence evolutionary changes.

Reference: Khan, M. G.: Heart Disease Diagnosis and Therapy. Baltimore, Williams & Wilkins, 1996.

3–17. (**C**) Bed rest is used to conserve energy, and ACE inhibitors are used to decrease afterload. Corticosteroids may be given for progressive myocarditis. Antiarrhythmic agents are contraindicated in myocarditis because of their negative inotropic and proarrhythmic effects. In sustained ventricular dysrhythmias, amiodorone is used instead of lidocaine because it does not depress the myocardium.

Reference: Khan, M. G.: Heart Disease Diagnosis and Therapy. Baltimore, Williams & Wilkins, 1996.

3–18. (**B**) The normal PR interval is 0.12 to 0.20 second. Prolongation of the PR interval above 0.2 second indicates first-degree heart block.

Reference: Ruppert, S. D., Kernicki, J. G., Dolan, J. T.: Dolan's Critical Care Nursing: Clinical Management Through the Nursing Process. Philadelphia, F. A. Davis, 1996.

3–19. (**C**) Although decreased level of consciousness as a precipitating factor may place a patient at risk of aspiration, the extent of pulmonary injury is determined by the pH and volume of the aspirate, size of the particles aspirated, and presence of food and contaminated materials.

Reference: Alspach, J. G. (ed.): AACN Core Curriculum for Critical Care Nursing, 5th ed. Philadelphia, W. B. Saunders, 1998.

3–20. (**B**) The most important aspect in assessing renal trauma is to obtain as complete a history as possible. The clinician must rely on a high index of suspicion for renal trauma to avoid overlooking it, because other injuries may mask the clinical symptomatology of renal involvement. Actual signs and symptoms of renal trauma may not be evident for hours or even days after the injury. Performing primary and secondary surveys is important for all types of trauma, but they do not consistently yield information specific to the occurrence of renal trauma. The determination of the type of diagnostic testing to be completed will be based on the information gathered during the history and the surveys.

Reference: Smith, M. F.: Renal trauma: Adult and pediatric considerations. Crit. Care Nurs. Clin. North Am. 2:67–77, 1990.

3–21. (**D**) Normal carboxyhemoglobin values are less than 5%. A range of 15% to 20% is associated with headache and mild confusion. Ranges of 20% to 40% are associated with disorientation, fatigue, nausea, and visual changes. Hallucinations, combativeness, coma, and shock state are found with levels of 40% to 60%. Levels greater than 60%, if uncorrected, lead to death.

Reference: Demling, R. H.: Smoke inhalation injury. In Shoemaker, W. C., Ayres, S. M., Grenvik, A., Holbrook, P. R. (eds.): Textbook of Critical Care, 3rd ed. Philadelphia, W. B. Saunders, 1995.

3–22. (**C**) Carotid massage is a vagal maneuver that slows conduction from the atria to the AV node and increases AV nodal delay of the impulse to the ventricles. This generally slows tachycardias that are caused by impulses originating above the AV junction. AV junctional rhythms are therefore not slowed by carotid massage. Atrial flutter, atrial tachycardia, and Wolff-Parkinson-White rhythms originate above the AV junction.

Reference: Kinney, M. R., Packa, D. R.: Andreoli's Comprehensive Cardiac Care, 8th ed. St. Louis, Mosby–Year Book, 1996.

3–23. (**D**) A volvulus is a 180° twist in a bowel segment. The telescoping of one bowel segment into another is called intussusception. An outpocketing of the colonic lumen is diverticulitis. A colonic carcinoma generally is treated by surgery but is unrelated to a volvulus.

Reference: Doughty, D. B., Jackson, D. B.: Gastrointestinal Disorders. St. Louis, Mosby–Year Book, 1993.

3–24. (**B**) Hypercapnia, defined as a $PaCO_2$ greater than 45 mm Hg, is a potent vasodilating factor that would be of concern because it may predispose the patient to cerebral vasodilation and increased blood volume to brain tissue, resulting in increased intracranial pressure. Hypercapnia is often associated with hypoxia. A normal $PaCO_2$ is between 35 and 45 mm Hg. The urine specific gravity of 1.018 and serum sodium levels 140 mEq/L are within normal limits.

Reference: Hickey, J. V.: The Clinical Practice of Neurological and Neurosurgical Nursing, 3rd ed. Philadelphia, J. B. Lippincott, 1992.

3–25. (**C**) These are all normal reactions from the family of a critically ill patient and can affect how the family interacts with the nurse. The nurse cognizant of these behaviors can use this knowledge to intervene most effectively. When teaching, the fact that the family may not be able to concentrate and assimilate incoming information would have the most impact. The nurse can give simple explanations and written material that the family can refer to later when more able to concentrate. Explanations may need to be repeated several times, as well; and suggesting to the family that they take notes is another way to make teaching more effective.

Reference: Clochesy, J. M., Breu, C., Cardin, S., et al. (eds.): Critical Care Nursing, 2nd ed. Philadelphia, W. B. Saunders, 1996.

3–26. (**A**) Broad-spectrum antibiotics are administered for neutropenia (neutrophil count less than 500/μL) in patients with fever before the source of infection is documented by culture. Colony-stimulating factor (cytokines) that stimulates various blood cell components is best used when neutropenia is expected (i.e., after cytoxic chemotherapy).

Reference: Alspach, J. G. (ed.): AACN Core Curriculum for Critical Care Nursing, 5th ed. Philadelphia, W. B. Saunders, 1998.

3–27. (**C**) In freshwater aspiration, water rapidly enters the circulation, resulting in hemodilution. Fluid in the alveoli increases the diffusion pathway, resulting in hypoxemia. Hypercapnia also occurs from impaired diffusion of CO_2. Both hypoxemia and hypercapnia produce acidosis. Thus, the pathophysiologic changes include hypoxemia and tissue hypoxia, hypoxic brain injury with cerebral edema, hypercapnia, and acidemia.

Reference: Alspach, J. G. (ed.): AACN Core Curriculum for Critical Care Nursing, 5th ed. Philadelphia, W. B. Saunders, 1998.

3–28. (**A**) Chronic aspiration pneumonia occurs with repeated aspiration of infected pharyngeal secretions. Tube feeding through a nasogastric tube frequently allows regurgitation of feedings followed by bacterial multiplication. Use of a PEG tube diminishes the chance of regurgitation and subsequent infected secretions. Corticosteriod therapy is indicated after chronic aspiration has developed. Prophylactic antibiotic therapy, in the absence of a definitive organism, is avoided because it may actually foster growth of resistant organisms.

Reference: Kinney, M. R., Packa, D. R., Dunbar, S. B. (eds.): AACN's Clinical Reference for Critical Care Nursing, 3rd ed. St. Louis, Mosby–Year Book, 1993.

3-29. (**B**) Presence of glucose in the secretions is highly suggestive of regurgitation of tube feedings but is not specific for aspiration. It can also occur in the presence of blood from gastritis or esophageal/gastric ulcers that have some bleeding. Food coloring (generally blue) in tube feedings helps assess whether silent aspiration of the tube feeding is occurring through an incompetent larynx. Presence of blue food coloring in tracheal secretions is therefore very specific for aspiration. A chest radiograph may show areas of pneumonia, but it is not necessarily due to aspiration. A swallowing study would be useful to evaluate ability to eat but would not help to establish if the patient has aspirated.

Reference: Alspach, J. G. (ed.): AACN Core Curriculum for Critical Care Nursing, 5th ed. Philadelphia, W. B. Saunders, 1998.

3-30. (**C**) Aspirin is contraindicated in burn patients because it acts to inhibit prostaglandin synthesis, thereby decreasing renal blood flow and urine output. Aspirin may produce gastric erosion if given in large doses over a prolonged period of time. Aspirin does not produce vasodilation or increased capillary permeability.

Reference: Roberts, S. L.: Multisystem deviations. In Critical Care Nursing: Assessment and Intervention. Stamford, Conn., Appleton & Lange, 1996.

3-31. (**D**) Torsades des pointes is a form of ventricular tachycardia characterized by QRS complexes of changing amplitude that appear to twist around the isoelectric line. Supraventricular tachycardias and accelerated idioventricular rhythms are generally regular in rhythm with normal contour to the QRS and a consistent QRS axis.

Reference: Braunwald, E., (ed.): Heart Disease: A Textbook of Cardiovascular Medicine. Philadelphia, W. B. Saunders, 1997.

3-32. (**D**) Magnesium sulfate in doses of 2 to 3 g is effective in suppressing torsades des pointes even in patients with normal magnesium levels. The exact mechanism is unknown, but it is believed that magnesium's calcium blocking effect may suppress automaticity. Amiodarone, sotolol, and lidocaine all prolong the QT interval and may perpetuate the dysrhythmia.

Reference: Braunwald, E. (ed.): Heart Disease: A Textbook of Cardiovascular Medicine. Philadelphia, W. B. Saunders, 1997.

3-33. (**A**) Hypokalemia and hypoxemia predispose to ventricular dysrhythmias and should be prevented. Cardiac surgical patients are prone to hypoxemia and hypokalemia because of extracorporeal circulation effects, anesthesia, and hemodilution. Lidocaine boluses are appropriate to suppress premature ventricular contractions but will not prevent them unless a constant infusion is also initiated. Asynchronous ventricular pacing predisposes to R on T phenomena, which may lead to ventricular tachycardia or fibrillation.

Reference: Ruppert, S. D., Kernicki, J. G., Dolan, J. T.: Dolan's Critical Care Nursing, 2nd ed. Philadelphia, F. A. Davis, 1996.

3-34. (**A**) The major difference in physical findings is that the trachea is deviated toward the injured side with an open pneumothorax and away from the injured side with a tension pneumothorax.

Reference: Alspach, J. G. (ed.): AACN Core Curriculum for Critical Care Nursing, 5th ed. Philadelphia, W. B. Saunders, 1998.

3-35. (**B**) Insertion of a large-gauge needle in the second intercostal space at the midclavicular line on the affected side will relieve the pressure. A chest tube should then be inserted as soon as possible. Neither bronchoscopy nor thoracoscopy is indicated for this condition.

Reference: Kinney, M. R., Packa, D. R., Dunbar, S. B. (eds.): AACN's Clinical Reference for Critical Care Nursing, 3rd ed. St. Louis, Mosby–Year Book, 1993.

3–36. (**D**) *Intracranial hemorrhage* is a nonspecific broad term that refers to any bleeding into the cranium. One of the most significant complications that can arise from this hemorrhage is rebleeding; thus interventions are tailored to reduce this risk. These interventions include the use of short- rather than long-acting sedatives to prevent agitation and restlessness, because long-acting sedatives may mask subtle changes in level of consciousness. Platelet-aggregating agents such as aspirin are contraindicated because they increase the risk for rebleeding. If vital signs permit, the head of the bed is maintained at about 30° to aid in venous drainage. Maintaining a quiet, dimly lit environment prevents sudden changes or surges in blood pressure. These sudden blood pressure alterations may increase the risk of rebleeding by disrupting the clot that forms on the vessel wall.

Reference: Clochesy, J. M., Breu, C., Cardin, S., et al. (eds.): Critical Care Nursing, 2nd ed. Philadelphia, W. B. Saunders, 1996.

3–37. (**B**) When enteral nutrients are withheld, mucosal atrophy and impaired mucosal barrier function dramatically diminish the immunologic function of the gastrointestinal tract. Early enteral feedings have an important role in supporting the gut as an immune organ. The elimination of pathogenic organisms, promotion of phagocytosis of foreign material by macrophages, and clearing the blood of bacterial endotoxin are contributions of the liver to immune protection.

Reference: Phillips, M. C., Olson, L. R.: The immunologic role of the gastrointestinal tract. Crit. Care Nurs. Clin. North Am. 5:107–120, 1993.

3–38. (**D**) Definitive treatment for this dysrhythmia (third-degree atrioventricular block) in an 80-year-old patient is a permanent pacemaker. A transcutaneous pacemaker may be used until the patient is able to have a permanent pacemaker inserted. A temporary transvenous pacemaker may be a more comfortable alternative for the patient than the transcutaneous pacemaker while the patient is awaiting permanent pacemaker implant. Atropine boluses are given when the patient is symptomatic and awaiting further therapy, such as a temporary transvenous or transcutaneous pacemaker.

Reference: Ruppert, S. D., Kernicki, J. G., Dolan, J. T.: Dolan's Critical Care Nursing, 2nd ed. Philadelphia, F. A. Davis, 1996.

3–39. (**D**) Verapamil is used in the treatment of supraventricular dysrhythmias. It causes an increase in atrioventricular nodal delay, which slows and may terminate supraventricular dysrhythmias. Lidocaine, procainamide, and bretyllium are indicated for ventricular dysrhythmias. Lidocaine and procainamide suppress ventricular dysrhythmias by decreasing ventricular automaticity. In addition, procainamide slows ventricular conduction. Both lidocaine and bretyllium increase the ventricular fibrillation threshold.

Reference: Kinney, M. R., Packa, D. R.: Andreoli's Comprehensive Cardiac Care, 8th ed. St. Louis, Mosby–Year Book, 1996.

3–40. (**A**) In the patient with acute renal failure, signs of hypervolemia include tachycardia, hypertension, bounding pulses, a paradoxic pulse, increasing pulmonary artery pressures, and cardiac output/cardiac index. These signs are hallmarks of fluid volume overload that results from the kidney's inability to excrete fluid.

Reference: Carlson, K. K.: Continuous renal replacement therapies. *In* Urban, N. A., Krumberger, J. M., Winkelman, C. (eds.): Guidelines for Critical Care Nursing. St. Louis, Mosby–Year Book, 1995.

3–41. (**B**) Burn patients are prone to stress diabetes secondary to altered carbohydrate metabolism. The hypermetabolism that follows burn injury increases the need for insulin, and the patient may not be able to produce sufficient amounts, thus leading to hyperglycemia. This is especially true when the patient is receiving supplemental feedings. The patient may transiently require insulin coverage to regulate hyperglycemia. While keeping accurate records is important, it will not determine serum glucose level. Excess salt intake does not produce polyuria, nor does a urinary tract infection cause thirst.

Reference: Roberts, S. L.: Multisystem deviations. *In* Critical Care Nursing: Assessment and Intervention. Stamford, Conn., Appleton & Lange, 1996.

3–42. (**B**) The carotids should be auscultated before carotid massage. If a bruit is auscultated, a different vagal maneuver should be attempted. The artery is palpated gently at first, and then firmer pressure is applied in a circular motion. Both sides are never massaged at the same time to prevent decreasing cerebral blood supply.

Reference: Braunwald, E. (ed.): Heart Disease: A Textbook of Cardiovascular Medicine. Philadelphia, W. B. Saunders, 1997.

3–43. (**A**) Sotolol decreases the defibrillation threshold and prolongs the ventricular refractory period, which decreases the energy level requirements to terminate ventricular fibrillation. Long-term amiodarone administration increases the defibrillation threshold due to its metabolite effects; therefore, patients require higher energy levels for defibrillation. Verapamil increases the defibrillation threshold, although the mechanism is unclear. Procainamide has no effect on defibrillation threshold.

Reference: Manz, M., Jung, W., Luderitz, B.: Interactions between drugs and devices: Experimental and clinical studies. Am Heart J 127:978–983, 1994.

3–44. (**B**) A chest radiograph will determine if lead fracture or migration of the electrode has occurred. The 12-lead ECG will detect whether ischemia or necrosis at the electrode or patch site has occurred, which would prevent depolarization of myocardium. Many medications increase the defibrillation threshold, which may require the programming of higher defibrillation energy in the ICD. Some of the medications that increase the defibrillation threshold include class IB and IC agents amiodarone and verapamil. Application of a magnet to the ICD generator turns the device on or off. We already know that the device is on because it fired appropriately. If the device did not fire, then application of the magnet would be appropriate to determine if the device was off, thus preventing it from terminating the dysrhythmia.

Reference: Kinney, M. R., Packa, D. R., Dunbar, S. B.: AACN's Clinical Reference for Critical Care Nursing, 3rd ed. St. Louis, Mosby–Year Book, 1993.

3–45. (**A**) Initial management of a prolonged bronchopleural fistula is to attach a Heimlich valve to the chest tube and drain the tube to a bag. This allows greater patient mobility and facilitates discharge home. A pleurodesis may be performed, although it is usually reserved for patients with repeated spontaneous pneumothoraces. Thoracotomy may be used, but only after other measures are unsuccessful.

Reference: Kersten, L. D.: Comprehensive Respiratory Nursing: A Decision Making Approach. Philadelphia, W. B. Saunders, 1989.

3–46. (**C**) Physical assessment findings in pneumothorax include subcutaneous emphysema, decreased vocal fremitus, ipsilateral hyperresonance, decreased breath sounds, and tracheal deviation toward the affected side.

Reference: Alspach, J. G. (ed.): AACN Core Curriculum for Critical Care Nursing, 5th ed. Philadelphia, W. B. Saunders, 1998.

3–47. (**C**) The two major processes involved in acute respiratory failure are increased lung vascular water and impaired ventilation. Causes of increased lung vascular water include pulmonary edema and adult respiratory distress syndrome; those of impaired ventilation include neuromuscular disease, chronic obstructive pulmonary disease, pneumothorax, and cerebrovascular accident.

Reference: Alspach, J. G. (ed.): AACN Core Curriculum for Critical Care Nursing, 5th ed. Philadelphia, W. B. Saunders, 1998.

3–48. (**D**) A basal skull fracture extends into the anterior, middle, or posterior fossae at the base of the skull. This may cause injury to cranial nerves as well as a tearing of the dura mater, which may result in a cerebrospinal fluid (CSF) otorrhea or rhinorrhea that can lead to meningitis, a serious complication after head trauma. Anterior fossa fractures may result in bilateral periorbital ecchymoses (raccoon eyes) from bleeding into the sinuses and rhinorrhea, if the dura is torn. Middle fossa fractures are characterized by Battle's sign (a hemorrhagic area behind the ear after fracture) and CSF otorrhea. Otorrhea occurs if the dura is torn and the tympanic membrane is ruptured, causing leakage of CSF. A halo sign is a yellow ring that appears around bloody drainage from the ear or nose. Posterior fossa fractures result in epidural hematomas with resultant medullary failure and death if left untreated. Spinal cord injury, jugular venous compression, and seizures may all result from head trauma, but meningitis is the sequela that causes the greatest concern.

Reference: Barker, E. (ed.): Neuroscience Nursing. Mosby–Year Book, St. Louis, 1994.

3–49. (**C**) Thrombus formation with migration to the mesentery due to myocardial infarction and/or atrial fibrillation is the likely cause of mesenteric ischemia. Mesenteric embolectomy will be necessary and is very risky, owing to the recent myocardial infarction. Duodenal ulcers are treated with pyloroplasty and vagotomy. Regional ileitis with fistulas would be treated with a temporary ileostomy. Diverticulitis is treated with a transverse colostomy.

Reference: Quinn, A. D.: Acute mesenteric ischemia. Crit. Care Nurs. Clin. North Am. 5:171–175, 1993.

3–50. (**B**) Treatment of hypoglycemia depends on the clinical severity of the episode and on blood glucose measurements. Mild and moderate hypoglycemia can be treated with rapid-acting oral carbohydrates. A patient with intravenous access with severe hypoglycemia should receive 50% dextrose IV, which acts within 5 minutes. A response to IM or SQ glucagon usually takes 10 to 15 minutes but is appropriate if the patient is without intravenous access.

Reference: Macheca, M. K. Diabetic hypoglycemia: How to keep the threat at bay. Am. J. Nurs. 93(4):26–30, 1993.

3–51. (**A**) Symptoms are most likely due to gut-associated graft-versus-host disease (GVHD), and the guaiac positive finding indicates sloughing of internal intestinal mucosa. The diarrhea can result in fluid and electrolyte imbalances and, therefore, fluid replacement is indicated. Antibiotics are instituted with fever. Analgesics are indicated if cramping is associated with diarrhea. GVHD treatment usually involves immunosuppressive therapy.

References: Franco, T., Gould, D. A.: Allogenic bone marrow transplantation. Semin. Oncol. Nurs. 10:3–11, 1994.
Wujcik, D., Ballard, B., Camp-Sorrell, D.: Selected complications of allogenic bone marrow transplantation. Semin. Oncol. Nurs. 10:28–41, 1994.

3–52. (**C**) Increasing minute ventilation is the body's attempt to compensate for the increasing dead space and increasing carbon dioxide production associated with tracheobronchitis. As the condition worsens, dynamic compliance decreases and shunting and pulmonary edema increase.

Reference: Demling, R. H.: Smoke inhalation injury. *In* Shoemaker, W. C., Ayres, S. M., Grenvik, A., Holbrook, P. R. (eds.): Textbook of Critical Care, 3rd ed. Philadelphia, W. B. Saunders, 1995.

3–53. (**C**) A widening QRS complex, tachycardia, aberrant conduction, and bradycardia are possible side effects of dopamine administration. Decreased venous return and myocardial ischemia may be present but do not cause a widened QRS complex. Anaphylaxis does not affect the QRS complex.

Reference: Roberts, S. L.: Multisystem deviations. *In* Critical Care Nursing: Assessment and Intervention. Stamford, Conn. Appleton & Lange, 1996.

3–54. (**B**) Postprocedural care of laser myoplasty patients is similar to that for other angiographic procedures. There is a risk of septal rupture from deep laser troughs, dysrhythmias, and cardiac ischemia (causing decreased cardiac output). Cerebrovascular accident is not a common complication of percutaneous laser myoplasty.

Reference: Enfanto, P. A., Pieczek, A. M., Kelley, K., et al.: Percutaneous laser myoplasty: Nursing care implications. Crit. Care Nurs. 14 (3):94–101, 1994.

3–55. (**A**) Regardless of the patient's hemodynamic status, stimulation of the latissimus dorsi muscle begins 2 weeks after surgery so that the flap has time to heal. The patient may have been discharged before the initiation of stimulation.

Reference: Bove, L. A., Mancini, M. G., Duris, L., et al.: Nursing care of patients undergoing dynamic cardiomyoplasty. Crit. Care Nurs. 15 (3):96–104, 1995.

3–56. (**A**) Patients with chronic obstructive pulmonary disease may become psychologically dependent on the ventilator and fearful of the weaning process—especially if weaning has been unsuccessful in the past. Weaning parameters that predict successful weaning include ability to double the minute ventilation, spontaneous tidal volume greater than 5 ml/kg, and respiratory rate less than 35 breaths/min.

References: Alspach, J. G. (ed.): AACN Core Curriculum for Critical Care Nursing, 5th ed. Philadelphia, W. B. Saunders, 1998.
Kirsten, L. D.: Comprehensive Respiratory Nursing: A Decision Making Approach. Philadelphia, W. B. Saunders, 1989.

3–57. (**B**) Although all these weaning methods are viable options, pressure support ventilation provides consistent support while slowly reducing the ventilatory rate and providing positive reinforcement to the patient. T-tube trials tend to tire patients who have been ventilated for a long time, and the system provides no monitoring of rate or tidal volume. Intermittent mandatory ventilation provides support intermittently and monitoring is available, but patients can become fatigued breathing in between the ventilator breaths. Extubation ("sink or swim" method) is premature at this point but is generally used as a last resort or when the endotracheal tube is small and creates increased airway resistance and work of breathing.

References: Alspach, J. G. (ed.): AACN Core Curriculum for Critical Care Nursing, 5th ed. Philadelphia, W. B. Saunders, 1998.
Kirsten, L. D.: Comprehensive Respiratory Nursing: A Decision Making Approach. Philadelphia, W. B. Saunders, 1989.

3–58. (**A**) Septal rupture is indicated by the ECG changes indicating disruption of conduction through the right bundle. Septal defects will also cause holosystolic murmurs and lung congestion. Mitral valve rupture would cause a holosystolic murmur but would not cause bundle branch block. Aortic valve rupture would cause a diastolic murmur. Tricuspid valve rupture would cause systemic venous congestion but not pulmonary congestion.

Reference: Rosenthal, M. A., Ellis, J. I.: Cardiac and mediastinal trauma. Emerg. Med. Clin. North Am. 13:887–899, 1995.

3–59. (**D**) The goal of nutrition therapy in acute renal failure is to provide a balance between sufficient calories and protein to prevent catabolism. The typical renal failure patient is hypermetabolic and requires increased calories. The kidneys are unable to rid the body of wastes, fluid, and electrolytes; therefore, the renal failure patient's diet is typically fluid, potassium, sodium, and protein restricted. Restricting protein results in less urea and nitrogen as waste products of metabolism.

Reference: Carlson, K. K.: Acute renal failure. *In* Urban, N. A., Krumberger, J. M., Winkelman, C. (eds.): Guidelines for Critical Care Nursing. St. Louis, Mosby–Year Book, 1995.

3–60. (**D**) Treatment of metabolic acidosis is usually not instituted until the serum bicarbonate level drops below 15 mEq/L. Once the serum bicarbonate level drops below 15 mEq/L, only one half of the base deficit is replaced to avoid overcorrecting the pH. Administration of excessive sodium bicarbonate can cause tetany and lead to the development of pulmonary edema.

Reference: Carlson, K. K.: Acute renal failure. *In* Urban, N. A., Krumberger, J. M., Winkelman, C. (eds.): Guidelines for Critical Care Nursing. St. Louis, Mosby–Year Book, 1995.

3–61. (**B**) The presentation of a penetrating right upper quadrant flank injury with symptoms of peritonitis is classic for a combined duodenal/pancreatic injury. This combination accounts for 5% to 10% of abdominal injury. Signs of peritonitis include rigid abdomen, rebound tenderness with guarding, decreased or absent bowel sounds, and fever, chills, or nausea. Anatomically, the head of the pancreas is nestled in the duodenum and the secretory ducts of the pancreas enter the duodenum. Respiratory distress would be present if the lung had been penetrated. The stomach and descending colon are not anatomically associated with the right upper quadrant. The liver and gallbladder are partially shielded by the rib cage and are generally not associated with right upper quadrant/flank penetration injuries.

Reference: Lawrence, D. M.: Gastrointestinal trauma. Crit. Care Nurs. Clin. North Am. 5:127–140, 1993.

3–62. (**B**) The blood gas shows respiratory acidosis, which is common in patients with COPD. However, the low oxygen level in a clinically stable patient leads one to suspect an inaccurate blood gas; the most likely cause is a venous blood gas. There is no indication of either hypoventilation (the spontaneous tidal volume of 350 ml is close to normal) or cardiac failure.

Reference: Kirsten, L. D.: Comprehensive Respiratory Nursing: A Decision Making Approach. Philadelphia, W. B. Saunders, 1989.

3–63. (**D**) It is premature at this point to hold a conference, call the daughter-in-law, or have the chaplain involved. Patients with COPD can be very demanding (physically and emotionally). Family members or caregivers frequently use hospitalizations as a respite from the demands of caregiving. The most appropriate action, therefore, would be to call the patient's wife and discuss the family's wishes regarding how they would like to be involved in the patient's care.

References: Alspach, J. G. (ed.): AACN Core Curriculum for Critical Care Nursing, 5th ed. Philadelphia, W. B. Saunders, 1998.
Kirsten, L. D.: Comprehensive Respiratory Nursing: A Decision Making Approach. Philadelphia, W. B. Saunders, 1989.

3–64. (**C**) Pursed-lip breathing does not affect secretion clearance. Pursed-lip breathing does increase airway back pressure that may help to stabilize the open airways, slows breathing, and reduces the sensation of dyspnea.

Reference: Alspach, J. G. (ed.): AACN Core Curriculum for Critical Care Nursing, 5th ed. Philadelphia, W. B. Saunders, 1998.

3–65. (**A**) Autotransfusion of shed blood has fewer risks than packed cells. Risks of nonautologous transfusion include transfusion reaction and the potential for disease transmission. The laboratory results would be back by the time the fresh frozen plasma was defrosted. Plasmanate would offer volume expansion only, but the patient needs blood replacement.

Reference: Wright, J. E., Shelton, B. K.: Desk Reference for Critical Care Nursing. Boston, Jones & Bartlett, 1993.

3–66. (**D**) Ankle-brachial indexes of less than 0.50 indicate advanced occlusive disease. The normal ankle-brachial index is greater than 0.95. An ankle-brachial index of 0.94 to 0.50 indicates that claudication is present.

Reference: Moore, W.: Vascular Surgery: A Comprehensive Review. Philadelphia, W. B. Saunders, 1993.

3–67. (**D**) The kidneys receive one fourth of the cardiac output, and their function is a reflection of graft patency. Neurovascular integrity indicates graft patency and perfusion. Colonization and symptoms of infection generally take more than 24 hours to become evident.

Reference: Wright, J. E., Shelton, B. K.: Desk Reference for Critical Care Nursing. Boston, Jones & Bartlett, 1993.

3–68. (**A**) The usual range of dosage for urokinase infusion is 1000 to 4000 IU/min carefully titrated and delivered by infusion pump.

Reference: Fahey, V.: Vascular Nursing, 2nd ed. Philadelphia, W. B. Saunders, 1994.

3–69. (**A**) A shift of the oxyhemoglobin dissociation curve to the right causes oxygen to dissociate more readily from hemoglobin and diffuse to the tissues, not bind more tightly. A shift to the right occurs with acidosis.

Reference: Alspach, J. G. (ed.): AACN Core Curriculum for Critical Care Nursing, 5th ed. Philadelphia, W. B. Saunders, 1998.

3–70. (**B**) Obstructive shock occurs as a result of a mechanical barrier to blood flow that blocks oxygen delivery to the tissues. Obstructions that can cause obstructive shock include pulmonary thromboembolism, pericardial tamponade, tension pneumothorax, dissecting aortic aneurysm, and atrial myxoma. Respiratory compromise related to flail chest or bronchial edema, if of sufficient severity, produces hypoxia followed by cardiogenic shock.

Reference: Roberts, S. L.: Cardiac deviations. *In* Critical Care Nursing: Assessment and Intervention. Stamford, Conn., Appleton & Lange, 1996.

3–71. (**A**) Hypertension can cause graft rupture with resultant hemorrhage. Pressures are maintained below specified systolic readings to prevent this occurrence. Nitroglycerin will not prevent spasm from occurring, nor will it prevent embolization. Although tissue perfusion is enhanced by the nitroglycerin, this is not its primary goal and it cannot raise blood pressure to the specified target range.

Reference: Wright, J. E., Shelton, B. K.: Desk Reference for Critical Care Nursing. Boston, Jones & Bartlett, 1993.

3–72. (**A**) Status epilepticus is characterized by recurrent generalized seizure activity without consciousness being regained. These recurrent tonic-clonic (grand mal) seizures are generalized symmetric seizures that affect the whole body. Absence seizures (petit mal) are so named because the patient experiences a brief loss of contact with the environment. Akinetic seizures are manifested by a brief loss of muscle tone. Myoclonic seizures are sudden, brief muscular contractions that usually involve the arms.

Reference: Alspach, J. G. (ed.): AACN Core Curriculum for Critical Care Nursing, 5th ed. Philadelphia, W. B. Saunders, 1998.

3–73. (**B**) Unless contraindicated, early enteral nutrition in the patient who has sustained abdominal trauma will maintain and nourish the intestinal mucosa. This is crucial in the prevention of bacterial translocation leading to gram-negative sepsis. Inhibition of bile secretion, inadequate glutamine intake, and the hypermetabolic response are consequences of inadequate enteral nutrition that result in the impairment of gut mucosal protection mechanisms.

Reference: Romito, R. A.: Early administration of enteral nutrients in critically ill patients. AACN Clin. Issues 6(2):242–256, 1995.

3–74. (**D**) The left coronary artery supplies the anterior two thirds of the left ventricle, atrioventricular junction, and posterior one third of the septum. The right coronary artery supplies the sinoatrial node in 90% of people and the inferior wall of the myocardium. The lateral wall of the left ventricle is supplied by the left coronary artery.

Reference: Dossey, B. M., Guzzetta, C. E., Kenner, C. V.: Critical Care Nursing, Body–Mind–Spirit. Philadelphia, J. B. Lippincott, 1992.

3–75. (**A**) Diabetes insipidus results in the hyposecretion of antidiuretic hormone (ADH) from the posterior lobe of the pituitary gland. The increased urine output that results from diabetes insipidus is caused by the inability to conserve water because of the lack of ADH. Consequently, the urine is minimally concentrated, as evidenced by a very low urine specific gravity.

Reference: Counsel, C. M., Gilbert, M., Snively, C.: Management of the patient with a pituitary tumor. Dimens. Crit. Care Nurs. 15(2):75–81, 1996.

3–76. (**B**) Patients who have had cardiac surgery have pain from sternal incisions that may be difficult to distinguish from ischemic cardiac pain due to spasm or infarction. ST segment monitoring provides continuous visual monitoring of ST segment elevation or depression that can be an early warning of ischemia. ST segments are elevated in the leads over the area of ischemia and may be depressed over the reciprocal leads. Supraventricular and ventricular ectopy are best distinguished from analysis of the 12-lead ECG. The 12-lead ECGs are performed in the postoperative period to assess all myocardial changes as well as to differentiate ventricular from supraventricular dysrhythmias.

Reference: Thelan, L. A., Davie, J. K., Urden, L. D., Lough, M. E.: Critical Care Nursing, Diagnosis and Management, 2nd ed. St. Louis, Mosby–Year Book, 1994.

3-77. (**D**) CK-MB2/MB1 ratio of 2.0 is diagnostic for acute MI. CK-MB isoforms may be divided into two subforms: MB1 and MB2. They are normally equal in plasma (1:1), but in acute myocardial infarction, MB2 is released early while CK-MB levels may still be normal. Levels of CK MB2/MB1 equal to or greater than 1.5/1 are diagnostic for acute MI. The normal CK total is 96 to 140 U/L in females and 36 to 174 U/L in males. CPK-MB is measured in percent of total CPK, the normal being 0%.

Reference: Puleo, P. R., Meyer, D., Tawa, C. B., et al. (eds.): Use of a rapid assay of subforms of creatine kinase MB to diagnose or rule out acute myocardial infarction. N. Engl. J. Med. 331:561–566, 1994.

3-78. (**C**) Her symptoms and history point to respiratory distress syndrome as the most likely diagnosis. An amnionic fluid embolus is the likely cause. Pulmonary thromboembolus does not present as hypotension unless massive and, additionally, presents as pleuritic chest pain and fever. Cardiomyopathy would show cardiac signs; status asthmaticus would elicit wheezing or diminished breath sounds rather than crackles and CO_2 retention.

Reference: Alspach, J. G. (ed.): AACN Core Curriculum for Critical Care Nursing, 5th ed. Philadelphia, W. B. Saunders, 1998.

3-79. (**A**) PEEP is the most appropriate therapy at this point to correct the refractory hypoxemia. Negative-pressure ventilation would not be appropriate because it would not correct the severe hypoxemia. Hyperbaric oxygen might be indicated, but a carboxyhemoglobin level would need to be drawn to determine if it is necessary. A bronchoscopy may also be indicated to assess for any airway damage, but that would be considered as a diagnostic tool rather than as a treatment.

Reference: Alspach, J. G. (ed.): AACN Core Curriculum for Critical Care Nursing, 5th ed. Philadelphia, W. B. Saunders, 1998.

3-80. (**A**) Splanchnic hypoperfusion during shock can lead to subsequent acalculous cholecystitis and, infrequently, pancreatitis. Although the other choices can be complications of shock, the right upper quadrant would not be the expected location of pain.

Reference: Jones, K.: Shock. In Clochesy, J. M., Breu, C., Cardin, S., et al (eds.): Critical Care Nursing. Philadelphia, W. B. Saunders, 1996.

3-81. (**C**) Acute hemodialysis is indicated when the patient's blood urea nitrogen is greater than 100 mg/dl, creatinine is greater than 10 mg/dl, and the creatinine clearance is 5 to 7 ml/min. Other indications for acute hemodialysis include acute volume overload, uncontrolled hyperkalemia, uncontrolled acidosis, uremic encephalopathy, and pulmonary edema refractory to diuretics.

Reference: Carlson, K. K.: Acute renal failure. In Urban, N. A., Krumberger, J. M., Winkelman, C. (eds.): Guidelines for Critical Care Nursing. St. Louis, Mosby–Year Book, 1995.

3-82. (**C**) Wall motion abnormalities can be detected with echocardiography within 4 hours of an acute myocardial infarction (MI). Newly infarcted areas appear thickened due to edema and demonstrate decreased or altered motion on visualization by an echocardiogram. Non–Q wave MIs are not as easily visualized on an echocardiogram as transmural MIs, which affect the full thickness of the myocardium. Old MIs appear as thin-walled areas on the echocardiogram, and left ventricular aneurysms expand during systole.

Reference: Thelan, L. A., Davie, J. K., Urden, L. D., Lough, M. E.: Critical Care Nursing, Diagnosis and Management, 2nd ed. St. Louis, Mosby–Year Book, 1994.

3–83. (**D**) Typical findings in ventricular septal rupture are related to the left to right shunt produced and include large "v" waves in pulmonary artery tracings, increased oxygen saturation in the right ventricle, and a holosystolic murmur. In papillary muscle rupture, the "v" wave is large and a holosystolic murmur is present but right-sided oxygen saturation is normal. With right ventricular infarction, PCWP pressure is lower. In cardiogenic shock, an S_3 or S_4 would be noted but no change in right ventricular oxygen saturation would occur.

Reference: Thelan, L. A., Davie, J. K., Urden, L. D., Lough, M. E.: Critical Care Nursing, Diagnosis and Management, 2nd ed. St. Louis, Mosby–Year Book, 1994.

3–84. (**D**) Phenytoin (Dilantin) is a synthetic drug used as an anticonvulsant to inhibit the spread of seizure discharges within the nervous system. It is very effective for the control of seizures, but there are some precautions for its use. One major precaution that health care personnel, patients with seizures, and their families must know is that the drug should never be abruptly stopped or withdrawn because a seizure or status epilepticus may occur. Common side effects of phenytoin include gingival hyperplasia, megaloblastic anemia, blood dyscrasias, and decreased serum folate levels. Toxic effects include peripheral neuropathy.

Reference: Hickey, J. V.: The Clinical Practice of Neurological and Neurosurgical Nursing, 3rd ed. Philadelphia, J. B. Lippincott, 1992.

3–85. (**B**) H_2 blockers such as cimetidine, ranitidine, and famotidine are frequently used to block the histamine stimulation of gastric acid–secreting cells. Ethanol decreases gastric mucus thickness and stimulates histamine release. Salicylates inhibit bicarbonate secretion. Corticosteroids decrease mucus production and increase acid secretion.

Reference: Prevost, S. S., Oberlie, A.: Stress ulceration in the critically ill patient. Crit. Care Nurs. Clin. North Am. 5:163–169, 1993.

3–86. (**A**) Assessment of hemodynamic stability as well as oxygenation parameters such as arterial blood gases are priorities to determine readiness to wean. Chest radiographic findings may be helpful but do not always correlate directly with the clinical picture. Spirometry and pulmonary function tests are not performed on intubated patients, although certain portions of the tests are measured as weaning parameters.

Reference: Knebel, A. R.: Ventilator weaning protocols and techniques: Getting the job done. AACN Clin. Issues 7:550–559, 1996.

3–87. (**C**) Slowly decreasing the mechanical ventilation rate would be the appropriate first step in weaning. Weaning by other means would be inappropriate at this time because the patient's tidal volume is low, respiratory rate is high, vital capacity is low, MVV should be at least double the minute ventilation before initiating weaning, and MIP should be more than -20 cm H_2O. All indications, then, are that she is not ready to wean at this point. A T-tube trial therefore would be premature. Getting her out of bed would increase her oxygen requirements, so dangling or resistive range of motion with physical therapy could be an initial step during the weaning process to ensure tolerance. It is also premature to transfer her to a special weaning unit/hospital because she is not ready to be weaned and a trial of weaning has not yet been attempted.

Reference: Tobin, M. J. (ed.): Principles and Practice of Mechanical Ventilation. New York, McGraw-Hill, 1994.

3–88. (**D**) At this point, transfer to a special weaning unit/facility could be considered. Her weaning process seems to have plateaued, and weaning units/facilities are set up to maximize rehabilitation and weaning. These units have been shown to reduce length of stay, improve mortality, and decrease costs. Her SIMV rate is low, but her weaning parameters are still inadequate. Her saturation falls when getting to a chair, so ambulation is premature at this point. Her weaning parameters are still inadequate to attempt a T-tube trial, and decreasing the mechanical ventilatory rate has only succeeded in dropping the rate to 6.

Reference: Kersten, L. D.: Comprehensive Respiratory Nursing: A Decision Making Approach. Philadelphia, W. B. Saunders, 1989.

3–89. (**D**) Papillary muscle rupture almost always occurs after an inferoposterior or posterolateral myocardial infarction. The posterior papillary muscle receives its blood supply from the posterior descending branch of the right coronary artery or the dominant left coronary artery, occlusion of which causes inferoposterior or posterolateral myocardial infarction. The anterior papillary muscle has a dual blood supply from the left anterior descending and the circumflex arteries, making rupture or ischemia uncommon. These arteries supply the lateral and anterior walls as well. The inferior wall is supplied by the right coronary artery and the posterior wall is supplied by both the right and left coronary arteries.

Reference: Rich, M.: Therapy for acute myocardial infarction. Clin. Geriatr. Med. 12:141–161, 1996.

3–90. (**B**) Nutrition is not a priority during the initial phase because treatment priorities are to find and treat the source of sepsis. Once the patient is hemodynamically stable, nutritional support is essential to meet the increased energy demands associated with the shock syndrome. High-protein, low-fat, isotonic enteral feedings are preferred, but clinical status may require temporary parenteral support.

Reference: Clochesy, J. M.: Patients with systemic inflammatory response syndrome. *In* Clochesy, J. M., Breu, C., Cardin, S., et al. (eds.): Critical Care Nursing. Philadelphia, W. B. Saunders, 1996.

3–91. (**D**) Patients with acute head injury initially are hyperventilated to decrease cerebral edema. Hyperventilation decreases the $PaCO_2$, which results in vasoconstriction in the cerebral vasculature. Patients with asthma, respiratory distress syndrome, and acute lung injury may benefit from this therapy and be able to lower mean airway pressures, thus reducing the risk of volutrauma.

Reference: Wilmoth, D. F., Carpenter, R. M.: Preventing complications of mechanical ventilation: Permissive hypercapnia. AACN Clin. Issues 7:473–481, 1996.

3–92. (**B**) Although blood, inotropic agents, and fluid therapy may all be indicated, the most appropriate intervention is PEEP, which will correct the refractory hypoxemia and acidosis. Administration of blood would increase the oxygen-carrying capacity and transport if the hemoglobin level is decreased or the cardiac output is low. Fluid administration would be indicated to increase cardiac output and thus oxygen transport. Inotropic agents are given when the intravascular volume is adequate, yet the cardiac output remains low.

References: Alspach, J. G. (ed.): AACN Core Curriculum for Critical Care Nursing, 5th ed. Philadelphia, W. B. Saunders, 1998.
Kirsten, L. D.: Comprehensive Respiratory Nursing: A Decision Making Approach. Philadelphia, W. B. Saunders, 1989.

3–93. (**C**) Ticlodipine (Ticlid) and dipyridamole are both antiplatelet agents, although dipyridamole has less antiplatelet activity than aspirin. Warfarin (Coumadin) and heparin do not affect platelets directly. Enteric-coated aspirin may ease stomach upset, but if a patient cannot take aspirin due to allergy, he or she should not take enteric-coated aspirin either.

Reference: Ruppert, S. D., Kernicki, J. G., Dolan, J. T.: Dolan's Critical Care Nursing: Clinical Management Through the Nursing Process. Philadelphia, F. A. Davis, 1996.

3–94. (**B**) Third-degree (complete) AV block associated with inferior wall myocardial infarction is often transient, but when third-degree AV block occurs with anterior wall myocardial infarction, it is usually permanent, and thus a permanent pacemaker implant is indicated.

Reference: Kinney, M. R., Packa, D. R., Dunbar, S. B.: AACN's Clinical Reference for Critical Care Nursing, 3rd ed. St. Louis, Mosby–Year Book, 1993.

3–95. (**D**) Intracranial pressure may be monitored by several methods, including the intraventricular, intraparenchymal, subarachnoid, and, less frequently, the epidural method. Normal ICP is generally less than 10 mm Hg, with pressures between 10 and 20 mm Hg considered to be mildly to moderately elevated. ICPs greater than 20 mm Hg are considered severely elevated. Normal CPP is about 70 mm Hg. A calculated CPP of less than 70 mm Hg (mean arterial pressure minus ICP) denotes diminished perfusion related to an increase in ICP.

References: Alspach, J. G. (ed.): AACN Core Curriculum for Critical Care Nursing, 5th ed. Philadelphia, W. B. Saunders, 1998.
Clochesy, J. M., Breu, C., Cardin, S., et al. (eds.): Critical Care Nursing, 2nd ed. Philadelphia, W. B. Saunders, 1996.

3–96. (**A**) Also called plateau waves or Lundberg waves, A waves are waveforms that represent elevations of intracranial pressure (ICP) between 50 and 100 mm Hg. A waves last between 5 and 20 minutes and are usually associated with advanced stages of intracranial hypertension. B and C waves correspond to respiratory and arterial pressure changes, respectively, but are generally not considered significant in relation to ICP. D waves are not seen on the ICP monitor.

Reference: Alspach, J. G. (ed.): AACN Core Curriculum for Critical Care Nursing, 5th ed. Philadelphia, W. B. Saunders, 1998.

3–97. (**D**) The treatment plan must be scrutinized for elements that will cause false results when monitoring for occult blood in gastric juice or stool. Antacids in gastric juice commonly cause false-negative results on guaiac testing. Cimetidine, aspirin, and iron supplements cause a false-positive result on the Hemoccult-type slide guaiac test.

References: Prevost, S. S., Oberlie, A.: Stress ulceration in the critically ill patient. Crit. Care Nurs. Clin. North Am. 5:163–169, 1993.
Yamada, T. (ed.): Textbook of Gastroenterology, 2nd ed. Philadelphia, J. B. Lippincott, 1995.

3–98. (**A**) Patients with anterior infarcts are more prone to left ventricular failure. Nitroglycerin decreases preload and blood volume and therefore should decrease signs of failure. Fluid restriction does not remove the fluid. Sodium restriction without preload reduction such as nitrates or diuretics will not decrease pulmonary congestion. Performance of a 12-lead ECG is not a treatment.

Reference: Kinney, M. R., Packa, D. R., Dunbar, S. B.: AACN's Clinical Reference for Critical Care Nursing, 3rd ed. St. Louis, C. V. Mosby, 1993.

3–99. (**A**) The arterial blood pressure reflects the adequacy of fluid administration if the patient responds rapidly and maintains a mean arterial pressure of 60 mm Hg or greater. If the patient has evidence of heart failure, the pulmonary artery wedge pressure is maintained at 12 to 18 mm Hg. Indirect measurements of adequate volume replacement and correction of septic insult include a urine output greater than 20 ml/hr and arterial blood lactate levels less than 2.2 mmol/dL.

Reference: Jones, K.: Shock. *In* Clochesy, J. M., Breu, C., Cardin, S., et al. (eds.): Critical Care Nursing. Philadelphia, W. B. Saunders, 1996.

3–100. (**A**) This collection of signs and symptoms are the defining characteristics of SIADH, which results in water intoxication. This is reflected in the nursing diagnosis of fluid volume excess. Thought processes are altered related to fluid volume excess and cerebral edema, not confusion and ICU psychosis. If the patient's condition goes untreated, impaired gas exchange may become a relevant nursing diagnosis, but the symptoms do not indicate this problem yet.

Reference: Alspach, J. G. (ed.): AACN Core Curriculum for Critical Care Nursing, 5th ed. Philadelphia, W. B. Saunders, 1998.

3–101. (**C**) Acute rejection is primarily a cellular immune response that is mediated by T lymphocytes, and it is currently the only type of transplant rejection that can be effectively treated. Chronic graft rejection is mediated by both B and T lymphocytes but primarily from a humoral immune response. Hyperacute rejection can be prevented by ensuring ABO blood group compatibility and by lymphocyte crossmatching.

Reference: Wahrenberger, A.: Pharmacologic immunosuppression: Cure or curse? Crit. Care Nurs. Q. 17(4):27–36, 1995.

3–102. (**B**) The Glasgow Coma Scale (GCS) is an internationally recognized standardized assessment tool that evaluates level of consciousness, the most sensitive indicator of cerebral function. The patient's best responses in three areas, eye opening, motor response, and verbal response, are graded, and then the scores are summed. Scores range from a low of 3 to a high of 15, with 15 being normal.

Reference: Clochesy, J. M., Breu, C., Cardin, S., et al. (eds.): Critical Care Nursing, 2nd ed. Philadelphia, W. B. Saunders, 1996.

3–103. (**C**) Right ventricular myocardial infarction is highly associated with inferior wall myocardial infarctions because both the right ventricle and the inferior wall receive their blood supply from the right coronary artery. Therefore, assessment of changes in right precordial ECG leads is suggested.

Reference: Proulx, R., Guidetti, K., Bagg, A., Marchette, L.: Detection of right ventricular myocardial infarction. Crit. Care Nurs. 12(6):50–59, 1992.

3–104. (**A**) Aspirin and heparin prevent thrombosis by their antiplatelet and antithrombin activity. Nitroglycerin dilates coronary arteries and ACE inhibitors prevent vasoconstriction, but they have no effect on thrombus development.

Reference: Braunwald, E. (ed.): Heart Disease: A Textbook of Cardiovascular Medicine. Philadelphia, W. B. Saunders, 1997.

3–105. (**D**) The first step should be to check the transducer level because it is the most frequently manipulated equipment. Second, the nurse would inspect for leaks, blood, or air bubbles. The skin-to-tip distance can alert the nurse if the catheter has migrated. The most expensive measure for the patient is to take a chest radiograph to determine where the tip of the catheter is located.

Reference: Boggs, R. L., Wooldridge-King, M. (eds.): AACN Procedure Manual for Critical Care, 3rd ed. Philadelphia, W. B. Saunders, 1993.

3–106. (**B**) Pneumothoraces occur because of a difference between alveolar and interstitial pressures. The larger the difference, the more likely a pneumothorax is to occur. Atelectasis would impair the transmission of pressure to the alveolus, and a pneumothorax is less likely to occur. Alpha$_1$-antitrypsin deficiency and COPD may increase the risk of pneumothorax in select patients but would not increase the risk in the respiratory distress patient population in general.

Reference: Marini, J. J.: New options for the ventilatory management of acute lung injury. New Horizons 1:489–503, 1993.

3–107. (**C**) Isolation for tuberculosis should be continued until a satisfactory clinical and bacterial response to the drug therapy is achieved. Drug therapy lasts a year or more, even beyond negative sputum cultures. A definitive positive sputum culture can take 4 to 8 weeks to manifest.

Reference: Kinney, M. R., Packa, D. R., Dunbar, S. B. (eds.): AACN's Clinical Reference for Critical Care Nursing, 3rd ed. St. Louis, Mosby–Year Book, 1993.

3–108. (**B**) The most appropriate treatment of headache is to reduce the nitroglycerin, give appropriate analgesia for the headache, and then titrate the nitroglycerin slowly upward. Relief of the headache is important because pain increases the sympathetic response, which may induce further decreases in myocardial perfusion.

Reference: Olson, H. G., Aronow, W. S.: Medical management of stable and unstable angina in the elderly with CAD. Clin. Geriatr. Med. 12:121–137, 1996.

3–109. (**D**) Enteral nutrients are a key factor in preventing bacterial translocation from the gut to the circulation, leading to sepsis. Narcotics and bed rest contribute to constipation. A hypermetabolic state occurs when enteral feeding is withheld. Hypoplasia of the intestinal mucosa will occur in the absence of enteral nutrition, even when total parenteral nutrition is in place.

Reference: Lawrence, D. M.: Gastrointestinal trauma. Crit. Care Nurs. Clin. North Am. 5:127–140, 1993.

3–110. (**C**) Lipids are limited to 10% to 15% of the total caloric requirements to provide essential fatty acids while at the same time avoiding fatty liver and cholecystitis complications. Lesser amounts of lipids would delay healing.

Reference: Roberts, S. L.: Multisystem deviations. *In* Critical Care Nursing: Assessment and Intervention. Stamford, Conn., Appleton & Lange, 1996.

3–111. (**C**) Coronary air embolism is usually a self-limiting complication; however, it may result in myocardial infarction. To ensure adequate arterial oxygenation until the embolus resolves, 100% oxygen is delivered. Patient position should be maintained so that the affected leg is maintained without flexion. Vasoactive medications are maintaining hemodynamic stability. The patient is being monitored for ST changes, indicating ischemia and making immediate performance of 12-lead ECG unnecessary.

Reference: Kern, M. J., Deligonul, U.: The Interventional Cardiac Catheterization Handbook. St. Louis, Mosby–Year Book, 1996.

3–112. (**D**) Decreased stroke volume related to loss of atrial kick may be contributing to the patient's decreased mental status and hypotension. Insertion of a transvenous atrioventricular sequential pacemaker would restore atrial kick. Transthoracic pacing would not restore atrial kick and may make the patient more confused and combative because of the discomfort associated with pacemaker discharge. Atropine administration may be used as a bridge to the use of a pacemaker in acute myocardial infarction, but it is not necessary if the cardiologist is available to insert the pacemaker and the blood pressure is stable. Bypass surgery may be performed when the patient is stable after a cardiac catheterization has been performed.

Reference: Ruppert, S. D., Kernicki, J. G., Dolan, J. T.: Dolan's Critical Care Nursing; Clinical Management Through the Nursing Process. Philadelphia, F. A. Davis, 1996.

3–113. (**B**) An abdominal support will help support the patient's abdomen when coughing or taking a deep breath. Arterial blood gas analysis may be useful but is expensive and invasive. A pulse oximeter would be more appropriate for continued monitoring. Suction equipment and a nasal trumpet are not necessary unless she is unable to mobilize secretions.

Reference: Alspach, J. G. (ed.): AACN Core Curriculum for Critical Care Nursing, 5th ed. Philadelphia, W. B. Saunders, 1998.

3–114. (**C**) This patient's obesity and abdominal surgery predispose her to hypoventilation. In addition, she is at risk for atelectasis from the hypoventilation. Thus she retains carbon dioxide, leading to a respiratory acidosis and hypoxia, which will further the acidosis.

Reference: Alspach, J. G. (ed.): AACN Core Curriculum for Critical Care Nursing, 5th ed. Philadelphia, W. B. Saunders, 1998.

3–115. (**D**) Assisting the patient to make changes in a positive manner will aid the patient to continue the changes enforced in the hospital, even if the patient is in denial. The role of the nurse is to reinforce and clarify medical information given. It would be more appropriate for the nurse to respond to the denial by encouraging the patient to discuss findings with the physician than to confront the patient with this evidence. Doing so may cause the patient to block out all of the information the nurse is attempting to impart that would help the patient change behaviors. Involving both the family and the patient in educational endeavors is important. Educating the family and not the patient may disrupt the family member's ability to make necessary changes. Repetition is a valuable device used in teaching, but it does not affect motivation. For a patient in denial, the patient may "tune out" the repeated phrases. Enabling the patient to see that he has already accommodated change will make the changes easier to accept and encourage the patient to continue the changed behaviors.

Reference: Manson, J. E., Ridker, P. M., Gaziano, J. M., Hennekens, C. H.: Prevention of Myocardial Infarction. New York, Oxford University Press, 1996.

3–116. (**C**) Q waves in leads II, III, aVF and ST segment elevation in lead V_1 indicate a right ventricular myocardial infarction. Low blood pressure and elevated creatine kinase totals also indicate acute myocardial infarction. Treatment of right ventricular infarction requires fluid maintenance to improve preload to maintain cardiac output. Nitroglycerin is not generally used in right ventricular myocardial infarction because its vasodilatory effects decrease preload. Q waves signify necrosis, which does not resolve within 8 hours.

Reference: Khan, M. G.: Heart Disease Diagnosis and Therapy. Baltimore, Williams & Wilkins, 1996.

3–117. (**D**) Prinzmetal's angina is caused by coronary artery spasm. Beta blockers have been identified as a cause of increasing spasm in patients with Prinzmetal's angina. New onset of rest angina is classified as unstable angina, whereas rest pain in Prinzmetal's angina typically follows a chronic pattern, occurring at night. Both Prinzmetal's angina and unstable angina are associated with ST segment elevation during pain episodes, although ST segment depression is also common in unstable angina.

Reference: Khan, M. G.: Heart Disease Diagnosis and Therapy. Baltimore, Williams & Wilkins, 1996.

3–118. (**B**) Diabetes insipidus is caused by a decreased secretion of antidiuretic hormone (ADH). Patients with this syndrome excrete copious amounts of dilute urine of as much as 10 L/day. Urine specific gravity is low (1.001 to 1.005), patients complain of polyuria, and their serum osmolarity is elevated. After traumatic brain injury, patients may experience central diabetes insipidus as a result of injury to the hypothalamus. Nephrogenic diabetes insipidus is unrelated to traumatic brain injury. Treatment of diabetes insipidus focuses on replacing lost fluids, administering ADH, monitoring urinary output and specific gravity, and monitoring electrolyte values. The syndrome of inappropriate secretion of antidiuretic hormone (SIADH) is characterized by a low serum osmolarity, dilutional hyponatremia, and decreased urinary output with a concomitant increased specific gravity. Treatment of SIADH focuses on fluid restriction, replacement of sodium with a hypertonic saline solution, and loop diuretics for diuresis.

Reference: Hickey, J. V.: The Clinical Practice of Neurological and Neurosurgical Nursing, 3rd ed. Philadelphia, J. B. Lippincott, 1992.

3–119. (**A**) Inotropic agents are administered to stimulate cardiac function. Vasopressors and fluid restrictors will compromise tissue perfusion, including cardiac perfusion. Hypertonic fluids are contraindicated because of the fluid shifts that will produce congestive heart failure as preload increases.

Reference: Shoemaker, W. C.: Diagnosis and treatment of the shock syndromes. *In* Shoemaker, W. C., Ayres, S. M., Grenvik, A., Holbrook, P. R. (eds.): Textbook of Critical Care, 3rd ed. Philadelphia, W. B. Saunders, 1995.

3–120. (**B**) Grey Turner's sign is characterized by periumbilical ecchymosis and may indicate retroperitoneal hematoma, a potential complication of femoral catheter insertion. Chvostek's and Trousseau's signs are seen in patients with hypocalcemia and hypomagnesemia. Kernig's sign is seen in patients with meningeal irritation.

Reference: Carlson, K. K.: Continuous renal replacement therapies. *In* Urban, N. A., Krumberger, J. M., Winkelman, C. (eds.): Guidelines for Critical Care Nursing. St. Louis, Mosby–Year Book, 1995.

3–121. (**D**) A bleeding duodenal ulcer that has not responded to conventional therapy would be treated with pyloroplasty and vagotomy. Mesenteric ischemia secondary to embolus would respond to embolectomy. Temporary ileostomy is used to rest the bowel for regional ileitis and Crohn's disease. Diverticulitis is treated with transverse colostomy.

References: Doughty, D. B., Jackson, D. B.: Gastrointestinal Disorders. St. Louis, Mosby–Year Book, 1993.
Prevost, S. S., Oberlie, A.: Stress ulceration in the critically ill patient. Crit. Care Nurs. Clin. North Am. 5:163–169, 1993.

3–122. **(B)** His symptoms and history are consistent with community-acquired pneumonia, which occurs in patients who are at risk, such as the elderly or immunosuppressed. Nosocomial pneumonia develops within 3 to 5 days of discharge from the hospital. The causative organisms are different for community-acquired pneumonia than for nosocomial pneumonia. His history of having a recent cold suggests the causative agent could be *Staphylococcus aureus*. The fever and type of sputum production are not consistent with pulmonary embolus, edema, or congestive heart failure.

Reference: American Thoracic Society: Guidelines for the initial management of adults with community-acquired pneumonia: Diagnosis, assessment of severity, and initial antimicrobial therapy. Am. Rev. Respir. Dis. 148:1418–1426, 1993.

3–123. **(D)** Twenty to 40% of the population are colonized with methacillin-resistant *Staphylococcus aureus,* and institutions are a common site for transmission of this organism between individuals. The patient has not exhibited symptoms of shock or pulmonary embolus, and it is unlikely that he has developed a superinfection so soon.

Reference: Kersten, L. D.: Comprehensive Respiratory Nursing: A Decision Making Approach. Philadelphia, W. B. Saunders, 1989.

3–124. **(A)** The retirement home may not accept him back until the methacillin-resistant *S. aureus* infection has been eliminated. Financial status should not be an issue for discharge planning because he already was placed in the home. It is unknown at this time what effect his illness will have on his ability to do activities of daily living or need for oxygen, so these are premature considerations.

Reference: Kersten, L. D.: Comprehensive Respiratory Nursing: A Decision Making Approach. Philadelphia, W. B. Saunders, 1989.

3–125. **(C)** Precipitating events leading to diabetic ketoacidosis consist of the following in order of their frequency: (1) infection, (2) omission or inadequate use of insulin, (3) new-onset diabetes, and (4) miscellaneous events. A complete blood cell count is important to assess for infection. A white blood cell count greater than 25,000/mm^3 with a left shift indicates bacterial infection. An increased anion gap is associated with diabetic ketoacidosis but is not reliable for diagnosis and does not point to etiology. Although chloride values help with the evaluation of fluid status and severity of acidosis, this value is complicated by a variety of states and patients present with varying degrees of hyperchloremia. Patients with diabetic ketoacidosis and abdominal pain may have normal amylase values, and patients with elevated amylase may be asymptomatic. Recently, hyperamylasemia has been demonstrated to be a feature of nondiabetic metabolic acidosis and is due to an increase in nonpancreatic amylase isozyme.

References: Civetta, J. M., Taylor, R. W., Kirby, R. R. (eds.): Critical Care, 2nd ed. Philadelphia, J. B. Lippincott, 1992.
Kitabchi, A. E., Wall, B. M.: Diabetic ketoacidosis. Med. Clin. North Am. 79:9–37, 1995.

3–126. **(B)** Hypoxemia (Pao_2 = 60 mm Hg) stimulates production of erythropoietin in the kidney, augmenting RBC synthesis. A secondary polycythemia develops as demonstrated by an increase in RBCs and hemoglobin only. Polycythemia vera (one of the myeloproliferative syndromes) usually demonstrates increased RBCs, WBCs, hemoglobin, and platelets. Idiopathic thrombocytopenic purpura, an autoimmune disorder, typically demonstrates laboratory values of reduced hemoglobin, hematocrit, and platelets.

Reference: Alspach, J. G. (ed.): AACN Core Curriculum for Critical Care Nursing, 5th ed. Philadelphia, W. B. Saunders, 1998.

3–127. (**B**) ST segment depression is more common in stable than in unstable angina. ST segment elevation in two or more leads is considered diagnostic for myocardial ischemia. ST segment elevation signifies ischemia in both stable and unstable angina. ST segment depression may also occur in chronic stable angina. Q waves signify that infarction has occurred.

Reference: Matrisciano, L.: Unstable angina: An overview. Critical Care Nurse, 12(12):30–40, 1992.

3–128. (**C**) T wave inversion is present in the anterior (V_{2-6}) and lateral (I, aVL) leads, which is common during anginal episodes in patients with unstable angina and is often associated with either ST segment elevation or depression (as noted in V_{4-5}). These ECG changes resolve with pain relief. Sinus node dysfunction or atrioventricular block is not indicative of unstable angina. There are no Q waves in this ECG.

Reference: Braunwald, E. (ed.): Heart Disease: A Textbook of Cardiovascular Medicine. Philadelphia, W. B. Saunders, 1997.

3–129. (**D**) Patients who have had a cardiac transplant or who have diabetic neuropathy require more subtle assessment of myocardial ischemia. Patients with neuropathy have diminished pain sensation. Nerves are severed in the transplanted heart so that angina is not experienced. Shortness of breath, dyspnea on exertion, or symptoms of left ventricular failure may be the only early clues to coronary ischemia. Persons with scleroderma and chronic renal failure are prone to unstable angina because of the vascular abnormalities associated with these conditions. They experience angina because they do not have nerve pathology.

Reference: Blake-Inada, L., Goldschlager, N.: Unstable angina: Strategies to minimize myocardial injury. Postgrad Med. 100:139–154, 1996.

3–130. (**B**) The breakdown of protein occurs in hyperdynamic metabolic states such as septic shock. As proteins are broken down, urea is produced. Initiation of nutritional support to achieve positive nitrogen balance will correct the problem. The kidneys are functioning; therefore, electrolyte, diuretic, and fluid volume therapy are not indicated.

Reference: Haak, S. W., Richardson, S. J., Davey, S. S.: Alterations in cardiovascular function. *In* Huether, S. E., McCance, K. L. (eds.): Understanding Pathophysiology. St. Louis, C. V. Mosby, 1996.

3–131. (**B**) Stable patients on pharmacologic therapy with unstable angina do not require emergent percutaneous transluminal coronary angioplasty.

Reference: Blake-Inada, L., Goldschlager, N.: Unstable angina: Strategies to minimize myocardial injury. Postgrad. Med. 100:139–154, 1996.

3–132. (**B**) Transtentorial herniation is most often associated with epidural and acute subdural hematoma formation because diffuse brain swelling shifts the intracranial structures. In transtentorial herniation, the medial aspect of the temporal lobe (also called the uncus) shifts toward the midline until finally shifting over the edge of the tentorium cerebelli. Herniation syndromes are a rostral to caudal (head to tail) event that manifests as Cushing's reflex associated with increasing intracranial pressure (i.e., increased arterial blood pressure with widened pulse pressure, bradycardia, and altered respiratory patterns). Deep, regular, sustained respirations (hyperpnea) is termed *central neurogenic hyperventilation* and is the characteristic respiratory pattern associated with transtentorial herniation; thus, a patient with an acute subdural hematoma with respiratory changes has, most likely, experienced a transtentorial herniation. Although respiratory changes could occur as a result of any intracranial pathology, tonsillar (medullary) herniation results from the contents of the cerebellum displacing through the foramen magnum causing brain stem disruption. Vasospasm is a sudden, transient contraction of cerebral vessels and is most often caused by an aneurysm, not a subdural hematoma. Hydrocephalus is an increased volume of cerebrospinal fluid (CSF) most often resulting from obstruction to the CSF by such things as mass lesions or impaired reabsorption of CSF from the subarachnoid space caused by meningeal irritation, not subdural hematoma.

Reference: Alspach, J. G. (ed.): AACN Core Curriculum for Critical Care Nursing, 5th ed. Philadelphia, W. B. Saunders, 1998.

3–133. (**C**) Although the first line of defense to pathogens in the gastrointestinal tract is the secretion of hydrochloric acid, fungal organisms such as *Candida* can survive at a pH of 1. Gram-negative organisms, gram-positive organisms, and oral microflora are very sensitive to gastric acidity.

Reference: Lord, L. M., Say, H. C.: The role of the gut in critical illness. AACN Clin. Issues 5:450–458, 1994.

3–134. (**B**) The typical signs and symptoms of an acute asthma attack are bilateral inspiratory and expiratory wheezing, increased respiratory rate, and accessory muscle use. Sputum production is minimal, white, thick, and sticky. Rales and rhonchi occur with fluid and mucus in the alveoli and airways and are not characteristic of an acute asthma attack.

Reference: Kersten, L. D.: Comprehensive Respiratory Nursing: A Decision Making Approach. Philadelphia, W. B. Saunders, 1989.

3–135. (**A**) Inhaled nitric oxide is used to reduce airway resistance by relaxing bronchial smooth muscle. Inverse ratio ventilation would result in hyperinflation and barotrauma because mucus blocks the removal of air. Permissive hypercapnia is used with caution in the elderly because it may be difficult to regulate the level of carbon dioxide. Pressure support ventilation would not be appropriate because her lungs are stiff and would necessitate high intrathoracic pressures with the risk of barotrauma and cardiovascular depression.

Reference: Zapol, W. M., Hurford, W. E.: Inhaled nitric oxide in the adult respiratory distress syndrome and other lung diseases. New Horizons 1:638–650, 1993.

3–136. (**A**) Administration of sublingual nitroglycerin should be implemented immediately after the 12-lead ECG is obtained. If sublingual nitroglycerin is ineffective, intravenous nitroglycerin is administered. If intravenous nitroglycerin is ineffective, morphine sulfate is given. If these pain relief measures are ineffective, the patient will then be placed on heparin as a treatment for myocardial ischemia to prevent and/or treat clot formation.

Reference: Blake-Inada, L., Goldschlager, N.: Unstable angina: Strategies to minimize myocardial injury. Postgrad. Med. 100:139–154, 1996.

3–137. (**A**) Application of manual pressure proximal to the insertion site is the most effective intervention because the angle at which the sheath is introduced generally punctures the artery proximal to the skin site. The sheath for PTCA is arterial so distal pressure will not slow bleeding. Sandbags may be applied after manual pressure has stopped visible bleeding to maintain tamponade.

Reference: Tracy, M. F., Hadlich, E. N., Fiebiger, C., Ruffing, B.: Developing nursing guidelines for the PTCA patient. Dimens. Crit. Care Nurs. 11(2):108–113, 1992.

3–138. (**A**) Wellen's syndrome is a form of unstable angina. Typical ECG changes noted in Wellen's syndrome are deeply inverted, symmetric T waves with little or no ST segment elevation in leads V_2 and V_3. Treatment with thrombolytics is not appropriate unless ST segment elevation is greater than 2 mm or there is no relief of chest pain with aggressive nitroglycerin therapy. If nitroglycerin is ineffective in relief of pain, heparin therapy may then be instituted.

Reference: Wu, K. T., Baker-Carpenter, K.: ST-T segment changes in a patient with ECG evidence that suggests stenosis of the proximal left anterior descending artery. Crit. Care Nurs. 16(6):56–58, 1996.

3–139. (**D**) Optimal therapeutic goals for patients in septic shock include cardiac index 50% greater than normal, oxygen consumption 30% greater than normal, and a circulating blood volume that is 500 ml in excess of normal values. This hypermetabolic response is present in survivors versus nonsurvivors of life-threatening critical illnesses. These supranormal values reflect the body's response to the increased metabolic rate associated with sepsis.

Reference: Shoemaker, W. C.: Diagnosis and treatment of the shock syndromes. In Shoemaker, W. C., Ayres, S. M., Grenvik, A., Holbrook, P. R. (eds.): Textbook of Critical Care, 3rd ed. Philadelphia, W. B. Saunders, 1995.

3–140. (**C**) All of the options listed are potential complications of hypophosphatemia. In prolonged hypophosphatemia, platelet dysfunction and decreased white blood cell phagocytic activity occur. Hypoxia, ataxia, and fatigue are potential early complications of hypophosphatemia.

Reference: Baer, C. L.: Fluid and electrolytes. In Kinney, M. R., Packa, D. R., Dunbar, S. B. (eds.): AACN's Clinical Reference for Critical-Care Nursing, 3rd ed. St. Louis, Mosby–Year Book, 1993.

3–141. (**B**) Health care personnel are at high risk for herpetic whitlow, a herpes simplex virus that affects the fingers. Using two gloves helps to prevent cross-contamination among health care personnel, patients, and respiratory equipment. Hepatitis is generally contracted through blood transmission. All intubated patients are at risk for pneumonia and aspiration irrespective of using gloves, but not health care workers.

Reference: Kirsten, L. D.: Comprehensive Respiratory Nursing: A Decision Making Approach. Philadelphia, W. B. Saunders, 1989.

3–142. (**C**) Virchow's triad of risk factors for venous thrombosis includes blood stasis, alterations in blood coagulation, and vessel-wall abnormalities. Anemia is not a risk factor for venous thrombosis.

Reference: Alspach, J. G. (ed.): AACN Core Curriculum for Critical Care Nursing, 5th ed. Philadelphia, W. B. Saunders, 1998.

3–143. (**D**) The definitive test for pulmonary embolism is the pulmonary angiogram because it is more sensitive and specific to detect blockage of the pulmonary vascular system. Both the ventilation/perfusion scan and angiogram are invasive tests in which intravenous dye is used; thus an allergic reaction may occur with either. Both tests must be performed in the radiology department.

Reference: Kinney, M. R., Packa, D. R., Dunbar, S. B. (eds.): AACN's Clinical Reference for Critical Care Nursing, 3rd ed. New York, McGraw-Hill, 1993.

3–144. (**B**) Cerebral vasospasm is often treated with triple-H therapy (hypervolemia, hemodilution, and hypertension) along with calcium channel blockers. Because this therapy has a risk of pulmonary complications such as pulmonary edema, it is advisable for the patient to have placement of hemodynamic lines to evaluate the efficacy of treatment. Whereas a central venous catheter is adequate for the otherwise healthy young adult, a 57-year-old patient or one with pre-existing cardiovascular compromise would benefit most from the pulmonary artery measurements to rule out any complications. An intraventricular catheter is not required for these patients.

Reference: Alspach, J. G. (ed.): AACN Core Curriculum for Critical Care Nursing, 5th ed. Philadelphia, W. B. Saunders, 1998.

3–145. (**A**) Tarry, melanotic stools are characteristic of an upper gastrointestinal tract hemorrhage. A prolonged, ventilator-dependent, hemodynamically unstable ICU stay predisposes this patient to stress ulcers, which are now bleeding. Bile duct obstruction eliminates bile pigments from the stool, which leaves feces clay colored. Pancreatic erosion produces a characteristic silver-colored stool. Mesenteric ischemia produces a foul-smelling, mucoid, blood-tinged stool.

References: Doughty, D. B., Jackson, D. B.: Gastrointestinal Disorders. St. Louis, Mosby–Year Book, 1993.
Yamada, T. (ed.): Textbook of Gastroenterology, 2nd ed. Philadelphia, J. B. Lippincott, 1995.

3–146. (**D**) The effective outcome of therapy for unstable angina is evidenced by the absence of clinical and ECG changes indicating increasing ischemia. Reduction in the frequency of pain episodes would also indicate effective therapy. Relief of pain with nitroglycerin indicates a successful intervention for an anginal episode, but multiple episodes of angina indicate a need for further definitive treatment. Anginal episodes are generally caused by local reductions in myocardial oxygen supply, which are evidenced by ECG changes such as ST depression or inversion of T waves, which are typically seen in the patient with unstable angina during pain episodes. The presence of Q waves would indicate infarction. Absence of anginal episodes would indicate achievement of treatment goals.

Reference: Kinney, M. R., Packa, D. R.: Andreoli's Comprehensive Cardiac Care, 8th ed. St. Louis, Mosby–Year Book, 1996.

3–147. (**A**) Q waves without ST segment elevation in leads V_1 through V_3 indicate the site of an old infarction. Q waves may remain present permanently after infarction and would not be affected by current therapy. ST segment elevation in leads II, III, and aVF is indicative of inferior wall injury. Inferior ischemia may progress to posterior or right ventricular ischemia. Right ventricular ischemia is indicated by ST segment elevation in lead V_1. Posterior wall ischemia is indicated by tall R waves and ST segment depression in leads V_1 and V_2.

Reference: Chulay, M., Guzzetta, C., Dossey, B.: AACN Handbook of Critical Care Nursing. Stamford, Conn., Appleton & Lange, 1997.

3–148. **(C)** In right bundle branch block the QRS complex has a triphasic pattern in V_1 and V_6. In V_1 it typically has an rSR′ pattern. Left bundle branch block produces a slurred S wave in V_1. Both left and right bundle branch blocks have a QRS duration of greater than or equal to 0.12 second. In left bundle branch block, the QRS complex is negative in V_1 and positive in V_6.

Reference: Kinney, M. R., Packa, D. R., Dunbar, S. B.: AACN's Clinical Reference for Critical Care Nursing, 3rd ed. St. Louis, Mosby–Year Book, 1993.

3–149. **(A)** Vasopressors produce uneven and unpredictable maldistributions of blood flow while at the same time exerting an inotropic action that increases cardiac index. The smallest dose possible to maintain MAP greater than 60 mm Hg is recommended to avoid masking inadequate blood volume and tissue perfusion deficits. Urine output, SVR, and PCWP are only indirect measures of vasopressor effects.

Reference: Shoemaker, W. C.: Diagnosis and treatment of the shock syndromes. *In* Shoemaker, W. C., Ayres, S. M., Grenvik, A., Holbrook, P. R. (eds.): Textbook of Critical Care, 3rd ed. Philadelphia, W. B. Saunders, 1995.

3–150. **(D)** The major cause of fluid loss in DKA is osmotic diuresis, which is brought about by excess excretion of glucose in the urine. Because of this and the fact that it is very easy to test urine for glucose, this should be evaluated first. SIADH results in fluid retention, decreased urine output, weight gain, and hyponatremia. Diabetes insipidus is totally unrelated to DKA and is seen most frequently with neurosurgery or neurologic trauma and the resultant effects on antidiuretic hormone.

Reference: Kitabchi, A. E., Wall, B. M.: Diabetic ketoacidosis. Med. Clin. North Am. 79:9–37, 1995.

3–151. **(C)** All of these values may be altered in DIC with elevations in thrombin, FDP, and D-dimer levels and a reduction in platelet levels. FDP elevation is due to increased plasmin, but it does not distinguish between the breakdown products of fibrinogen and fibrin; it only indicates the presence and activity of plasmin. D-Dimer is a laboratory test that uses monoclonal antibodies to measure fibrin-specific degradation products created as plasmin degrades fibrin that has been cross-linked through a thrombin-initiated activity. Thus, D-dimer represents thrombin and plasmin generation. This is thought to represent an advantage over conventional measurement of FDP because D-dimer does not detect fibrinogen or its degradation products.

Reference: Bell, T.: Disseminated intravascular coagulation: Clinical complexities of aberrant coagulation. Crit. Care Nurs. Clin. North Am. 5:389–410, 1993.

3–152. **(C)** The 8-second ventricular pause demonstrates that this patient has carotid sinus hypersensitivity and should be instructed in methods to prevent vagal stimulation such as avoidance of tight neck collars, straining at stool, and rapid head movements. Instructing the patient in vagal maneuvers to terminate SVT may cause the patient to develop asystole. Cough CPR produces vagal stimulation. Calcium channel blockers are contraindicated in patients with carotid hypersensitivity unless necessary for other conditions such as angina. Most patients with carotid sinus hypersensitivity require permanent pacemaker implant.

Reference: Khan, M. G.: Heart Disease Diagnosis and Therapy. Baltimore, Williams & Wilkins, 1996.

3–153. **(C)** The appropriate treatment is to reprogram the pacemaker from DDD to VVI. DDD pacemakers pace, sense, and respond to both atrial and ventricular activity. In addition, DDD pacemakers track the atrial rate and respond to increases in atrial activity by increasing the ventricular rate to correspond with the atrial rate. A VVI pacemaker paces, senses, and responds only to ventricular activity. Because the DDD pacemaker tracks the atrial rate and supplies a ventricular beat if it does not occur, patients with atrial fibrillation or flutter require reprogramming so that the atrial activity is not sensed and rapid paced ventricular rhythms are avoided. DDD pacemakers will track to their preset upper rate. In the example, the upper rate is 140. Synchronized cardioversion is suggested for regular rhythms such as atrial flutter, not irregular rhythms such as atrial fibrillation. Digoxin loading takes approximately 24 hours to produce effects. Although digoxin normally slows the ventricular rate by prolonging atrioventricular nodal refractoriness and depression of Purkinje fiber automaticity, the DDD pacemaker, if not reprogrammed, will continue to respond to the rapid atrial activity.

Reference: Furman, S., Hayes, D. L., Holmes, D. R.: A Practice of Cardiac Pacing. Mount Kisco, N.Y., Futura Publishing, 1993.

3–154. **(A)** The atrial pacing spike should occur at the end of the VA interval. The AV interval or AV delay is a programmed interval to allow time for atrial emptying. In many pacemakers this delay is programmed to be longer after paced atrial beats to allow patient conduction to occur. The AV interval added to the VA interval equals the basic pacing rate in milliseconds.

Reference: Furman, S., Hayes, D., Holmes, D. R.: A Practice of Cardiac Pacing, 3rd ed. Mount Kisco, N.Y., Futura Publishing, 1993.

3–155. **(C)** Right ventricular failure is demonstrated by lowered left ventricular and pulmonary capillary wedge pressures. Failure of the right ventricle results in decreased forward flow to the lungs and increased back-pressure into the venous system, resulting in clear lungs and jugular venous distention. Pulsus alternans is a symptom of left ventricular failure.

Reference: Kinney, M. R., Packa, D. R.: Andreoli's Comprehensive Cardiac Care, 8th ed. St. Louis, Mosby–Year Book, 1996.

3–156. **(A)** A spinal cord injury between T1 and L2 causes paraplegia with varying loss of intercostal and abdominal muscle function. In the acute phase, cardiac output is diminished, owing to the loss of sympathetic outflow caused by the transection and vasodilation, with a decreased venous return and hypotension. Bradycardia is also a result of the sympathetic blockade. Typically, vital capacity (normal = 4 to 5 L) and tidal volume (normal = 500 ml) are diminished as a result of hypoventilation in injuries below C4.

Reference: Alspach, J. G. (ed.): AACN Core Curriculum for Critical Care Nursing, 5th ed. Philadelphia, W. B. Saunders, 1998.

3–157. **(B)** The initial patient condition and laboratory results suggest hepatic failure with probable evolving encephalopathy. Serum alkaline phosphatase, aspartate aminotransferase and alanine aminotransferase would be anticipated to evaluate for hepatic failure. In pancreatitis, the initial blood glucose would be elevated. Amylase and lipase levels would be evaluated for pancreatitis. Gastric aspirate for pH and blood are collected to evaluate for gastric ulceration. Without a history of abdominal trauma, peritoneal lavage is not appropriate.

Reference: Kucharski, S. A.: Fulminant hepatic failure. Crit. Care Nurs. Clin. North Am. 5:141–151, 1993.

3–158. (**C**) Jugular venous pressure more than 3 to 4 cm above the sternal angle is considered elevated. Right-sided heart failure is the most frequent cause of abnormally increased venous pressures. Right ventricular failure may be preceded by left ventricular failure. In hypovolemia the neck veins are flat.

Reference: Ruppert, S. D., Kernicki, J. G., Dolan, J. T.: Dolan's Critical Care Nursing: Clinical Management Through the Nursing Process. Philadelphia, F. A. Davis, 1996.

3–159. (**A**) Although the mechanism is not known, the risk of precipitating convulsions increases when flumazenil is administered for benzodiazepine overdose with tricyclic antidepressant co-ingestion. The drug interaction does not precipitate arrhythmias, hypertensive crisis, or jaundice.

Reference: Clancy, C. and Litovitz, T. L.: Poisoning. *In* Shoemaker, W. C., Ayres, S. M., Grenvik, A., Holbrook, P. R. (eds.): Textbook of Critical Care, 3rd ed. Philadelphia, W. B. Saunders, 1995.

3–160. (**C**) The administration of mannitol, an osmotic diuretic, causes excessive sodium in the extracellular fluid, resulting in hypernatremia. Hyperkalemia may be caused by potassium-sparing diuretics. Hypokalemia and hyponatremia may be caused by loop diuretics, methylxanthines, and thiazide diuretics.

Reference: Baer, C. L.: Fluid and electrolytes. *In* Kinney, M. R., Packa, D. R., Dunbar, S. B. (eds.): AACN's Clinical Reference for Critical-Care Nursing, 3rd ed. St. Louis, Mosby–Year Book, 1993.

3–161. (**C**) Placing the patient on the left side with head down traps the air in the right atrium and away from the pulmonary artery. Placing the patient with head up will allow the air to go into the pulmonary artery, where it can occlude the vessel and result in cardiovascular collapse. Placing the patient on the right side with the head down may allow air to travel past the tricuspid valve and right ventricle, into the pulmonary artery.

Reference: Kinney, M. R., Packa, D. R., Dunbar, S. B. (eds.): AACN's Clinical Reference for Critical Care Nursing, 3rd ed. St. Louis, Mosby–Year Book, 1993.

3–162. (**D**) The symptoms of pulmonary fibrosis related to amiodarone use include a dry cough, fever, bluish skin discoloration, and patchy infiltrates on a chest radiograph. Pneumonia appears on a radiograph as an area of consolidation and is associated with the development of fever. A side effect of angiotensin converting enzyme inhibitor administration is a persistent, dry cough but is not related to the development of radiographic changes. The radiograph demonstrates minimal failure, which would not produce a cough.

Reference: Kupersmith, J., Deedwania, P. C.: The Pharmacologic Management of Heart Disease. Baltimore, Williams & Wilkins, 1997.

3–163. (**B**) Although the primary problem is excess fluid volume, priority should be given to airway compromise and the potential for impaired gas exchange. Assessment and implementation activities should focus on the potential for lack of adequate oxygenation. Correction of impaired gas exchange will improve exercise tolerance. Infection generally causes increases in heart rate, which would increase myocardial oxygen demand.

Reference: Wright, J. E., Shelton, B. K.: Desk Reference for Critical Care Nursing, Boston, Jones & Bartlett, 1993.

3–164. (**A**) Aggressive diuresis may cause hypovolemia, hypomagnesemia, hypokalemia, and hyponatremia. Hypomagnesemia, hypokalemia, and hypovolemia predispose to digoxin toxicity. This patient has medication orders, which should maintain his potassium level in the normal range of 3.5 to 5.0 mEq/L. Cardiac cachexia may occur in chronic heart failure when shortness of breath from lung congestion and anorexia from decreased perfusion prevent adequate nutrition.

Reference: Ruppert, S. D., Kernicki, J. G., Dolan, J. T.: Dolan's Critical Care Nursing: Clinical Management Through the Nursing Process. Philadelphia, F. A. Davis, 1996.

3–165. (**A**) Oropharyngeal angioedema is the only absolute contraindication to the use of ACE inhibitors in left ventricular failure. Cough is a nuisance but not a reason to discontinue ACE inhibitors unless associated with symptoms of failure. Many patients with heart failure tolerate a slightly lower systolic blood pressure than 90 mm Hg.

Reference: Konstam, M., Dracup, K., Baker, D., et al.: Heart Failure: Evaluation and Care of Patients with Left-Ventricular Systolic Dysfunction. Clinical Practice Guideline No. 11. ACHPR publication No. 94–0612. Rockville, Md.: Agency for Health Care Policy and Research, Public Health Service, U.S. Department of Health and Human Services, June 1994.

3–166. (**D**) Renal dose dopamine increases renal blood flow and potentiates the effect of diuretics. Continuous infusion of furosemide is more effective in some patients than bolus dosing, particularly when used with renal dose dopamine. Thiazide diuretics such as hydrochlorthiazide act on the distal tubule, whereas loop diuretics such as furosemide act on the loop of Henle. Combination therapy is frequently more effective in promoting diuresis than single-medication therapy. Ultrafiltration is an invasive approach to preload reduction in patients who do not respond to diuretic therapy. Ultrafiltration may take the form of dialysis, in which only fluid and not electrolytes are removed. Forms of ultrafiltration can also be used continuously at the bedside, including continuous arteriovenous hemofiltration.

Reference: Crawford, M. H.: Current Diagnosis and Treatment in Cardiology. Norwalk, Conn., Appleton & Lange, 1995.

3–167. (**D**) Hypokalemia and hypomagnesemia are associated with aggressive diuresis. Symptoms of hypomagnesemia include tetany, weakness, vertigo, confusion, paresthesias, anorexia, nausea, hypotension, and dysrhythmias. Hypokalemia causes ventricular irritability, "u" waves, prolonged QT and PR intervals, as well as muscle weakness. Lidocaine is generally used when PVCs occur at a rate of 6 or more per minute, are coupled, or are multifocal.

Reference: Crawford, M.: Diagnosis and Treatment in Cardiology. Norwalk, Conn., Appleton & Lange, 1995.

3–168. (**B**) A crisis is a state of emotional disequilibrium characterized by the absence of one or more balancing factors. The three balancing factors necessary to avoid a crisis include (1) an accurate perception of the event, (2) utilization of usual coping mechanisms, and (3) adequate situational supports. Crises may occur if an individual has a distorted or inaccurate perception of the diagnosis, has inadequate coping mechanisms, or lacks the situational support necessary to deal with the stressor. The two major types of crises are maturational and situational. The inability to deal with the stressor causes disequilibrium. If any one of the balancing factors is absent, an individual may experience a crisis. The goal of treatment in a crisis is to restore the patient to the pre-crisis state.

Reference: Caine, R. M., Bufalino, P. M. (eds.): Nursing Care Planning Guides for Adults, 2nd ed. Baltimore, Williams & Wilkins, 1991.

3–169. (**C**) Level of consciousness is the most important index of severity of hepatic encephalopathy. Serum ammonia level does *not* correlate well with severity of encephalopathy. Papilledema is rarely observed. The electroencephalogram may show generalized slowing with hepatic encephalopathy, but this is an unreliable index for severity.

Reference: Kucharski, S. A.: Fulminant hepatic failure. Crit. Care Nurs. Clin. North Am. 5:141–151, 1993.

3–170. (**A**) Exchange transfusion involves the removal of circulating blood and the infusion of red blood cells and plasma products. Although of limited use, it may be indicated as a last resort in life-threatening cases of methemoglobinemia from ingestion of dapsone or nitrites to remove the abnormal hemoglobin. Methemoglobin cells are too large to be removed by either plasmapheresis or hemodialysis. Peritoneal dialysis promotes osmotic exchange, not hemoglobin removal.

Reference: Clancy, C., Litovitz, T. L.: Poisoning. *In* Shoemaker, W. C., Ayres, S. M., Grenvik, A., Holbrook, P. R. (eds.): Textbook of Critical Care, 3rd ed. Philadelphia, W. B. Saunders, 1995.

3–171. (**B**) Her symptoms suggest that she had a pulmonary embolus the previous day that was undetected. Her coexisting pulmonary disease, age, and diabetes place her at an increased risk for embolism. Virchow's triad identifies risk factors for pulmonary embolus: venous stasis (bed rest, diabetes), hypercoagulability (COPD), and damage to vessel wall (surgery on foot). Patients with COPD are hypoxemic; and as a compensatory mechanism, erythropoietin release is increased, which increases the hemoglobin level and maintains oxygen transport. The embolus caused a pulmonary infarct, which then necrosed and bled. It is too early in her course to suspect pneumonia and unlikely in the absence of symptoms such as fever and sputum production. It is also unlikely that she has tuberculosis because the symptoms would have been present before surgery and not appear suddenly afterward. Heart failure produces frothy blood-tinged sputum, which this patient does not have.

Reference: Alspach, J. G. (ed.): AACN Core Curriculum for Critical Care Nursing, 5th ed. Philadelphia, W. B. Saunders, 1998.

3–172. (**D**) The usual range of dosage for captopril is 6.25 to 50 mg three times a day; however, captopril is generally withheld in patients receiving diuretic therapy. Its administration is closely monitored in patients with low urinary sodium who are on vasoactive medications such as dobutamine and nitroglycerin. The systolic blood pressure is within the parameters of the physician orders for nitroglycerin administration and the blood pressure will rise when the captopril is discontinued.

Reference: Wright, J. E., Shelton, B. K.: Desk Reference for Critical Care Nursing, Boston, Jones & Bartlett, 1993.

3–173. (**C**) For persistent volume overload, it is suggested that a trial of nitrates and hydralazine be instituted. Metolazone is also a potent diuretic. Combination diuretic therapy with medications that act on different sites in the kidney may be more effective than monotherapy. Propranolol is contraindicated in patients with volume overload because it decreases the force of contraction and slows heart rate, which may worsen failure.

Reference: Konstam, M., Dracup, K., Baker, D., et al.: Heart Failure: Evaluation and Care of Patients with Left-Ventricular Systolic Dysfunction. Clinical Practice Guideline No. 11. ACHPR publication No. 94–0612. Rockville, Md.: Agency for Health Care Policy and Research, Public Health Service, U.S. Department of Health and Human Services, June 1994.

3–174. (**C**) The arterial blood gas is the best evaluation parameter of respiratory function. The chest radiograph gives insight into lung congestion. Respiratory rate may be affected by a wide range of medications and other central nervous system effects. Oxygen saturation should be evaluated in light of blood gas results for treatment purposes.

Reference: Khan, M. G.: Heart Disease Diagnosis and Therapy. Baltimore, Williams & Wilkins, 1996.

3–175. **(B)** Intravenous insulin should be continued until ketoacidosis is resolved. Usually the patient's blood sugar level decreases before ketones are eliminated, and dextrose is added to fluids so the insulin drip can be continued. Ketoacidosis may resolve and intravenous insulin may be discontinued before or after the patient tolerates food. Of course, glucose monitoring is still necessary once a diet is resumed to ensure adequate subcutaneous insulin to prevent a relapse. Although the pH is usually above 7.3 before insulin is discontinued, this is because the ketoacidosis is resolved and ketones are negative.

Reference: Leovitz, H. E.: Diabetic ketoacidosis. Lancet 345:767–772, 1995.

3–176. **(D)** DIC occurs when the underlying pathologic condition triggers overstimulation of the normal coagulation mechanism, resulting in excessive fibrinolysis. Research indicates that in DIC the extrinsic pathway may be affected more than the intrinsic pathway. Prothrombin is synthesized in the liver and converted to thrombin in the final stages of the clotting pathway. Its altered production does not appear to be a factor in DIC.

References: Alspach, J. G. (ed.): AACN Core Curriculum for Critical Care Nursing, 5th ed. Philadelphia, W. B. Saunders, 1998.
Bell, T.: Disseminated intravascular coagulation: Clinical complexities of aberrant coagulation. Crit. Care Nurs. Clin. North Am. 5:389–410, 1993.

3–177. **(C)** TTP occurs in adults (women more often than men) and usually in the fourth decade of life. Although the etiology of TTP is unclear, in some patients the disease is reported in conjunction with an infection. In TTP, some activation of the coagulation cascade exists but is usually not enough to prolong the PT and PTT. Platelets, Hgb, and Hct are usually decreased in TTP; lactate dehydrogenase, fibrin split products, and bilirubin levels are increased. In DIC, serum laboratory alterations include decreased platelet and fibrinogen levels and prolongation of the PT and PTT. Leukemia is a cancer of white cells that is diagnosed by a high white blood cell count, low red cell indices, low platelets, and cell typing with bone marrow biopsy. Upper respiratory tract infections can be viral or bacterial in origin and are usually diagnosed by clinical signs of fever, sore throat, and nasal congestion (with or without drainage).

References: Alspach, J. G. (ed.): AACN Core Curriculum for Critical Care Nursing, 5th ed. Philadelphia, W. B. Saunders, 1998.
Kajs-Wyllie, M.: Thrombotic thrombocytopenic purpura: Pathology, treatment, and related nursing care. Crit. Care Nurs. 15(6):44–51, 1995.

3–178. **(D)** *Astereognosis* is the inability to recognize objects placed in the hand without aid of visual cues. *Hemianopia* is blindness in half of the visual fields. *Dressing apraxia* is the inability to dress one's self properly. *Autotopagnosia* is the inability to recognize or localize various parts of the body. *Anosognosia* is the lack of awareness of neurologic deficit (e.g., hemiplegia).

Reference: Alspach, J. G. (ed.): AACN Core Curriculum for Critical Care Nursing, 5th ed. Philadelphia, W. B. Saunders, 1998.

3–179. **(C)** One of the most severe problems associated with PCP overdose is hypertensive crisis. Because PCP causes systemic vasoconstriction, it is treated with potent antihypertensive medications such as nitroprusside. PCP does not affect cardiac conduction, renal function, or muscle mass.

Reference: Schnoll, S. H.: Drug abuse, overdose and withdrawal syndromes. *In* Shoemaker, W. C., Ayres, S. M., Grenvik, A., Holbrook, P. R. (eds.): Textbook of Critical Care, 3rd ed. Philadelphia, W. B. Saunders, 1995.

3–180. **(D)** During intravenous magnesium replacement therapy the patient must be monitored for the development of respiratory depression and heart block. If the infusion of magnesium is too rapid the patient may experience flushing, hypoventilation, and sinus bradycardia. This may progress to the development of heart block and eventually cardiac arrest.

Reference: Innerarity, S. A.: Electrolyte emergency in the critically ill renal patient. Crit. Care Clin. North Am. 2:89–99, 1990.

3–181. **(C)** Cholelithiasis (gallstone disease) and alcoholism account for 70% to 80% of underlying pathology for acute pancreatitis. Foreign travel, mushroom poisoning, and blood transfusions are causes of fulminant hepatitis and hepatic failure.

References: Krumberger, J. M.: Acute pancreatitis. Crit. Care Nurs. Clin. North Am. 5:185–202, 1993. Urban, N., et al.: Guidelines for Critical Care Nursing. St. Louis, Mosby–Year Book, 1995.

3–182. **(A)** Streptokinase and urokinase work by activating plasminogen, a fibrinolytic enzyme precursor. Blocking fibrinogen prevents the clot from dissolving and promotes further clotting. Activation of fibrin occurs farther down the clotting cascade, and streptokinase has no effect at that level. Fibrin split products are released as the clot dissolves.

Reference: Kinney, M. R., Packa, D. R., and Dunbar, S. B. (eds.): AACN's Clinical Reference for Critical Care Nursing, 3rd ed. St. Louis, Mosby–Year Book, 1993.

3–183. **(D)** Although amiodarone has controlled the atrial dysrhythmias, signs of pulmonary fibrosis evidenced by patchy infiltrates, fever, and dry cough necessitate discontinuing this medication. The cough associated with captopril is persistent, not occasional, and not associated with radiographic changes or fever. Pulmonary congestion has greatly improved with the diuretic action of furosemide. The chest radiographic findings indicating severe failure, such as interstitial and perivascular edema, have cleared to minimal bibasilar interstitial edema.

Reference: Kupersmith, J., Deedwania, P. C.: The Pharmacologic Management of Heart Disease. Baltimore, Williams & Wilkins, 1997.

3–184. **(D)** A chest radiograph will give information on cardiac size, integrity of the aorta, pulmonary congestion, and presence of pleural effusions. In patients with chronic hypertension, hypertrophy of the left ventricle enlarges the cardiac silhouette. If the cardiac silhouette is normal, pheochromocytoma or some other cause of the hypertensive episode should be explored. MRI would not be performed until the patient's blood pressure has stabilized, and only if focal symptoms were present. Pheochromocytoma is not likely from the assessment because there was no change in the blood pressure with position changes, and patients with catecholamine excess are usually agitated, not somnolent. The patient had equal blood pressures in both arms and no complaints of chest or back pain, making aortic dissection unlikely.

Reference: Khan, M. G.: Heart Disease Diagnosis and Therapy. Baltimore, Williams & Wilkins, 1996.

3–185. **(B)** Severe hypertension may cause renal failure, cerebrovascular accident, or dissection of an aortic aneurysm. Pheochromocytoma is a tumor of the adrenal medulla that secretes excessive levels of catecholamines, which may cause malignant hypertension, but it is not a potential complication of hypertension.

Reference: Khan, M. G.: Heart Disease Diagnosis and Therapy. Baltimore, Williams & Wilkins, 1996.

3–186. (**C**) If the concentration of sodium nitroprusside is 50 mg in 250 ml, the concentration is 200 μg in each milliliter. Because delivery is based on time, 200 divided by 60 (minutes) gives the microgram per minute rate of 3.3 μg/min. The patient is receiving 15 ml/hr so 15 is multiplied by 3.3 to determine the actual dose of 49.5 μg/min.

Reference: Khan, M. G.: Heart Disease Diagnosis and Therapy. Baltimore, Williams & Wilkins, 1996.

3–187. (**B**) Control of blood pressure with an oral antihypertensive agent is a goal of aggressive therapy and is necessary for transfer to a lower level of care. It is easy for patients to be compliant with the medication regimen in the hospital; a more appropriate outcome would be that the patient demonstrates behavior indicating he will be compliant with medications after discharge. Renal complications may be chronic changes related to chronic hypertension and have no bearing on immediate transfer from the unit.

Reference: Thelan, L. A., Davie, J. K., Urden, L. D., Lough, M. E.: Critical Care Nursing, Diagnosis and Management, 2nd ed. St. Louis, Mosby–Year Book, 1994.

3–188. (**D**) One of the hallmarks of cardiac tamponade is equalization of the central venous pressure (CVP) and pulmonary capillary wedge pressure (PCWP) pressures due to the constriction of both the right and left ventricles. Papillary muscle rupture would cause elevation of the PCWP but the effect on the right side of the heart and CVP would be late findings. Anterior wall myocardial infarction would cause symptoms of left-sided heart failure. Pulmonary embolism would not cause an increase in the PCWP.

Reference: Ruppert, S. D., Kernicki, J. G., Dolan, J. T.: Dolan's Critical Care Nursing, 2nd ed. Philadelphia, F. A. Davis, 1996.

3–189. (**D**) In cardiogenic shock, IABP insertion is indicated before surgery, angioplasty, or diagnostic angiography. The IABP reduces afterload and cardiac work and increases diastolic pressure, which improves coronary perfusion. The balloon is inserted before other invasive measures to stabilize the patient and improve outcomes. IABP insertion may be performed as the sole measure to treat cardiogenic shock in the patient with acute myocardial infarction.

Reference: Khan, M. G.: Heart Disease Diagnosis and Therapy. Baltimore, Williams & Wilkins, 1996.

3–190. (**D**) Sodium bicarbonate therapy is efficacious in the management of the central nervous system effects of cyclic antidepressant overdose, although the exact mechanism of action is not clear. Alkalinization of the serum is also effective in reversing QRS prolongation, ventricular arrhythmias, and hypotension associated with cyclic antidepressant ingestion. There is no clinical evidence to support administration of sodium bicarbonate for overdose by a benzodiazepine, cocaine, or acetaminophen.

Reference: Clancy, C., Litovitz, T. L.: Poisoning. *In* Shoemaker, W. C., Ayres, S. M., Grenvik, A., Holbrook, P. R. (eds.): Textbook of Critical Care, 3rd ed. Philadelphia, W. B. Saunders, 1995.

3–191. (**B**) Inflammation and edema of the airways have been recognized as the primary pathologic processes in asthma. Anti-inflammatory drugs, especially inhaled corticosteroids, are considered the most effective long-term preventive medication "controllers" for asthma. Short-acting beta$_2$ agonists and theophyllines (bronchodilators) are considered "relievers" because they provide quick relief of bronchoconstriction. Antihistamines only provide symptomatic control secondary to allergies.

References: Expert Panel Report II: Guidelines for the Diagnosis and Management of Asthma. Bethesda, Md., National Institutes of Health, 1997. Global Initiative for Asthma (GINA): Pocket Guide for Asthma Management and Prevention: A Pocket Guide for Physicians and Nurses. Bethesda, Md., National Institutes of Health, 1995.

3–192. (**C**) Pain is an often overlooked phenomenon in the patient who has experienced a stroke. It is not true that medication is unnecessary because the patient may be experiencing other painful events (e.g., associated with treatments, muscle or joint pain). Narcotic analgesics, however, are contraindicated because they may dilate cerebral blood vessels, thus increasing intracranial pressure. After a cerebrovascular event, the head of the bed may be positioned either flat (if the patient experienced an embolic or thromboembolic stroke) or it may be elevated to enhance venous blood flow. Hyperdilution with intravenous solutions may be ordered to reduce blood viscosity. Percutaneous endoscopic gastrostomy tubes are the preferred route for feeding the patient with dysphagia.

Reference: Barker, E. (ed.): Neuroscience Nursing. St. Louis, Mosby–Year Book, 1994.

3–193. (**C**) Somatostatin successfully decreases intestinal motility and reduces endocrine/exocrine pancreatic secretion. Lactulose promotes fecal nitrogen excretion in fulminant hepatic failure. Neomycin enemas suppress enteric flora biotransformation of nitrogen and are used to treat hepatic encephalopathy. Papaverine hydrochloride is a smooth muscle relaxant that is used to dilate arterioles in mesenteric ischemia.

References: Krumberger, J. M.: Acute pancreatitis. Crit. Care Nurs. Clin. North Am. 5:185–202, 1993.
Kucharski, S. A.: Fulminant hepatic failure. Crit. Care Nurs. Clin. North Am. 5:141–151, 1993.
Quinn, A. D.: Acute mesenteric ischemia. Crit. Care Nurs. Clin. North Am. 5:171–175, 1993.

3–194. (**B**) Coronary angioplasty may salvage myocardium in acute myocardial infarction by restoring coronary blood flow. Open-heart surgery carries a very high mortality in cardiogenic shock. Intravenous ACE inhibitors and calcium antagonists are contraindicated because they may worsen shock. ACE inhibitors may prevent compensatory vasoconstriction from supporting blood pressure. Calcium channel blockers have negative inotropic effects and cause bradycardia and hypotension, which may reduce coronary circulation.

Reference: Khan, M. G.: Heart Disease Diagnosis and Therapy. Baltimore, Williams & Wilkins, 1996.

3–195. (**D**) In cardiogenic shock improved circulation is demonstrated by improved cardiac output, decreased systemic vascular resistance, and increased pulse pressure (decreased afterload). A decrease in dysrhythmias demonstrates improved coronary artery perfusion, which may be influenced by vasodilation of the coronary arteries and/or improved systemic blood pressure.

Reference: Kinney, M. R., Packa, D. R.: Andreoli's Comprehensive Cardiac Care, 8th ed. St. Louis, Mosby–Year Book, 1996.

3–196. (**C**) A widened, notched, bifid, or flat-topped P wave is seen in mitral stenosis due to left atrial enlargement. P mitrale is found in 90% of patients with significant mitral stenosis. As the left atrium increases in size to accommodate blood unable to pass through the stenotic valve during atrial systole, the electrical impulses have further to travel and result in the appearance of a wider P wave on the ECG. Right atrial enlargement appears late in mitral valve dysfunction after right ventricular failure has occurred. Atrioventricular junction delay would cause a longer PR interval but not a wider P wave. Right ventricular dysfunction, not left ventricular dysfunction, occurs with mitral valve stenosis.

Reference: Kinney, M. R., Packa, D. R., Dunbar, S. B.: AACN's Clinical Reference for Critical Care Nursing, 3rd ed. St. Louis, Mosby–Year Book, 1993.

3–197. (**C**) Patients with mitral stenosis often have concomitant heart failure and right ventricular failure, which contraindicates beta blockade. Prophylactic antibiotics are suggested before any invasive procedure to reduce the risk of endocarditis. Anticoagulation is necessary to prevent embolism because atrial fibrillation due to left atrial hypertrophy may mobilize mural thrombi.

Reference: Kinney, M. R., Packa, D. R., Dunbar, S. B.: AACN's Clinical Reference for Critical Care Nursing, 3rd ed. St. Louis, Mosby–Year Book, 1993.

3–198. (**C**) Atenolol is a cardioselective beta blocker that interferes with depolarization, leading to widening QRS complex and depressed cardiac output. Transvenous pacing, intra-aortic balloon pump, or cardiopulmonary bypass may be implemented to provide support. Calcium is indicated with calcium channel blocker, not beta blocker, overdose. Glucagon, not glucose, is administered for its positive inotropic and chronotropic action. Beta blockers do not materially affect potassium levels.

Reference: Clancy, C., and Litovitz, T. L.: Poisoning. *In* Shoemaker, W. C., Ayres, S. M., Grenvik, A., Holbrook, P. R. (eds.): Textbook of Critical Care, 3rd ed. Philadelphia, W. B. Saunders, 1995.

3–199. (**D**) Patients receiving large amounts of blood and blood products are susceptible to a transient but profound hypomagnesemia due to the presence of citrate. Citrate is used to prevent the coagulation of stored blood and interferes with renal magnesium reabsorption. Hypercalcemia is primarily associated with malignancies. Hypokalemia occurs from low potassium intake, excess renal excretion, excessive gastrointestinal loss, and excessive integumentary loss. Causes of hyperphosphatemia include increased phosphate intake, acute and chronic renal failure, and neoplastic disease.

Reference: Workman, M. L.: Magnesium and phosphorus: The neglected electrolytes. AACN Clin. Issues Crit. Care Nurs. 3:655–663, 1992.

3–200. (**D**) The goal of treatment of diabetic ketoacidosis is to reverse ketoacidosis, which is best evaluated by measurement of serum ketones and pH. Measuring glucose tells nothing about the acidosis but is done during treatment to prevent a precipitous decrease and the complications associated with a rapid drop in serum glucose.

Reference: Leovitz, H. E.: Diabetic ketoacidosis. Lancet 345:767–772, 1995.

Annotated Bibliography

CARDIOVASCULAR

Ahrens, T. S., Taylor, L. A.: Hemodynamic Waveform Analysis. Philadelphia, W. B. Saunders, 1992.
This text gives a thorough explanation of hemodynamic waveforms and a large number of examples of the different waveforms and pathologic processes. The test-yourself sections are extremely helpful.

Baas, L. (ed.): Essentials of Cardiovascular Nursing. Gaithersburg, Md., Aspen Publications, 1991.
Emphasis is placed on the psychosocial aspects of patient care in this good basic text on cardiovascular nursing. Nursing care plan formats and pathophysiology, clinical presentation, and outcome-oriented care are used to present different cardiovascular problems.

Braunwald, E., Mark, D. B., Jones, R. H., et al.: Unstable Angina: Diagnosis and Management. Clinical Practice Guideline Number 10. ACHPR Publication No. 94–0602. Rockville, Md.: Agency For Health Care Policy and Research and the National Heart, Lung and Blood Institute, Public Health Service, U.S. Department of Health and Human Services. March 1994.
The ACHPR guidelines give comprehensive information and a review of current literature on the topic. They also provide the clinician with useful assessment and treatment algorithms.

Braunwald, E. (ed.): Heart Disease: A Textbook of Cardiovascular Medicine. Philadelphia, W. B. Saunders, 1997.

Daily, E. K., Schroeder, J. S.: Techniques in Bedside Hemodynamic Monitoring, 5th ed. St. Louis, Mosby–Year Book, 1994.
This will always be the basic text for understanding hemodynamic monitoring. The latest edition includes measurement of oxygenation and circulatory assist.

Darovic, G. O.: Hemodynamic Monitoring: Invasive and Noninvasive Clinical Application, 2nd ed. Philadelphia, W. B. Saunders, 1995.
This text is extremely comprehensive in outlining the assessment and treatment of cardiovascular patients. It is somewhat misleading in its description as a hemodynamic monitoring text because it gives so much more information on treatment modalities and assessment than its name implies.

Dossey, B. M., Guzzetta, C. E., Kenner, C. V.: Critical Care Nursing, Body–Mind–Spirit. Philadelphia, J. B. Lippincott, 1992.
This text utilizes a nursing process format and the authors' unique nursing theory to present the care of critically ill patients. The case studies are helpful examples of patient presentations, and the care plans are excellent.

Fahey, V.: Vascular Nursing, 2nd ed. Philadelphia, W. B. Saunders, 1994.

This is the definitive nursing text on assessment, care, and surgical interventions for the patient with vascular disease.

Furman, S., Hayes, D. L., Holmes, D. R.: A Practice of Cardiac Pacing. Mount Kisco, N.Y., Futura Publishing Company, 1993.
This text has everything you always wanted to know about the new generation of pacemakers. It explains timing cycles, hemodynamics, and practical considerations such as drug–device interactions.

Khan, M. G.: Heart Disease Diagnosis and Therapy. Baltimore, Williams & Wilkins, 1996.
This is a medical textbook that does not provide insight to nursing care but does completely describe the diagnosis and treatment of cardiac pathologic processes. It is especially helpful in the area of medications, their indications as well as their effects. The assessment of patients and the symptoms of cardiac disease are well described along with the specific diagnostic tests, their findings and rationale.

Kinney, M. R., Packa, D. R.: Andreoli's Comprehensive Cardiac Care, 8th ed. St. Louis, Mosby–Year Book, 1996.
This test is an excellent review of cardiac anatomy and physiology, dysrhythmia interpretation, and treatment. An overview is also presented of the cure of cardiac patients, pacemakers, cardiac surgery, and cardiac rehabilitation.

Kinney, M. R., Packa, D. R., Dunbar, S. B.: AACN's Clinical Reference for Critical Care Nursing, 3rd ed. St. Louis, Mosby–Year Book, 1993.
A comprehensive critical care text for experienced critical care nurses. The text uses a systems format to outline patient care problems typically found in critical care units. It provides pathophysiology as well as rationale for different treatment modalities.

Konstam, M., Dracup, K., Baker, D., et al.: Heart Failure: Evaluation and Care of Patients with Left-Ventricular Systolic Dysfunction. Clinical Practice Guideline No. 11. ACHPR publication No. 94–0612. Rockville, Md.: Agency for Health Care Policy and Research, Public Health Service, U.S. Department of Health and Human Services, June 1994.
The ACHPR guidelines give comprehensive information and a review of current literature on the topics. They also provide the clinician with useful assessment and treatment algorithms.

Mandel, W.: Cardiac Arrhythmias, Their Mechanisms, Diagnosis and Management, 3rd ed. Philadelphia, J. B. Lippincott, 1995.
This is an advanced text on cardiac dysrhythmias for those who really want to understand the causes of cardiac dysrhythmias and why differ-

ent therapies are effective. The chapters on pace-makers and cardiac dysrhythmias after cardiac surgery are particularly useful and informative.

Phalen, T.: The 12-Lead ECG in Acute Myocardial In-farction. St. Louis, Mosby–Year Book, 1996.
This very easy-to-understand text on 12-lead ECG interpretation and acute myocardial in-farction also gives case studies for practice as well as many 12-lead practice ECGs. For nurses who work in institutions with dedicated coronary care units, the non-CCU nurse will find this book very helpful.

Ruppert, S. D., Kernicki, J. G., Dolan, J. T.: Dolan's Critical Care Nursing: Clinical Management Through the Nursing Process. Philadelphia, F. A. Davis, 1996.
This text includes major organ pathophysiology and treatment. It presents current information along with case studies and comprehensive care plans. Included in the text are chapters on pa-tient education, family and patient interaction, and critical care of the elderly.

Thelan, L. A., Davie, J. K., Urden, L. D., Lough, M. E.: Critical Care Nursing, Diagnosis and Management, 2nd ed. St. Louis, Mosby–Year Book, 1994.
This text is presented in a systems format. Each system is presented by first describing physiology, assessment parameters, and diagnostic proce-dures. Specific disorders are presented next, along with technological, surgical, and medical management modalities. Each unit ends with a chapter on nursing management that includes case studies and nursing care plans for specific problems and therapies.

Wright, J. E., Shelton, B. K.: Desk Reference for Criti-cal Care Nursing. Boston, Jones & Bartlett, 1993.
The chapters are easy to follow and comprehen-sive. It also allows the reader to self-test using the sample questions at the beginning and end of each chapter.

PULMONARY

Alspach, J. G. (ed.): AACN Core Curriculum for Critical Care Nursing, 5th ed. Philadelphia, W. B. Saun-ders, 1998.
Updated edition presented in nursing process for-mat with nursing diagnosis, interventions, and evaluation is an excellent reference for both be-ginning and advanced critical care nurses.

Boggs, R. L., Wooldridge-King, M. (eds.): AACN Proce-dure Manual for Critical Care, 3rd ed. Philadelphia, W. B. Saunders, 1993.
Reference manual for critical care procedures based on research has standards listed for all critical care patients.

Dellinger, R. P. (ed.): Adult respiratory distress syn-drome: Current considerations in future directions. New Horizons 1(4):463–650, 1993.
This reference on physiology and treatment of ARDS discusses new therapies in terms of their physiologic basis and future directions for recog-nition, treatment, and outcome.

Demling, R. H. (ed.): Acute respiratory failure. New Horizons 1(3):361–462, 1993.
This reference on physiology and treatment of acute respiratory failure discusses acute respira-tory failure secondary to blunt chest trauma,

smoke inhalation, aspiration, and cerebral injury.

Expert Panel Report II: Guidelines for the Diagnosis and Management of Asthma. Bethesda, Md., Na-tional Asthma Education Program, National Insti-tutes of Health, 1997.
Guideline report issued by the Expert Panel on Asthma Education discusses treatment guide-lines for mild, moderate, and severe asthma as well as guidelines for treatment in the home, emergency department, and intensive care unit. A patient education booklet is also available from the NIH.

Global Initiative for Asthma: Pocket Guide for Asthma Management and Prevention. Bethesda, Md., Na-tional Institutes of Health, 1995.
An overview of diagnosing and controlling asthma is provided. Asthma medications are re-viewed and the "long-term control" and "quick relief" classification of medications is introduced. Factors involved in noncompliance with therapy, a major factor in the increase in mortality sec-ondary to asthma, are discussed.

Kersten, L. D.: Comprehensive Respiratory Nursing: A Decision Making Approach. Philadelphia, W. B. Saunders, 1989.
This text is an excellent resource for pulmonary nursing care. Although new therapies and inter-ventions are not discussed, basic nursing man-agement of the ventilator patient from ICU to home is covered. Graphs and tables are plentiful and help to explain physiology, signs, and symp-toms. Also discussed are psychosocial and reha-bilitation aspects of respiratory care.

Kinney, M. R., Packa, D. R., Dunbar, S. B. (eds.): AACN's Clinical Reference for Critical Care Nurs-ing, 3rd ed. St. Louis, Mosby–Year Book, 1993.
Comprehensive text for all critical care nurses is an excellent reference of physiology and patho-physiology integrated with nursing care.

Morris, A., Chapman, R.: Wedge pressure confirmation by aspiration of pulmonary capillary blood. Crit. Care Med. 13:736–741, 1985.
Classic study discusses confirming the accuracy of the pulmonary capillary wedge pressures by aspiration of a pulmonary capillary blood gas.

Shapiro, B. A., Peruzzi, W. T., Templin, R.: Clinical Application of Blood Gases, 5th ed. St. Louis, C. V. Mosby, 1994.
An excellent reference for reviewing blood gases and physiology associated with oxygen transport, this updated edition discusses bedside, noninva-sive, and laboratory measurements of blood gases and provides case studies. It is directed to physi-cians, nurses, and respiratory therapists.

Tobin, M. J. (ed.): Principles and Practice of Mechanical Ventilation. New York, McGraw-Hill, 1994.
This text is an excellent resource for ventilatory history, physiology, and patient management. Airway management, noninvasive ventilator management, and complications of therapy are discussed.

West, J. B.: Respiratory Physiology: The Essentials, 5th ed. Baltimore, Williams & Wilkins, 1995.
Classic text on pulmonary physiology is compre-hensive yet easy to read and understand.

West, J. B.: Pulmonary Pathophysiology: The Essen-tials, 4th ed. Baltimore, Williams & Wilkins, 1992.

A companion for the physiology text, this text discusses disease states and the pathophysiology associated with the diseases. Therapy is covered, but not in depth.

MULTISYSTEM

Bartz, C.: Families in critical care: Environment, needs, and barriers to care. *In* Shoemaker, W. C., Ayres, S. M., Grenvik, A., Holbrook, P. R. (eds.): Textbook of Critical Care, 3rd ed. Philadelphia, W. B. Saunders, 1995.

Intensive care units are reviewed from the family's perspective. A comprehensive review of literature is provided along with successful nursing interventions to support family members.

Caine, R. M.: Patients with burns. *In* Clochesy, J. M., Breu, C., Cardin, S., et al. (eds.): Critical Care Nursing. Philadelphia, W. B. Saunders, 1996.

Principles of burn care from pre-hospital through rehabilitation are reviewed, with a focus on the emergent and acute phases of care.

Clancy, C., Litovitz, T. L.: Poisoning. *In* Shoemaker, W. C., Ayres, S. M., Grenvik, A., Holbrook, P. R. (eds.): Textbook of Critical Care, 3rd ed. Philadelphia, W. B. Saunders, 1995.

Ingestion of toxic substances and medications is discussed in relation to their effects and treatment.

Clochesy, J. M.: Patients with systemic inflammatory response syndrome. *In* Clochesy, J. M., Breu, C., Cardin, S., et al. (eds.): Critical Care Nursing. Philadelphia, W. B. Saunders, 1996.

The etiology of SIRS, its effect on various systems, and interventions to correct the problem are described while providing supportive interim measures.

Demling, R. H.: Management of the burn patient. *In* Shoemaker, W. C., Ayres, S. M., Grenvik, A., Holbrook, P. R. (eds.): Textbook of Critical Care, 3rd ed. Philadelphia, W. B. Saunders, 1995.

The author reviews epidemiology of the problem, current medical management, and in-depth pathophysiology.

Demling, R. H.: Smoke inhalation injury. *In* Shoemaker, W. C., Ayres, S. M., Grenvik, A., Holbrook, P. R. (eds.): Textbook of Critical Care, 3rd ed. Philadelphia, W. B. Saunders, 1995.

Types of inhalation injury, the body's response to the insult, and appropriate medical therapy are presented in detail, along with extensive review of research studies describing a variety of responses and treatment.

Goodwin, S. R., Boysen, P. G., Modell, J. H.: Near-drowning: Adults and children. *In* Shoemaker, W. C., Ayres, S. M., Grenvik, A., Holbrook, P. R. (eds.): Textbook of Critical Care, 3rd ed. Philadelphia, W. B. Saunders, 1995.

Salt versus fresh water near-drowning sequelae are discussed. Treatments from early field interventions through such complex modalities as hyperbaric oxygen therapy are reviewed.

Haak, S. W., Richardson, S. J., Davey, S. S.: Alteration in cardiovascular function. *In* Huether, S. E., McCance, K. L. (eds.): Understanding Pathophysiology. St. Louis, Mosby–Year Book, 1996.

In addition to a comprehensive review of the anatomy and physiology of the cardiovascular system, a review of pathophysiology is discussed in the context of appropriate interventions to correct various cardiovascular problems.

Jones, K.: Shock. *In* Clochesy, J. M., Breu, C., Cardin, S., et al. (eds.): Critical Care Nursing. Philadelphia, W. B. Saunders, 1996.

Types of shock are discussed, with their etiology and treatment, in addition to expected outcomes.

Kravitz, M.: Burn injuries. *In* Copstead, L. C.: Perspectives on Pathophysiology. Philadelphia, W. B. Saunders, 1995.

How burns of the skin produce systemic responses, including major alterations in the immune system, is described. The systemic pathophysiology is discussed along with appropriate interventions.

Roberts, S. L.: Multisystem deviations. *In* Critical Care Nursing: Assessment and Intervention. Stamford, Conn., Appleton & Lange, 1996.

Multiple trauma and the interaction of injured systems on each other are discussed in relation to correcting the interrelated pathophysiology and priorities for treatment.

Schnoll, S. H.: Drug abuse, overdose and withdrawal syndromes. *In* Shoemaker, W. C., Ayres, S. M., Grenvik, A., Holbrook, P. R. (eds.): Textbook of Critical Care, 3rd ed. Philadelphia, W. B. Saunders, 1995.

Toxic ingestion of pharmaceutical and illicit drugs produces system responses that are presented in sections by drug type. The effects of cessation/withdrawal are also discussed, along with appropriate medical interventions.

Shoemaker, W. C.: Diagnosis and treatment of the shock syndromes. *In* Shoemaker W. C., Ayres, S. M., Grenvik, A., Holbrook, P. R. (eds.): Textbook of Critical Care, 3rd ed. Philadelphia, W. B. Saunders, 1995.

The etiology of shock syndromes, the different systemic responses each elicits, and their treatment are discussed in clinical detail and supported with review of research literature.

Wilson, R. F.: Thoracic injuries. *In* Shoemaker, W. C., Ayres, S. M., Grenvik, A., Holbrook, P. R. (eds.): Textbook of Critical Care, 3rd ed. Philadelphia, W. B. Saunders, 1995.

The mechanisms of thoracic injury, their local and systemic effects, and appropriate interventions are described.

NEUROLOGIC

Alspach, J. G. (ed.): AACN Core Curriculum for Critical Care Nursing, 5th ed. Philadelphia, W. B. Saunders, 1998.

Excellent, comprehensive review presenting detailed information on critical care nursing provides an appropriate synthesis of essential knowledge of the critical care patient experiencing neurologic and neurosurgical disorders. Presented in nursing process format, the text is organized in outline form to facilitate understanding.

Barker, E. (ed.): Neuroscience Nursing, St. Louis, Mosby–Year Book, 1994.

Comprehensive and well-written text that discusses neuroscience in an easy-to-understand format. Chapters present comprehensive pathophysiology, interventions, and rehabilitation concepts.

Caine, R. M., Bufalino, P. M. (eds.): Nursing Care Planning Guides for Adults, 2nd ed. Baltimore, Williams & Wilkins, 1991.

> This is a valuable resource for nurses who provide care in a variety of acute and rehabilitative settings for the patient with neurologic and neurosurgical disorders. The text provides a thorough discussion of the nursing process because it relates to patients with specific medical-surgical problems. The patient as an individual with social and family roles is emphasized throughout.

Clochesy, J. M., Breu, C., Cardin, S., et al. (eds.): Critical Care Nursing, 2nd ed. Philadelphia, W. B. Saunders, 1996.

> This excellent comprehensive text is for nurses who have been involved in critical care for a number of years. Pathophysiology is presented thoroughly as it relates to basic neurologic function and various neurologic disorders. Numerous tables and illustrations are used to enhance understanding. This book is directed at the advanced clinician desiring detailed information related to critical care nursing.

Feldman, Z., Kanter, M. J., Robertson, C. S., et al.: Effect of head elevation on intracranial pressure and cerebral blood flow in head-injured patients. J Neurosurg 77:651–652, 1992.

> This article reviews the traditional practice of elevating the head of the bed to lower intracranial pressure in head-injured patients. Elevation to 30° has been shown to significantly reduce intracranial pressure in the majority of patients.

Fortune, J. B., Feustal, P. J., Weigle, C. G., Popp, A. J.: Continuous measurement of jugular venous oxygen saturation in response to transient elevations of blood pressure in head-injured patients. J Neurosurg 80:461–468, 1994.

> Article presents research on the use of continuous bulb jugular venous oxygen saturation (SjO_2) in patients after head injury. Effects of this measurement were correlated with impaired or lost autoregulatory responses after traumatic brain injury.

Hickey, J. V.: The Clinical Practice of Neurological and Neurosurgical Nursing, 3rd ed. Philadelphia, J. B. Lippincott, 1992.

> This comprehensive text on neurologic and neurosurgical conditions has excellent tables and illustrations and presents complex material in an understandable manner.

Zornow, M. H., Prough, D. S.: Fluid management in patients with traumatic brain injury. New Horizons 3:488–498, 1995.

> An overview is presented of commonly administered rehydrating intravenous fluids to the patient experiencing traumatic brain injury. Hyperosmolar, hypo-osmolar, hypertonic crystalloid, hypertonic saline, colloid, and crystalloid fluids are reviewed. Fluid restriction parameters, once thought to be the mainstay of treatment for the traumatic brain–injured patient, are also discussed.

GASTROINTESTINAL

Aragon, D., Parson, R.: Multiple organ dysfunction syndrome in the trauma patient. Crit. Care Nurs. Clin. North Am. 6:873–881, 1994.

> The complex physiology of multiple organ failure is clearly explained. Appropriate monitoring, prevention, and treatment modalities are defined.

Chesla, C. A., Stannard, D.: Breakdown in the nursing care of families in the ICU. Am. J. Crit. Care 6:64–71, 1997.

> Observation of the nursing care of families of ICU patients results in the description of recurrent lapses in family care. Anecdotes of common nurse/patient/family interactions make this a powerful source for developing strong, therapeutic interventions for families.

Doughty, D. B., Jackson, D. B.: Gastrointestinal Disorders. St. Louis, Mosby–Year Book, 1993.

> This text is an excellent reference for all categories of gastrointestinal disorders. Although not specifically oriented to critical care, the pathophysiology is relevant for patients with acute, chronic, and co-morbid gastrointestinal diseases.

Felver, L.: Patient–environment interactions in critical care. Crit. Care Nurs. Clin. North Am. 7:327–335, 1995.

> This article describes the impact of the critical care environment on the biologic, psychologic, and sociologic patterns of the critically ill patient. A theoretic basis for modifying the plan of care to promote maintenance of patient's rhythms is provided.

Gupta, P. K., Al-Kawas, F. H.: Acute pancreatitis: Diagnosis and management. Am. Fam. Physician 52:435–443, 1995.

> A thorough presentation of the medical diagnosis and treatment of acute pancreatitis includes not only the expected course of the critically ill phase but also describes expected patient progression to home.

Kerber, K.: The adult with bleeding esophageal varices. Crit. Care Nurs. Clin. North Am. 5:153–162, 1993.

> In a superb Critical Care Nursing Clinics issue dedicated to the gastrointestinal system, bleeding esophageal varices are described along with the appropriate course of care. Of particular benefit is the discussion of causes of bleeding esophageal varices.

Kimbrell, J. D.: Acquired coagulopathies. Crit. Care Nurs. Clin. North Am. 5:453–458, 1993.

> This excellent reference makes clear the multiple sources for acquired coagulopathies in the critically ill patient. Coagulation pathways are described with practical assessment and clinical implications.

Klein, D.: Physiologic response to traumatic shock. AACN Clin. Issues Crit. Care Nurs. 1:508–521, 1990.

> Specific considerations for the patient's response to traumatic shock are presented succinctly. Comparison to other categories of shock is also included.

Krumberger, J. M.: Acute pancreatitis. Crit. Care. Nurs. Clin. North Am. 5:185–202, 1993.

> The detection, monitoring, and treatment of acute pancreatitis in the critically ill are described. Pathophysiology and prognosis are key components of the review.

Kucharski, S. A.: Fulminant hepatic failure. Crit. Care. Nurs. Clin. North Am. 5:141–151, 1993.

> The author reviews the critical care challenges in fulminant hepatic failure. Causes of and clinical

differences between chronic and acute hepatic failure are discussed.

Lawrence, D. M.: Gastrointestinal trauma. Crit. Care Nurs. Clin. North Am. 5:127–140, 1993.
The implications of traumatic critical injury to the gastrointestinal tract are reviewed with a clear presentation of mechanism of injury and likely complications.

Lord, L. M., Say, H. C.: The role of the gut in critical illness. AACN Clin. Issues 5:450–458, 1994.
An excellent analysis of the gastrointestinal system in critical illness is provided along with specific implications of gut malfunction for each body system. System equilibrium, immunology, injury, and interventions are discussed.

Luckmann, J., Sorensen, K. C. (eds.): Medical Surgical Nursing, 4th ed. Philadelphia, W. B. Saunders, 1993.
This classic medical-surgical nursing textbook thoroughly covers anatomy, physiology, disease process, medical therapeutics, and nursing management for the adult. It is well indexed and well illustrated.

Mueller, C. et al.: Parenteral nutritional support of a patient with chronic mesenteric artery occlusive disease. Nutr. Clin. Pract. 8(2):73–77, 1993.
The pros, cons, and process for effective parenteral nutritional support are presented with specific implications for the patient with mesenteric artery occlusive disease.

Neal, M. C., Paquette, M., Mirch, M. (eds.): Nursing Diagnosis Care Plans for DRGs. Venice, Calif., General Medical Publishers, 1990.
A well-indexed care plan reference addresses both the diagnostic-related groups (DRGs) and nursing. The contributors provide an updated and practical perspective on the integration of nursing into the health system.

Prevost, S. S., Oberlie, A.: Stress ulceration in the critically ill patient. Crit. Care Nurs. Clin. North Am. 5:163–169, 1993.
The differential diagnosis of stress ulceration and the currently recommended therapeutics are reviewed. This article provides a particularly clear presentation of pathophysiology.

Phillips, M. C., Olson, L. R.: The immunologic role of the gastrointestinal tract. Crit. Care Nurs. Clin. North Am. 5:107–120, 1993.
Although the complex immunology of the gastrointestinal tract is not as well understood by most nurses as it should be, this presentation is particularly thorough yet understandable. A clear review is provided of nutritional implications in maintaining gut function.

Quinn, A. D.: Acute mesenteric ischemia. Crit. Care Nurs. Clin. North Am. 5:171–175, 1993.
Acute mesenteric ischemia is one of the most critical gastrointestinal disorders. Nursing care priorities, medical care, and surgical treatment options are described.

Romito, R. A.: Early administration of enteral nutrients in critically ill patients. AACN Clin. Issues 6:242–256, 1995.
The author provides a thorough analysis of the controversy of when and whether to use enteral nutrients in critical illness. An up-to-date research basis for all recommendations is included.

Scher, H. E.: Chest pain: Developing rapid assessment skills. Orthop. Nurs. 14(3):30–34, 1995.
The many sources of chest pain are compared and contrasted, with associated nursing implications for each.

Toto, K. H., Yucha, C. B.: Magnesium: Homeostasis, imbalances, and therapeutic uses. Crit. Care Nurs. Clin. North Am. 6:767–781, 1994.
The sources of magnesium imbalance(s) in critical illness as well as the appropriate therapeutic interventions are presented clearly, making this a valuable resource as the importance of magnesium balance to recovery emerges.

Urban, N., et al.: Guidelines for Critical Care Nursing. St. Louis, Mosby–Year Book, 1995.
A comprehensive critical care nursing text in a very practical table/outline format fosters rapid access to information.

Yamada, T. (ed.): Textbook of Gastroenterology, 2nd ed. Philadelphia, J. B. Lippincott, 1995.
This classic medical textbook of the gastrointestinal system has in-depth reviews of each topic, including some of the more obscure diagnoses.

RENAL

Acute Renal Failure

Baer, C. L.: Acute renal failure. In Kinney, M. R., Packa, D. R., Dunbar, S. B. (eds.): AACN's Clinical Reference for Critical-Care Nursing, 3rd ed. St. Louis, Mosby–Year Book, 1993.
An excellent resource for the care of the critically ill patient with acute renal failure, this comprehensive resource includes discussion of anatomy, physiology, pathophysiology, and nursing care planning for the critically ill patient.

Beckman, N. J., Schell, H. M., Calixto, P. R., Sullivan, M. M.: Kidney transplantation: A therapeutic option. AACN Clin. Issues Crit. Care Nurs. 3:570–584, 1992.
This article examines the role of transplantation as a therapeutic treatment modality in the management of renal failure. It provides supplemental information for the practitioner requiring further information on the risks and benefits of renal transplantation.

Binkley, L. S., Whittaker, A.: Erythropoietin use in the critical care setting. AACN Clin. Issues Crit. Care Nurs. 3:640–649, 1992.
Erythopoietin is a commonly used medication in the management of anemia resulting from renal failure. This article discusses the physiology of erythropoiesis, the pathophysiology of anemia, and the mechanism of action, uses for, and limitations of erythopoietin.

Douglas, S.: Acute tubular necrosis: Diagnosis, treatment, and nursing implications. AACN Clin. Issues Crit. Care Nurs. 3:688–697, 1992.
Acute tubular necrosis is the most common cause of acute renal failure. This resource provides a comprehensive review of the causes, pathophysiology, and diagnosis of ATN. There is an excellent review of the essential principles for preventing the development of ATN.

Owen, W. F., Lazarus, J. M.: Hemodialysis in acute renal failure. In Lazarus, J. M., Brenner, B. (eds.): Acute Renal Failure, 3rd ed. New York, Churchill Livingstone, 1993.
This chapter is an excellent resource for understanding acute renal failure and provides an ex-

tensive review of this patient care management option.

Peschman, P.: Acute hemodialysis: Issues in the critically ill. AACN Clin. Issues Crit. Care Nurs. 3:545–557, 1992.

This article reviews the principles and process of hemodialysis. There is an extensive discussion on the physiologic responses of the body to the hemodialysis procedure, including a good review of disequilibrium syndrome.

Price, C. A.: An update on continuous renal replacement therapies. AACN Clin. Issues Crit. Care Nurs. 3:597–604, 1992.

A good primer on renal replacement therapy, this article reviews the principles of continuous renal replacement therapy, including vascular access, anticoagulation, dialysate, and fluid balance. There is a review of the indications for therapy, complications of therapy, and the responsibilities of the critical care nurse.

Smith, L. J.: Peritoneal dialysis in the critically ill patient. AACN Clin. Issues Crit. Care Nurs. 3:558–569, 1992.

This article provides an extensive review of the physiologic basis and the peritoneal dialysis process. Included is a discussion of the essential equipment and the potential complications of this therapeutic modality.

Toto, K.: The kidney in multiple organ dysfunction syndrome. *In* Secor, V. H. (ed.): Multiple Organ Dysfunction and Failure: Pathophysiology and Clinical Implications, 2nd ed. St. Louis, Mosby–Year Book, 1996.

This chapter is an excellent reference for the practitioner who requires an in-depth discussion of the pathophysiology of acute tubular necrosis. The pathophysiologic development of multisystem organ failure and the current trends in the management of individual system dysfunction are detailed.

Tucker, S. M., Canobbio, M. M., Paquette, E. V., Wells, M. F. (eds.): Patient Care Standards: Collaborative Practice Planning Guides, 6th ed. St. Louis, Mosby–Year Book, 1996.

This text is a good resource for planning the care of the patient with renal system dysfunction and/or electrolyte dysfunction. It uses the nursing process as the framework for ascertaining nursing care priorities.

Urban, N. A., Greenlee, K. K., Krumberger, J. M., Winkelman, C. (eds.): Guidelines for Critical Care Nursing. St. Louis, Mosby–Year Book, 1995.

An excellent clinical resource for planning the care of the critically ill patient and family, this book provides a comprehensive plan of care, based on the patient acuity. It serves as an excellent guide to prioritizing patient care needs from admission through discharge.

Renal Trauma

Cook, L.: Genitourinary Injuries and Renal Management. *In* Cardona, V. D., Hurn, P. D., Mason, P. J., Scanlon-Schilpp, A. M. (eds.): Trauma Nursing: From Resuscitation Through Rehabilitation, 2nd ed. Philadelphia, W. B. Saunders, 1994.

This book is a primary resource on trauma and the management of trauma. The genitourinary/renal chapter provides a comprehensive review of

the management of this type of trauma, including assessment findings, diagnostic testing, and therapeutic interventions.

Smith, M. F.: Renal trauma: Adult and pediatric considerations. Crit. Care Clin. North Am. 2:67–77, 1990.

This article is an excellent resource on the identification and initial management of the patient experiencing renal trauma. There is an in-depth review of assessment findings, diagnostic testing, interventions, and potential complications of this type of trauma. It provides this essential information for both the adult and pediatric patient populations.

Wright, J. E., Shelton, B. K. (eds.): Desk Reference for Critical Care Nursing. Boston, Jones & Bartlett, 1993.

The section on renal trauma in this comprehensive resource on the care of the critically ill patient discusses pathophysiology, assessment findings, and nursing standards of care.

Life-Threatening Electrolyte Imbalances

Baer, C. L.: Fluid and electrolyte balance. *In* Kinney, M. R., Packa, D. R., Dunbar, S. B. (eds.): AACN's Clinical Reference for Critical-Care Nursing, 3rd ed. St. Louis, Mosby–Year Book, 1993.

Managing fluid and electrolyte balance in the critically ill patient provides the critical care nurse with a complex challenge. This primer on fluid and electrolyte balance discusses the physiology, pathophysiology, and interventions for the management of electrolyte balance.

Hawthorne, J. L., Schneider, S. M., Workman, M. L.: Common electrolyte imbalances associated with malignancy. AACN Clin. Issues Crit. Care Nurs. 3:714–723, 1992.

This article provides an extensive discussion of hypercalcemia, especially in patients with malignancies. There is a good review of the etiology, manifestations, patient care management, and nursing considerations.

Kelso, L. A.: Fluid and electrolyte disturbances in hepatic failure. AACN Clin. Issues Crit. Care Nurs. 3:681–685, 1992.

The patient with hepatic failure provides the critical care nurse with unique issues related to fluid and electrolyte management. This article provides an in-depth discussion of ascites and the electrolyte imbalances of sodium, potassium, calcium, magnesium, and chloride.

Mendyka, B. E.: Fluid and electrolyte disorders caused by diuretic therapy. AACN Clin. Issues Crit. Care Nurs. 3:672–680, 1992.

A comprehensive review is provided of function of the kidney and the physiologic basis of each classification of diuretic. There is a discussion of the electrolyte disorders associated with the use of diuretics, especially hypokalemia and hyponatremia, followed by an extensive review of the nursing care of patients receiving diuretics.

Tucker, S. M., Canobbio, M. M., Paquette, E. V., Wells, M. F. (eds.): Patient Care Standards: Collaborative Practice Planning Guides, 6th ed. St. Louis, Mosby–Year Book, 1996.

This good resource for planning the care of the patient with electrolyte dysfunction uses the nursing process as the framework for ascertaining nursing care priorities.

Urban, N. A., Greenlee, K. K., Krumberger, J. M., Winkelman, C. (eds.): Guidelines for Critical Care Nursing. St. Louis, Mosby–Year Book, 1995.
> *This textbook is an excellent clinical reference for planning the care of the critically ill patient and family. It establishes a comprehensive plan of care based on the acuity of the patient and facilitates prioritizing patient care needs from admission through discharge.*

Vaska, P. L.: Fluid and electrolyte imbalances after cardiac surgery. AACN Clin. Issues Crit. Care Nurs. 3:664–671, 1992.
> *This article is a good resource to review common electrolyte imbalances seen in the postoperative period due to the use of cardiopulmonary bypass. There is an extensive review of the alterations in sodium, potassium, and calcium due to bypass, hypothermia, fluid shifts, and the stress of surgery.*

Workman, M. L.: Magnesium and phosphorus: The neglected electrolytes. AACN Clin. Issues Crit. Care Nurs. 3:655–663, 1992.
> *An in-depth review of the management of magnesium and phosphorus imbalances is provided in this article, which discusses the role of these electrolytes in the maintenance of critical physiologic functions, especially in the myocardial tissue. There is a review of the patients at risk for the development of increased or decreased electrolyte levels.*

ENDOCRINE

Alspach, J. G. (ed.): AACN Core Curriculum for Critical Care Nursing, 5th ed. Philadelphia, W. B. Saunders, 1998.
> *This is the primary text on which the content for the CCRN examination is based. It includes much of the relevant physiology, clinical symptomatology, nursing diagnoses, and nursing interventions on which critical care nursing practice is founded.*

Boylan-Starks, L.: Hypoglycemic hemiplegia: A case study. Heart Lung 24:330–332, 1995.
> *Informative article discusses an unusual presentation of hypoglycemia and offers a review of symptoms for this disorder.*

Bryce, J.: S.I.A.D.H. Nursing 24(4):33, 1994.
> *A concise review of S.I.A.D.H. symptoms, nursing interventions, and treatment is presented.*

Civetta, J. M., Taylor, R. W., Kirby, R. R. (eds.): Critical Care, 2nd ed. Philadelphia, J. B. Lippincott, 1992.
> *This comprehensive reference covers physiology and management of disease processes in the critically ill.*

Clochesy, J. M., Breu, C., Cardin, S., et al. (eds.): Critical Care Nursing, 2nd ed. Philadelphia, W. B. Saunders, 1996.
> *An excellent compilation of multidimensional knowledge related to the critically ill is provided in this textbook.*

Counsel, C. M., Gilbert, M., Snively, C.: Management of the patient with a pituitary tumor. Dimens. Crit. Care Nurs. 15(2):75–81, 1996.
> *An extensive overview is presented of patient management and nursing care for patients with pituitary tumors.*

Kitabchi, A. E., Wall, B. M.: Diabetic ketoacidosis. Med. Clin. North Am. 79:9–37, 1995.
> *This in-depth review of diabetic ketoacidosis includes pathogenesis, diagnosis, evaluation, treatment, follow-up, and complications.*

Leovitz, H. E.: Diabetic ketoacidosis. Lancet 345:767–772, 1995.
> *The emergency management of diabetic ketoacidosis is presented.*

Lipsky, M. S.: Management of diabetic ketoacidosis. Am. Fam. Physician 49:1607–1612, 1994.
> *The diagnosis, causes, and management of diabetic ketoacidosis are reviewed.*

Lorber, D.: Nonketotic hypertonicity in diabetes mellitus. Med. Clin. North Am. 79:39–52, 1995.
> *This article details pathophysiology, diagnosis, presentation, treatment, and prevention of hyperglycemic hyperosmolar nonketotic coma.*

Macheca, M. K.: Diabetic hypoglycemia: How to keep the threat at bay. Am. J. Nurs. 93(4):26–30, 1993.
> *Nursing aspects, symptoms, and management of hypoglycemia are reviewed.*

Service, F. J.: Hypoglycemia. Med. Clin. North Am. 79:1–8, 1995.
> *This article is a comprehensive presentation of hypoglycemia and includes the physiology, risk factors, clinical presentation, treatment, and sequelae.*

HEMATOLOGY/IMMUNOLOGY

Clochesy, J. M., Breu, C., Cardin, S., et al. (eds.): Critical Care Nursing, 2nd ed. Philadelphia, W. B. Saunders, 1996.
> *This comprehensive text covers the body of knowledge of critical care nursing. The physiological basis of critical illness and the technological/supportive environment of critical care are addressed. Several chapters are specific to hematologic disorders, human immunodeficiency virus infection, and immunosuppression. Nursing assessment and clinical management of patients with coagulopathies are included. This updated edition adds chapters that address managed care, transitional care, and chronic illnesses as they relate to critical care nursing.*

Dacie, J. V., Lewis, S. M.: Practical Haematology, 8th ed. New York, Churchill Livingstone, 1995.
> *A laboratory reference, this source provides explanation of the technology behind laboratory testing, reference values, and standards. Standards are based on International Council for Standards in Haematology.*

Hudak, C. M., Gallo, B. M., Benz, J. J.: Critical Care Nursing: A Holistic Approach, 6th ed. Philadelphia, J. B. Lippincott, 1994.
> *The assessment and management of various disorders are discussed in this comprehensive text. Holism is the underlying philosophy, and there is an emphasis on the patient–nurse relationship and the ethical/legal implications of professional practice. Individual units include both the gastrointestinal system and the immunologic system. The units encompass discussion of the normal physiology of these systems as well as the pathophysiology. Transplantation issues specific to heart and kidney transplantation are included. Case studies and care plans are included for most disorders.*

Lee, G. R., Bithell, T. C., Foerster, J., et al.: Wintrobe's

Clinical Hematology, 9th ed. Philadelphia, Lea & Febiger, 1993.

Expansive text of the basic science of hematology has updated chapters in oncology and excellent references.

Rippe, J. M., Irwin, R. S., Fink, M. P., & Cerra, F. B. (eds.): Intensive Care Medicine, 3rd ed. Boston, Little, Brown, 1996.

The current edition of this excellent resource on many areas of critical care provides up-to-date information on transplantation, including immune system, immunosuppressive agents, diagnosis and treatment of infection and rejection, and management of the organ donor. Hematologic problems are discussed from the critical care perspective.

Sigardson-Poor, K. M., Haggerty, L. M.: Nursing Care of the Transplant Recipient. Philadelphia, W. B. Saunders, 1990.

This book is an excellent resource for nurses responsible for the care of transplant recipients. Solid organ transplant sections are presented as well as specific chapters devoted to transplant immunology, immunosuppression, and infec-
tions. Special attention is devoted to psychological, legal/ethical, and patient education issues surrounding transplantation.

Smith, S. L. (ed.): Tissue and Organ Transplantation: Implications for Professional Nursing Practice, St. Louis, C. V. Mosby, 1990.

Both solid organ and tissue transplantation are covered in this excellent resource on history of transplantation. Surgical techniques are described and integrated with postoperative care. Each chapter has an excellent reference list.

Thelan, L. A., Davie, J. K., Urden, L. D., Lough, M. E.: Textbook of Critical Care Nursing: Diagnosis and Management, 2nd ed. St. Louis, C. V. Mosby, 1994.

The new edition of this comprehensive reference on all body systems and alterations of human functioning across biopsychosocial realms includes chapters on transplantation and gerontology. One chapter is devoted to the evaluation and nursing care of recipients of solid organ transplants. An extensive review is presented of the immune system and the immunology of organ rejection. Up-to-date information is given on both the immunologic agents and immunosuppressive protocols. Patient education is also addressed.